# Cognitive Rehabilitation
## Conceptualization and Intervention

# Cognitive Rehabilitation
## Conceptualization and Intervention

Edited by
**Lance E. Trexler**
Community Hospital of Indianapolis
Indianapolis, Indiana

PLENUM PRESS • NEW YORK AND LONDON

Library of Congress, Cataloging in Publication Data

Main entry under title:

Cognitive rehabilitation.

"Proceedings of a Conference on Models and Techniques of Cognitive Rehabilitation, held January 28–30, 1981, in Indianapolis, Indiana"—T.p. verso.
Bibliography: p.
Includes index.
1. Brain damage—Complications and sequelae. 2. Cognitive disorders—Treatment. 3. Rehabilitation. I. Trexler, Lance E. II. Conference on Models and Techniques of Cognitive Rehabilitation (1981: Indianapolis, Ind.) [DNLM: 1. Brain injuries—Rehabilitation—Congresses. 2. Cognition disorders—Rehabilitation—Congresses W3 C7827 1981c/WL 341 C748c 1981]
RC387.5.C63 616.8 82-7619
ISBN 0-306-41016-8 AACR2

Proceedings of a Conference on Models and Techniques of Cognitive Rehabilitation, held January 28–30, 1981, in Indianapolis, Indiana


A Division of Plenum Publishing Corporation
233 Spring Street, New York, N.Y. 10013



Printed in the United States of America

# PREFACE

The present volume has come about through an awareness of the absence of any cohesive and substantive source on the treatment of cognitive dysfunction following brain insult. I initiated the development of our annual symposium Models and Techniques of Cognitive Rehabilitation, on which the present volume is based, so as to educate myself, as well as others, about the state of the art in modifying cognitive processes in the brain, injured. I became aware of the need for interventive strategies for the brain, injured while a graduate student. Brain functions had, for a long time, always fascinated me, but from an academic perspective. I was confronted with the clinical consequences of brain injury while administering batteries of neuropsychological tests, and this experience added another dimension to my interest in brain functions. I felt grossly inadequate because I was able to rather eloquently describe changes in brain-behavior relations with neuropsychological tests, but could only generate recommendations based solely on the use of compensatory strategies and occasionally on some unfounded, and probably naive, remedial guess. A literature search at this time yielded devastating, little information. The next several years were characterized by a pseudo-obsession, occurring at times without total awareness, with methods and techniques which might alter impaired brain-behavior relations. Completing graduate school, however, required that these thoughts take a secondary position relative to more typical graduate student thoughts. After completing all of my academic and clinical requirements, and after locating myself in an environment receptive to my ideas, I was then ready to learn. Hence, our symposium and this volume.

As an individual I constantly try to balance a need for empiricism with a need for clinical intervention. This same balancing needs to occur for cognitive rehabilitation. There is obviously a profound need to alter cognitive processing impairment characteristics of brain injury. Our best guess as to what interventive strategies are efficacious is not, however, enough. There continues to be a profound dearth of clinical evaluation research. This dearth has been offset in recent years by a small, albeit growing, body of continuing clinical evaluation research. It was the explicit intent of Models and Techniques of Cognitive Rehabilitation to address both concerns. It will become obvious to the reader that there are several different models or theoretical conceptualizations of the mechanisms of brain processes which give rise to cognitive functions. These theoretical assumptions are crucial, in that they dictate our approach to intervention. As a consequence, the clinician must struggle with these varying models. The extreme "neglect" of this struggle is characterized by the utilization of thoughtless cookbook techniques which increases the fragmentation of brain injured peoples' lives. Brain, injured people do not need further fragmentation. Rather, what brain, injured people need is someone who can understand the totality of their experience, both in terms of the disruption of brain-behavior relations and in terms of the emotional-social consequences and reactions. To achieve these ends, I believe it is the responsibility of the rehabilitation professional to adopt a model; one which can be both flexible and account for the variance in individual differences, and has the most supporting empirical evidence. An adequate model makes the methods of intervention obvious. These techniques or methods then must be evaluated, resulting in a confirmation or alteration of the model employed.

Rehabilitation, and especially cognitive rehabilitation, is in many respects a very young and empirically unsophisticated science. Cognitive rehabilitation derives its clinical and theoretical underpinnings primarily from clinical neuropsychology, the field of rehabilitation with all its components, and cognitive psychology. It is an explicit assumption, at least by the present author, that cognition underlies functionally all behavior, whether it be emotional, linguistic or purposeful and coordinated movement behavior. As a consequence, assessing and treating cognitive impairment is of concern, I believe, to all rehabilitation professionals. Cognition is not one of those components of a person which can be professionally fragmented. The whole patient goes from each therapist's office to the next.

I want to acknowledge especially Nancy D. Schmidt of Community Hospital who has had a significant impact on this volume, both covertly and overtly. As a cognitive rehabilitation therapist she has openly offered a keen clinical sensitivity, a great tolerance for times that were and, sometimes continue to be, quite ambiguous, and has contributed markedly to the shaping of our Cognitive Rehabilitation Program and the symposium in a manner that consistently resulted in an ultimate concern for the welfare of our patients and continual growth and change of our thinking. Indispensable to the development of our symposium and, hence, this volume were Nathan Aldrich and Cyd Pomerance whose behind the scenes work laid the foundation for these efforts. Sharon Steinhart, Seward Horner, Jerry Wesch, and

Sallie Potter have collectively created an environment responsive to the development of our program and symposium. Their management philosophy has been tremendously supportive. Further, my wife, Carol, deserves significant acknowledgement and much thanks for her untiring support and tolerance for the efforts herein invested.

Lance E. Trexler

Indianapolis, Indiana U.S.A.
September 1981

CONTENTS

# PART I: INTRODUCTORY CONSIDERATIONS

# INTRODUCTION

Lance E. Trexler, Ph.D.

Coordinator, Neuropsychology Service
Medical Psychology Department
Community Hospital of Indianapolis, Inc.

The extent to which the title of the present volume subsumes theory and treatment efforts which can be differentiated from traditional rehabilitation paradigms is a matter of debate. On one hand, "cognitive rehabilitation" may be considered to represent a new body of interventive strategies which serve to augment the rehabilitation professional's armamentarium designed to assault the consequences of brain dysfunction. This conceptualization may lead to the inference that cognitive rehabilitation concerns the treatment of a specific domain of the compromises associated with brain injury, depending upon one's definition of "cognition." In other words, conceptualizing cognitive rehabilitation as new treatment approaches which are additive to the more prototypical rehabilitation paradigm implies some professional discipline specificity. In this context, cognitive functioning, perhaps mistakenly, is commonly thought to concern "higher-level" mentalistic phenomena such as abstract thinking or reasoning, concept formation and problem-solving and consequently may fall largely within the general domain of psychology. Cognitive rehabilitation can, therefore, be viewed as a battery of interventive strategies designed to ameliorate circumscribed aspects (cognitive) of the consequences of brain injury.

Contrastingly, cognitive rehabilitation may be viewed as a shift in the rehabilitation paradigm in its entirity and thereby have implications for all involved disciplines. The principle philosophical underpinning of this belief holds rehabilitation as essentially a learning (or relearning) paradigm in conjunction with the treatment of medical illness or disease. As such, learning and relevant parameters of learning becomes the focus of rehabilitation. Moreover, all disciplines in rehabilitation facilities engage in therapeutic efforts to facilitate learning. In this context, cognition can be generally viewed as the processes and operations which subserve learning and, additionally, to the neuropsychologist concerns the quantitative and qualitative interaction of a number of central subsystems. The parallels between the neuropsychological investigation of cognition and concomitantly impairments of cognition, and information processing theory as investigated by cognitive psychologists may lay a foundation for an understanding of the cerebral processes and operations subserving learning. The relatively recent development of information processing theory (as reviewed by Bower and Hilgard, 1981) and the neuropsychological investigation of attention (see Luria, 1973 and Thatcher and John, 1977 for reviews) or memory (Cermak and Craik, 1979) exemplify such parallel lines of investigation. As a consequence, this growing base of information may clarify the relevant parameters of learning as well as the operations and processes of the central nervous system which subserve learning.

The implications of how one conceptualizes cognition are obvious. Assuming that cognitive processes concern only "higher-level" mental operations, not indifferent from Lurian notions of "thinking" (Luria, 1973, p.327) cognitive rehabilitation may represent a specialized area of empirical and clinical effort involving various and sundry types of psychologists. The inverse perspective implies that cognitive factors are relevant to all rehabilitation professionals. Consequently, how one conceptualizes cognitive rehabilitation has implications for (1) the scope of human behavior which it concerns and (2) the professional discipline which engages in the study and treatment of cognitive dysfunction.

The two differing herein described conceptualizations of cognitive rehabilitation are, in some ways, analogous to differing perspectives on functional neurology, namely the localizationist and the anti-localizationist positions. Early proponents of localization theory believed that a specific behavioral function was subserved by a circumscribed area of the cerebral cortex and that discrete lesions resulted in relatively discrete impairment. The anti-localizationist's position, most commonly associated with the work of Lashley (1929) was that a particular behavioral deficit could not be associated with a designated focal lesion and that "the nervous system was organized according to a hierarchy in which voluntary symbolic behaviors were mediated by the highest levels and stimulus-bound behaviors by the lowest" (Moscovitch, 1979, p.380) The reader is referred to Luria (1980) for an indepth discussion on the issue of localization of function in the human cerebral cortex. Nonetheless, one might question the extent to which cognitive processes are localizable, the answer depending upon one's definition of cognition. The implications of these assumptions and definitions extend to beliefs concerning treatment of cognitive disturbance following cerebral dysfunction and are related to the nature of the neuropathology under consideration. Assuming that specific behaviors are localizable, treatment may follow a deficit-specific approach, at least in the case of focal lesions. In the case of non-focal lesions, rehabilitative strategies may be considered to represent merely an additive process, addressing specific deficits one at a time. On the other hand, viewing brain-behavior relationships as systemically organized to subserve information processing, in general, suggests that rehabilitative strategies should address information processing capacity in context of the component processes, and their interaction, which subserve information processing. The critical issue, therefore, becomes defining the parameters through which information processing capacity can be facilitated.

It is probably the case, however, that neither of these positions adequately address the complexity of the functional organization of cerebral processes. Further, the configuration or patterning of behavioral-cognitive dysfunction probably differs between varying neuropathological groups (see Thomas and Trexler of the present volume). Nonetheless, it may not be a totally erroneous assumption that cerebral dysfunction affects general and specific dimensions of brain-behavior functioning and that an interaction between regions within and between the cerebral hemispheres subserves those normatively highly integrated behavioral-cognitive processes which become of concern clinically in rehabilitation settings following central dysfunction. It is for these reasons that a cookbook approach to the rehabilitation of cognitive dysfunction seems, at least to the present author, naive. Cognitive rehabilitation may be found to represent treatment efforts oriented at (1) the general information processing capability of the central nervous system, as particularly related to mechanisms of arousal, attention and memory; (2) the, relatively speaking, more specific consequences, such as dysphasia or perceptual disorders; and (3) in context of (1) and (2), the dynamic interaction of these intertwined processes and functions which eventuates in highly organized behavior. Consequently, cognitive rehabilitation may represent both a conceptual and interventive compilation extending from the field of psychology, specifically cognitive psychology and neuropsychology as well as an integral consideration to all professional disciplines intentful of facilitating learning for patients with dysfunction of the central nervous system.

Conceptualizing cognitive rehabilitation along the aforementioned lines brings about substantial problems with which rehabilitation professional must struggle. Initially, this conceptualization brings havoc to the discipline boundaries inherent in rehabilitation settings. The complexity and interrelatedness of brain-behavior relationships and the concomitant nature of cerebral dysfunction mandates an interdisciplinary effort. It is likely that activities of daily living are not divisible into autonomous functional repertoires of behavior (no more so than the neural substrate of language). Stated in an over-simplistic manner, the functional capacity of the central nervous system represents more than a mere sum of its parts.

The extent to which interdisciplinary models of care are implemented in rehabilitation settings may be most significantly related to the "cognitive flexibility" of the staff. Secondly, conceptualizing cognitive rehabilitation in the manner herein previously described suggests that no one treatment strategy will be totally applicable for more than one patient and would probably need to be modified frequently for that one patient as a function of changes in brain-behavior integrity associated with recovery and new learning. Thirdly, while there exists an impressive body of literature concerning the parameters of learning for humans with intact neural systems, the investigation of the relevant parameters of learning (research oriented at asking the question, how do people with brain dysfunction learn?) for persons with impaired cerebral functions is in its infancy; there is a dearth of basic applied research defining the parameters which would elucidate under what conditions central nervous system damaged patients learn and do not learn. In other words, the literature which would ascertain the extent to which models of abnormal cognitive functioning resembles models of normal human cognition does not exist. It seems unlikely that models of normal and dysfunctional cognition would be compatible. These problems of cognitive rehabilitation can only be addressed through further empirical investigation, especially that of factor analytic neuropsychological and information processing research with relevant clinical populations. Finally, the mere complexity of the topic, as predicated by this conceptualization of cognitive rehabilitation and the attempt to modify learning in a pathologic brain-behavior system, necessitates an unending self-examination and questioning of professional methodology, optimally through empirical research. The chapters which follow are an initial and humble attempt at beginning to address these problems.

## REFERENCES

Bower, G.H. and Hilgard, E.R. Theories of learning, Fifth edition. Englewood Cliffs: Prentice-Hall, 1981.

Cermak, L.S. and Craik, F.I. Levels of processing in human memory. Hillsdale, New Jersey: Lawrence Erlbaum, 1979.

Lashley, K.S. Brain mechanisms and intelligence. Chicago: University of Chicago Press, 1929.

Luria, A.R. The working brain. New York: Basic Books, 1973.

Luria, A.R. Higher cortical functions in man, Second edition. New York: Basic Books, 1980.

Moscovitch, M. Information processing and the cerebral hemispheres. In: M.G. Gazzaniga (Ed.), Handbook of behavioral neurobiology, Volume 2 on neuropsychology. New York: Plenum Press, 1979.

Thatcher, R.W. and John, E.R. Foundations of cognitive processes. Hillsdale, New Jersey: Lawrence Erlbaum, 1977.

# NEUROPSYCHOLOGICAL ASSESSMENT OF BRAIN BEHAVIOR RELATIONSHIPS: AN INTRODUCTION

William J. Lynch, Ph.D.

Director, Brain Injury Rehabilitation Unit
Veterans Administration Medical Center
Palo Alto, California

## INTRODUCTION

A fundamental principle of clinical neuropsychology is the belief that there is a discoverable relationship between brain function and observable behavior. The traditional approaches to inferring the status of the brain involved observation or the clinical neurologic examination. In the last 40 years, approaches utilizing a combination of psychometric and standardized clinical neurologic procedures have emerged. Beginning with the work of Halstead (1947) and Reitan (1966), and continuing with the efforts of Luria (1967) and Golden (1981), a proliferation of neuropsychologic batteries has taken place. In this presentation, I will focus upon the Halstead-Reitan battery, although Luria's formulations regarding brain functions will serve as a basis for this analysis.

### Basic Anatomical Considerations

The understanding of brain behavior relationships requires knowledge of brain structure and function as a starting point. The lateral view of the brain, as shown in Figure 1, contains many of the key landmarks of the human cerebral cortex. It is helpful to think of the brain functions as complex systems which are interrelated.

Luria (1967) felt that there were three basic functional units in the human brain: (a) an arousal or alerting system, (b) a sensory or input system, and (c) a motor or output system which included the higher, integrative functions such as planning, abstract reasoning, and judgement. The arousal system consists of structures in the brain stem (particularly the ascending reticular activating system) which maintain cortical activation. Alertness, attention, and

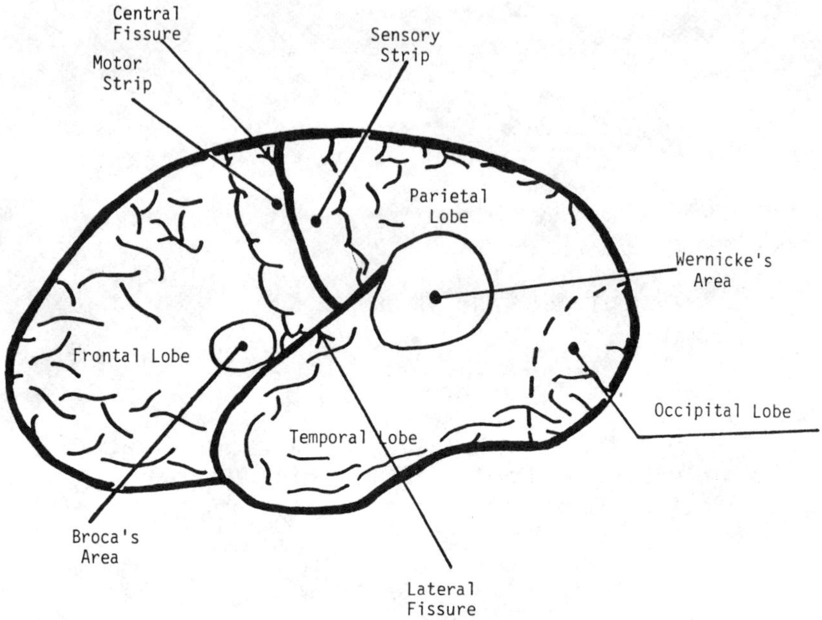


Figure 1. Lateral view of the brain (left hemisphere) with major landmarks.

concentration are dependent upon this system. And since virtually all cognitive activities require attention and concentration, problems at this level are critical to both diagnosis and prognosis.

Patients who suffer anoxic brain damage or certain toxic states (such as drug overdose) frequently display chronic problems with maintaining alertness, attention, and concentration. Their performance on formal testing is affected by their failure to properly attend to instructions or to maintain concentration on a task once it is begun. Clearly, memory retraining becomes nearly impossible with these patients until basic attentional deficits are addressed.

The second general unit contains the various sensory processing and integrating areas. Tactile, auditory and visual inputs are perceived and synthesized by the appropriate areas of the parietal, temporal, and occipital lobes, respectively. Accurate and timely detection and interpretation of sensory data presume proper functioning of the first functional unit.

Behavioral planning, anticipation, and execution constitute the role of the third functional unit. While the third unit consists of the frontal lobes, and therefore includes gross and fine motor functions, there are a number of capacities which are included in this dimension. Abstract reasoning, problem solving and logical analysis are among the higher level abilities which are mediated by the third functional unit. It is important to note that within each general unit are a number of specialized functions which in combination with other functional areas form the basis for complex psychological functions. These combinations or "functional systems" are the focus of analysis in Luria's scheme of assessment.

## NEUROPSYCHOLOGIC ASSESSMENT

It is the purpose of clinical neuropsychologic assessment to measure and evaluate the status of brain function as it is manifested in cognitive, sensory, motor and perceptual-motor abilities. The examination attempts to isolate intact, impaired, and lost-function abilities by systematically observing the patient's performance on structured tasks. In the following sections I will present the elements of neuropsychologic assessment according to the following seven catagories:

1. Mental Status and Memory Assessment
2. Sensory and Perceptual Assessment
3. Tactile-Spatial Perception Assessment
4. Language Assessment
5. Handedness and Motor Functions Assessment
6. Intellectual and Academic Achievement Assessment
7. Abstract Reasoning Assessment

### Mental Status and Memory Assessment

As I have noted above, a determination of the patient's level of alertness, attention, and concentration is a prerequisite to any type neuropsychologic assessment. While simple clinical observation is often informative, it is frequently necessary to obtain a more detailed and formal evaluation of mental status. There are a number of mental status forms available, although most tend to be either overly long (for example Strub and Black, 1977) or overly brief (for example Pfeiffer, 1975). The Galveston Orientation and Amnesia Test or GOAT (Levin, O'Donnell, and Grossman, 1979) is a newly developed examination which is designed specifically for traumatically head-injured persons. It is easily administered (10 minutes) and contains a profile on the record form for plotting the results of serial testing. It is especially useful for operationally defining the presence and course of posttraumatic amnesia (PTA).

Another brief mental status examination which I have found quite useful is the Mini-Mental State (MMS) examination by Folstein, Folstein, and McHugh (1975). The MMS requires about ten minutes to administer and contains a variety of items ranging from orientation to mental control to memory for three objects to rudimentary language abilities.

An added advantage of the MMS is the availability of norms for both controls and several clinical populations (psychiatric and organic). MMS results can be recorded on a graphic profile sheet in order to document longitudinal fluctuations in mental status.

The evaluation of memory requires a more elaborate test procedure than is typical of mental status examinations. The most widely used memory test is the Wechsler Memory Scale, or WMS (Wechsler, 1945) which includes the following subtests: Information, Orientation, Mental Control, Logical Memory, Digit Span, Visual Reproduction, and Associate Learning. The WMS yields a Memory Quotient which has a mean of 100 and a standard deviation of fifteen.

Although the Memory Quotient is a useful value, most clinicians find that a detailed subtest analysis, both from quantitative and qualitative standpoints, is necessary for a complete assessment of a patient's true memory capacity. Recently, Russell (1975) has published normative data for evaluating the results of delayed (30-minute) readministration of the Logical Memory and Visual Reproduction subtests of the WMS. It has been shown that a sizable proportion of patients with subtle memory disorders may be "missed" by the standard administration of the WMS, while the 30-minute delay format seems to be much more sensitive to these deficits. Other measures of visual (Benton, 1974) or auditory (Goldman, Fristoe, and Woodcock, 1974) memory are available for more specialzed purposes. Osborne and Davis (1978) have published norms for certain WMS subtests for various age groups. This allows the clinician to compare the patient's performance on each subtest to his/her age-peers so that apparent and actual deficits will not be confused.

Mental status and memory assessment serve several purposes in rehabilitation. First, it is primarily with such testing that the presence, extent, and type of dementia or memory disorder can be determined. Second, this testing allows the clinician to objectively assess alertness, attention and concentration so that appropriate therapeutic interventions can be initiated. For example, the need for either reality or memory retraining can be evaluated in a direct fashion. Finally, such structured testing can be readily used to establish baseline and follow-up levels of performance in these areas.

## Sensory and Perceptual Assessment

Most neuropsychologic batteries contain a cortical sensory-perceptual evaluation of some kind, whereas the traditional clinical neurologic examination includes a brief assessment of both cortical and spinal sensory systems. Cortical sensory functions include finger recognition, tactile perception of symbols, and tactile recognition of three dimensional objects (stereognosis). In addition, two-point texture and weight discriminations require cortical analysis. The ability to detect and identify bilateral simultaneous sensory (auditory, visual, or tactile) stimuli also requires higher level integration. Basic sensory functions such as unilateral detection of pain, temperature, vibration, sound, or light are not ordinarily considered "cortical" in nature.

The phenomenon of sensory extinction or suppression is the subject of debate regarding the exact nature of its etiology. Extinction is said to occur when the patient being confronted with bilateral simultaneous stimulation (auditory, visual, or tactile) consistently fails to detect the stimulus to one side of the body. This presumes normal response to unilateral stimuli. Whatever the cause, it appears that stimuli to the side of the body opposite a unilateral post-central brain lesion will typically fail to be perceived when they compete with stimuli opposite the normal hemisphere. This clinical observation has resulted in the inclusion of standard tests of extinction or suppression in most neuropsychologic batteries.

Sensory perceptual functions are evaluated on the Halstead-Reitan Battery by the following measures:

Tactile Perception. The basic ability to detect light touch to the back of either hand or to hand-and-face is evaluated, along with the ability to recognize double simultaneous stimulation. Failure to detect stimuli on one side of the body or the other is suggestive of post-central dysfunction in the contralateral cerebral hemisphere.

Finger Recognition. Finger recognition refers to the ability to correctly identify each of one's fingers by touch alone. This ability is tested by first blindfolding the patient and then by lightly touching each finger on each hand. Failure to correctly identify which finger is being touched may indicate dysfunction in the appropriate region of the parietal cortex contralateral to the side which evidenced deficit.

Tactile Symbol Recognition. The ability to perceive linquistic or numeric symbols which are traced on the skin is termed graphesthesia. Testing is carried out by tracing numbers or letters on the palm of the hand or fingertips. Failure to correctly identify numbers or letters may implicate the parietal lobe contralateral to the side of impairment.

Tactile Form Recognition. The ability to recognize both objects and shapes by touch alone is termed stereognosis. Testing typically consists of presenting the blindfolded patient with various objects or shapes which he or she is required to name. The difficulty with this approach is that patients with purely linquistic and not sensory deficits may be unable to name the objects correctly. If the patient fails to name objects placed in one hand, but not the other, the limiting factor cannot be a language disorder. When intactness of the language system is in doubt, the use of a matching format is advised. Here the patient feels the objects with one hand behind a screen and selects an identical object from among several on a panel

Table 1. Visual Field Defects and Corresponding Location of Lesion.

| Defect | Location of Lesion |
|---|---|
| 1. Loss of vision in one eye | Optic nerve, anterior to chiasm |
| 2. Loss of outer (temporal) half-field of each eye | Around chiasm, e.g. pituitary gland |
| 3. Loss of upper quadrant, same side for each eye | Temporal lobe (opposite to quadrant lost) |
| 4. Loss of half field, same side for each eye | Parietal lobe; occipital lobe |

in front of him or her. Consistent failure to recognize common objects by touch with one hand or the other is indicative of parietal lobe impairment in the contralateral cerebral hemisphere.

Visual Fields. Brain lesions which impinge upon the visual system result in characteristic alterations in the visual fields. Depending on the location of the lesion, the patient may lose all vision in one eye or portions of the visual fields in both eyes. The partial loss may be as small as a quadrant (quadrantopsia) or as large as half of the field. Whether the loss is on the left or right of each eye field, and whether it is a quadrant or a half-field loss will bear heavily upon the localizing information of a visual field loss.

Clinical assessment of the visual fields is carried out by confrontation. That is, the patient stands or sits at eye level with the examiner and covers one eye. He or she must then indicate detection of brief flashes from a penlight or finger movements at various points along the normal periphery of the visual field. Each eye is tested separately. While it is preferable to obtain a formal charting of the visual fields by perimetry, gross visual field impairments can be identified by the confrontation procedure. Table 1 presents a listing of common visual field defects along with corresponding likely lesion sites.

Auditory Perception. The ability to detect and discriminate among auditory signals is a prerequisite for normal verbal communication. Thus, prior to evaluating verbal intellectual skills, the clinician must assess the patient's ability to perform auditory discriminations. Presuming a normal audiometric examination, the patient's speech perception ability is evaluated. This can be accomplished by a number of means. The most basic approach is exemplified by the Goldman-Fristoe-Woodcock (GFW) Auditory Discrimination Test (1974). The patient is confronted with a series of pairs of pictures of like-sounding objects or scenes such as a "lake" and a "rake." A tape recorded voice then announces "Point to . . . lake," and the patient should then point to--or somehow indicate--which of the two pictures represents what has been heard. This same procedure is followed for 100 trials. A normal score indicates normal discrimination of speech sounds. An abnormal score may reflect impairment in the dominant temporal-parietal areas.

The Halstead Speech-Sounds Perception Test measures a similar ability but in a more obtuse fashion. The patient hears a nonsense word pronounced on a tape and selects from among four choices printed on an answer sheet for each of 60 trials. Nonverbal auditory discrimination is measured by the Seashore Rhythm Test. The patient is presented with 30 pairs of tonal patterns which are either identical or slightly different. The inability to correctly discriminate nonverbal auditory patterns is associated with temporal lobe dysfunction (probably more frequently in the minor cerebral hemisphere).

## Tactile-Spatial Perception Assessment

The evaluation of multiple modalities is helpful in determining the integrity of broad cortical association areas. One such test is the Tactual Performance Test or TPT. The TPT consists of an upright rectangular board containing ten variously-shaped indentations and ten like-shaped wooden blocks. The patient is required to replace all ten blocks, while blindfolded, with the preferred, nonpreferred, and both hands consecutively. Each performance is evaluated with regard to time and number of blocks replaced within the time limit (ten or fifteen minutes). In addition, after the blindfold has been removed, the patient is required to draw a picture of the board from memory. Attention is paid to both the number of shapes correctly recalled ("Memory" score) and the proper location of each shape ("Localization" score) with respect to the other shapes on the board. The TPT requires tactile discrimination, spatial perception, and motor performance. Tactile and spatial memory abilities are assessed by the Memory and Localization components of the TPT.

The fact that the patient is blindfolded during the unilateral performance trials permits the clinician to evaluate each cerebral hemisphere separately. It is expected that the patient will steadily improve his/her performance from one trial to the next.

The TPT is felt to assess the patient's ability to deal with a novel tactile/spatial problem, and to utilize accumulated knowledge to assist in solving this problem. Qualitative factors are significant as well. The patients' approach to the task in terms of strategy (methodical vs. haphazard), speed (rapid vs. plodding), recognition of errors (immediate vs. absent), or response to failure (minimal vs. catastrophic) are some of the variables which should be assessed.

With regard to brain-behavior relationships, the TPT is a complex measure. Test performance that is accurate but too slow, may reflect frontal lobe dysfunction. The examiner should refer to other motor function tests (Grip Strength, Finger Tapping) for corroboration of this hypothesis. Performance that is both inaccurate and slow may result from generalized cortical dysfunction. If the poor performance occurs with only one hand, the clinician should suspect impairment in the contralateral cerebral hemisphere. The dysfunction may be either anterior or posterior depending upon the presence or absence of associated motor deficit. Poor localization with adequate memory may implicate the postcentral area of the posterior nondominate hemisphere.

The TPT provides useful information regarding the patient's approach to new problems. Incidental learning and memory capacity, as well as certain spatial neglect syndromes, are frequently identified by the TPT.

Language Assessment

A complete neuropsychologic evaluation includes an assessment of the patient's ability to comprehend, process, and express language. Whereas thorough speech/language examinations are generally performed by speech pathologists, neuropsychologists typically employ some relatively brief screening device for detecting language disorders. Reitan (1966) uses the modified Halstead-Wepman Aphasia Screening Test (AST) which is a heterogeneous compilation consisting of 23 verbal, seven graphic, and three gestural items. Although termed an "Aphasia" Screening Test, the AST purports to assess various forms of dyspraxia, right-left confusion, and dysarthria. The common property of all measures of language function is the presentation of stimuli to the patient in order to assess his/her ability to comprehend, retain, or express information via speech, gestures, or writing. The various measures differ in the number and type of stimuli and the way in which performance is evaluated. While most language tests utilize a dichotomous or plus-minus scoring system, some such as the Porch Index of Communicative Ability or PICA (Porch, 1967) utilize a complex multidimensional scoring approach. The choice of scoring system depends primarily upon the clinician's needs for precision and reliability of scoring; and for serial testing, a multidimensional scoring system of some sort is recommended. For routine screening purposes, a plus-minus system is sufficient.

The importance of careful language assessment cannot be overemphasized. Aphasia is one of the few symptoms, if present, that can be considered definitely indicative (i.e., pathognomonic) of cerebral pathology. In right handed persons, the pathology will almost invariably be situated in the left cerebral hemisphere.

The type of language disorder can also assist in localizing the lesion responsible. For example, halting, telegraphic speech with relatively normal comprehension and right sided weakness is a pattern seen with lesions in the left cerebral hemisphere in the region of the third frontal convolution (Broca's Area). Likewise, when speech is fluent, yet dysphasic, with poor comprehension, but without any motor weakness on the right, a lesion in the posterior temporal-inferior parietal area (Wernicke's Area) should be suspected.

If both syndromes are present, either a widespread lesion which affects both anterior and posterior speech areas, or perhaps a disconnection of the anterior and posterior centers has taken place.

There is frequently a great deal of confusion surrounding the commonly used terms "Broca's" and "Wernicke's" or "fluent" and "nonfluent" aphasia. I would recommend adoption of topographical terms such as "anterior" and "posterior" to refer to the location of the lesion. This practice will immediately indicate where the lesion is presumed to be and will resolve the recurrent uncertainty of students and interns regarding the two major aphasic syndromes.

Put another way, one can divide most aphasic disorders into two major types: those which primarily involve linguistic expression or output (speaking, writing or gesturing) and those which involve comprehension or input of spoken, written or gestural information.

In rehabilitation, it is essential to identify both the intact and defective communicative systems. In this way, a rational program of retraining can be developed in which intact systems are utilized to assist in rehabilitating those which are impaired. And since all other components of the rehabilitation process depend in some fashion upon language, the importance of establishing a clear channel of communication cannot be overestimated.

## Handedness and Motor Functions Assessment

The determination of handedness is a first step in evaluating the patient's motor functions. The traditional manner of determining handedness involves observation of the patient's performance of such activities as writing, using tools, throwing a ball, or opening a door. It has been suggested by some that there are few individuals who are universally right-or left-handed. Estimates (Milner, Branch, and Rasmussen, 1964) are that between 90% and 95% of the population are right-handed, and that of these, about 98% are left-brain dominant for language. Of the left-handers, about 60% are also left-brain dominant for language, while the remaining 40% appear to have language mediated in the right cerebral hemisphere.

On the Halstead-Reitan battery, lateral preference is defined by the Lateral Dominance Examination, which takes into account such factors as hand preference for writing and strength of grip, foot preference for stepping or kicking, and eye preference for aiming or focusing upon nearby objects. The term "crossed dominance" refers to the situation in which the hand and eye preferences are incongruent. Swiercinsky (1977) has shown that crossed dominance tends to correlate with subnormal performance on neuropsychologic tests. It is also necessary to determine lateral preference prior to motor testing so that the patient can begin each test with the preferred hand or foot.

Evaluation of motor functions proceeds from gross to more refined motor skills. The individual tests are described in the following three sections.

Strength of Grip. Part of the clinical neurologic examination is the evaluation of manual strength. This is typically determined by asking the patient to firmly squeeze the hands or fingers of the examiner. A subjective estimate is then made regarding absolute strength (i.e., strong vs. weak), as well as relative strength of the two sides of the body. The neuropsychologist's rule of thumb, suggested originally by Reitan (1959), is that the preferred hand tends to be about 10% stronger than the nonpreferred hand in normal subjects. Whereas gross bilateral or unilateral weakness will be readily detected by the clinical method, more modest weakness will be less easily noted. Further, if one is interested in conducting serial evaluations, a more precise and objective measure is required.

The device employed by most neuropsychologists is the Hand dynamometer (available from Lafayette Instruments or the Stoelting Co.) which measures manual grip strength in kilograms. The patient squeezes the dynamometer alternately, with preferred, nonpreferred hands for four trials, yielding an average strength for each hand. With the dynamometer, exact determinations of grip strength, either at a given time or across a period of time, are possible. A significant finding could either be considerable weakness of the nonpreferred, as compared with the preferred, hand; or a tendency for the nonpreferred hand to be stronger than the preferred hand.

Weakness of grip may arise from noncerebral pathology, and thus the clinician should not be overly hasty in presuming brain dysfunction on the basis of unilateral or bilateral loss of grip strength. Such conditions as arthritis, improperly healed bone fractures, wrist sprains, muscular diseases, and cervical spinal disorders may significantly affect grip strength. Indeed, patients who are simply bedridden for more than a few days will begin to evidence weakness (bilateral) of their grips. If all of these possible sources of weakness can be ruled out, the cause of unilateral loss of grip strength is presumed to be impairment in or near the motor strip of the contralateral cerebral hemisphere. Upper body strength, as measured by Grip Strength, is useful in the performance of gross motor acts such as transferring with a bar, lifting, opening doors, and operating any kind of vehicle, including a wheelchair.

Finger and Foot Tapping Speed. Halstead (1947) originally included only dominant hand finger tapping speed in his neuropsychological test battery. Reitan (1966) later included both right and left hands in order to permit comparison of one side of the body with the other. Finger tapping speed is measured by a small telegraph-like key attached to a mechanical counter which is affixed to a board

(20 x 20 centimeters). The patient is instructed to hold his/her hand in the prone position, with forearm resting on the table and hand and fingertips (except for the index finger) touching the board. The patient then proceeds, on signal, to tap the key as rapidly as possible for ten seconds. Traditionally, five trials are obtained with each hand in alternating sequence. The mean, total, or best trial score is then used to determine the relative performance of the right and left hands.

Foot tapping speed has been added to the neuropsychologic battery in many settings as a means of assessing lower extremity motor performance for comparison with finger tapping speed. Foot tapping is assessed by means of an electric pedal device attached to a digital counter. As with finger tapping, the patient taps as rapidly as possible (while standing with heel on the floor) for ten seconds. And, as in finger tapping, the clinician is advised to first rule out noncortical causes for foot tapping problems.

The significance of impaired finger and foot tapping speeds is generally determined by comparing the relative efficiency of the two sides of the body, and by comparing the patient's relative proficiency on the two tasks. Patients with fairly "deep" or extensive lesions which interrupt efferent pathways from the motor cortex will evidence deficits on both finger and foot tapping speed. However, if the lesion is more circumscribed or is situated so that only a portion of the efferent pathways is affected, one may see a defect in only one of these tapping tests. For example, middle cerebral artery lesions affect the upper extremities more than the lowers; and the reverse is true of anterior cerebral artery involvement. Typically, <u>both</u> upper and lower extremities are affected to some degree, however.

In rehabilitation settings, it is useful to know how efficiently the patient performs on such tests as finger and foot tapping speed. Finger tapping reflects the speed and consistency with which the patient can carry out a simple, repetitive finger movement. Activity such as eating, dressing, and gross manual skills may require such movements. Foot tapping speed may indicate how proficient the patient is in the area of walking, climbing stairs, or driving (manipulating brake or clutch).

<u>Pegboard Tasks</u>. For the measurement of fine manipulative dexterity, there are two types of pegboards available commercially: The Purdue Pegboard and the Grooved Pegboard.

The Purdue Pegboard (marketed by Science Research Associates) consists of a flat (33 x 40 centimeters) board which is placed so that the shorter side faces the patient. At the top or distal end of the board are four concave round "dishes" in which are stored three types of metal objects: solid pins, washers, and collars. The pins are stored in the two outer dishes, while the collars and washers are stored in the center receptacles. Down the center of the board from the dishes to the patient are 25 pairs of small holes which will accomodate the pins. The task for the patient is to pick up pins (depending upon the hand used) and place them as rapidly as possible in the row of holes on that side within a 30-second time limit. Dominant and nondominant hands are evaluated. A third trial requires the patient to insert the pins simultaneously, in pairs. Then a total score is obtained.

Costa, Vaughn, Levita, and Farber (1963) have shown that the Purdue Pegboard can be used to predict the presence and laterality of brain damage in certain patients. Clearly, patients with cerebral dysfunction which does not involve the motor or visual system may perform quite normally on the Purdue Pegboard, and thus it should not be used as a determinant of the presence of brain damage.

The Grooved Pegboard (available from Lafayette Instruments) is a compact (ten x ten centimeters) portable device which consists of 25 holes arranged in five rows. Each hole contains a small notch which is designed to accommodate grooved metal pins which are provided in a large dish at the top of the board. The patient must insert the metal pin into each hole precisely by turning it so that the groove fits properly into the notch. Preferred and nonpreferred hand trials are obtained, with time to completion and errors (dropped pegs) being recorded for each.

Both the Purdue and Grooved Pegboards require coordination of visual input, proprioception, and precise motor output. Therefore, one cannot automatically assume motor dysfunction because of poor performance. Patients with impaired visual acuity, faulty extraocular movements, or poor positional sense may perform poorly on the pegboard tasks. Likewise, patients who have subcortical disease causing impaired attention or abnormal involuntary movements may obtain low scores. The information gained from the pegboard tasks may assist in determining the patient's general level of attention and concentration on a repetitive task. In addition, some of the finer aspects of dressing, such as buttoning or tying shoelaces require precise finger dexterity. And finally, patients who express an intent to work at small scale assembly or mechanical work may be prescreened with a pegboard task. It is typical during recovery for patients to evidence slower and less pronounced improvement on pegboard tasks than on other simpler tests of motor function.

## Intellectual and Academic Achievement Assessment

The evaluation of cognitive functions is an integral part of the neuropsychologic evaluation. The ability to recall specific information on command, as well as to comprehend the significance of social situations, to reason abstractly, or to express ideas clearly are among the abilities evaluated by psychometric intelligence tests. The Wechsler Adult Intelligence Scale, or WAIS (Wechsler, 1955), is the most frequently used individual intelligence test. The 11

Table 2. The WAIS Subtests and What They Measure.

| Subtest | What it Measures |
| --- | --- |
| Verbal: | |
| 1. Information | Recall of specific facts from long-term memory; extent of educational background. |
| 2. Comprehension | Practical judgment; social awareness; ability to reason toward a conclusion; abstract thinking. |
| 3. Arithmetic | Alertness, attention, concentration; knowledge of mathematic principles; ability to visualize numbers. |
| 4. Similarities | Abstract verbal reasoning; ability to attend to subtle details; associative thinking. |
| 5. Digit span | Alertness, attention, and concentration; auditory sequencing; immediate recall. |
| 6. Vocabulary | Verbal fluency; knowledge of word meanings. |
| Performance: | |
| 7. Digit symbol | Alertness, attention, concentration; ability to quickly learn new associations; eye-hand coordination. |
| 8. Picture completion | Visual alertness, visual scanning; ability to discriminate relevant from nonrelevant features. |
| 9. Block design | Visual organization (?); perceptive motor skills; constructional skills; appreciation of part-whole relationships; abstract nonverbal reasoning. |
| 10. Picture arrangement | Alertness to visual details; social awareness; visual sequencing. |
| 11. Object assembly | Perceptual organization, perception of part-whole relationships; ability to visualize end-result from component parts. |

subtests of the WAIS are divided into two general categories: Verbal and Performance. Table 2 contains a listing of the WAIS subtests along with a brief summary of what each measures.

The reader is referred to the excellent texts by Matarazzo (1972) and by Zimmerman and Woo-Sam (1973) for a more extensive review of the development, item composition, and statistical characteristics of the WAIS subtests.

The WAIS provides a great deal of useful information in evaluating the patient's neuropsychologic status. By knowing the patient's current intellectual level, treatment programs can be appropriately adjusted to accommodate his/her cognitive capacities. Specific subtest scores can reveal isolated problems in certain areas of intellectual functioning. For example, Massey (1968) has published forms which permit the calculation of "Deviation Quotients" for three principal WAIS factors: Verbal Comprehension, Memory and Freedom from Distractibility, and Perceptual Organization. This procedure allows the clinician to focus upon more meaningful cognitive or perceptual abilities than would be the case using only Verbal or Performance Intelligence Quotient (IQ) values.

Specific WAIS item responses may also be informative. Subtests such as Information, Comprehension, Similarities, and Vocabulary provide data regarding verbal memory, fluency, abstraction, and reasoning ability. The ease with which a patient defines a difficult word or identifies the principal similarity between two objects can reflect a degree of alertness and responsiveness which is helpful in the treatment process. The clinician should always take note of the quality of incorrect responses, as well. The magnitude of error may reveal a greater or lesser degree of pathology which will determine the type and intensity of treatment to be employed. Likewise, responses which are bizarre or totally inappropriate, or which indicate that the patient recognizes his/her inability to respond should be given separate attention.

In summary, the WAIS is probably the best psychometric intelligence test and should be employed whenever possible. The reader should be aware that the revised WAIS (WAIS-R) was published in the spring of 1981, and it now will be necessary to conduct new research on the utility of the WAIS-R as a measure of complex neuropsychologic abilities in rehabilitation settings.

With certain patients, such as those with motor weakness or expressive language problems, a different form of intelligence test is necessary. The Peabody Picture Vocabulary Test, or PPVT (Dunn, 1965) is probably the most frequently employed intelligence test in disabled populations. The PPVT has the advantage of being relatively brief, easily administered, objectively scored, and minimal in its verbal or motor requirements. Patients simply point to their choice from among four pictures, one of which represents a word spoken to them by the examiner.

Zimmerman and Woo-Sam (1973, p.33) report on a number of correlational studies between the PPVT and the WAIS. Correlations ranged from .61 to .91, with a median correlation in the upper .70's. Thus, the PPVT may be used as a substitute for the WAIS if one is merely concerned with global IQ measures.

Although the PPVT may be useful in predicting Verbal of Full Scale IQs, unfortunately, it is unidimensional and lacking in response variation. As a result, there is minimal opportunity to analyze specific intellectual operations such as verbal versus nonverbal abstraction, arithmetic skill, or memory. Its utility with disabled persons, however, is sufficient to outweigh these drawbacks.

Academic achievement is often an item of interest in evaluating higher cortical functions. Frequently, brain disorders affect the efficiency with which the patient deals with language or mathematic symbols. Since reading, writing, and calculating are skills which are required for independence, it is imperative that one determine at which level a patient is functioning in these primary areas. Aside from providing an additional measure of communicative abilities, achievement assessment helps to determine the level at which staff should attempt to interact with the patient. Thus, patients with normal reading skill may be expected to follow simple <u>written</u> instructions, whereas those who are reading at a lower-than-normal level may require simple, concrete <u>verbal</u> instructions.

There are two individually administered standardized achievement tests available widely. The most popular is the Wide Range Achievement Test, or WRAT (Jastak and Jastak, 1978). This test evaluates three areas of achievement: Reading (actually, single word recognition), Spelling, and Arithmetic. Each yields a raw score which is transformed into a grade equivalent. By referring to the appropriate age norms (the test range is from five to 64), the grade equivalent is transformed into either a standard score, percentile, or stanine. The standard scores include T-scores (Mean = 50; <u>SD</u> = ten), scaled score (Mean = ten; <u>SD</u> = three), or WAIS-type standard score (Mean = 100; <u>SD</u> = 15). By using these standard scores, a patient's performance relative to his/her peers can be obtained. In this fashion, persons with learning disabilities can be identified and assigned to appropriate remedial programs.

The Spelling and arithmetic subtests of the WRAT require the patient of write his/her responses. The patient must generate the correct response from memory. On the Reading subtest, the patient simply reads from a card containing letters and words of increasing difficulty. The more difficult words are such that they are not easily read phonetically if they are unfamiliar to the patient.

To accommodate the patient with expressive speech or motor deficits, a test format which minimizes the patient's output requirements is often desirable. The Peabody Individual Achievement Test, or PIAT (Dunn and Markwardt, 1970), provides a partial solution to this problem. The PIAT consists of five subtests: Mathematics, Reading Recognition, Reading Comprehension, Spelling, and General Information. In addition, a "Total Test" score is calculated by summing the raw scores from the five subtests. The raw scores are translated into grade equivalents as well as percentiles and standard scores.

What makes the PIAT so attractive for rehabilitation settings is the fact that it utilizes a multiple-choice format, whereby the patient must recognize the correct response from among similar alternatives. Thus, the patient need only point or somehow indicate his/her choice of response even on "Verbal" tests such as Spelling or Reading Comprehension, or on such complex tests as Mathematics.

Because the PIAT was not designed specifically for adults, it should not be used for determining exact percentiles or standard scores. However, it is quite useful for both screening and retraining purposes because of its simple output requirements.

Where possible, it is helpful to obtain both the WRAT and PIAT on each patient. Because of their similar content and dissimilar output modalities, the clinician can draw comparisons between performance on one test versus the other. For example, patients who cannot solve written mathematics problems on the WRAT, but who perform normally on the PIAT Mathematics subtest, may not have a mathematics problem at all. The limiting factor may be one of motor control of the pencil or an inability to discriminate the smaller numerals on the WRAT test form. In this same fashion, patients who write words incorrectly on the WRAT Spelling subtest, but who spell normally on the PIAT Spelling subtest may be suffering from a motor, rather than a language problem.

With regard to brain-behavior relationships, measures of intellectual functions and academic achievement do not fit neatly into a topographic scheme of brain functions. Due to the complexity of both the abilities and the way that they are measured, it is most likely that broad areas of the brain are involved in intellectual operations such as those assessed by the WAIS or WRAT. Deficits in learning which arise from problems with inhibiting or sustaining mental activity, comprehending abstract principles, or recognizing success or failure could well result from frontal lobe dysfunction. More specific problems such as impaired memory or attention span may result from temporal lobe, limbic, or brain stem malfunction. Difficulty with the symbolic significance of letters, words or numerals most likely results from more restricted brain dysfunction in the dominant cerebral hemisphere (parietal-temporal areas).

To summarize, information gained from intelligence and achievement is helpful for the following reasons:

1. It provides an objective estimate of the patient's current level of functioning in these areas.
2. By clinical interpretation of item and subtest variations, premorbid levels of functioning may be estimated.
3. Bearing in mind both current ability and premorbid

functioning, a realistic program of cognitive retraining can be implemented.

4. By becoming aware of the patient's current level of intellectual functioning, the staff can adjust the type, complexity, and frequency of all treatments to accommodate whatever cognitive strengths and weaknesses are present.

5. Finally, the use of objective intelligence and achievement measures permits more accurate determination of cognitive change during treatment.

## Abstract Reasoning Assessment

Although abstract reasoning is evaluated in various forms throughout the neuropsychologic assessment procedure, there is one measure which seems to approach conceptual reasoning more directly: the Halstead Category Test (Halstead, 1947). The Category Test consists of 208 slides, presented serially and grouped into seven subtests. The slides depict various shapes or designs, some of which are in color. Each subtest is organized according to some abstract principle, and it is the patient's task to discern the principle by the process of trial and error. The patient responds by indicating his/her choice from a response panel containing the numerals one through four. Each response is immediately reinforced either by a bell (correct) or a buzzer (incorrect). The concepts may be fairly simple--such as the number of figures seen--or fairly complex--such as the number of solid quarters present. To perform adequately on the Category Test, the patient must be able to see clearly and be able to indicate his/her response reliably by pulling a toggle switch or by pointing. No verbal response is required on the Category Test. Ideally, the patient begins each subtest by guessing; and then by a process of hypothesis testing, he/she arrives at a logical solution. The patient's behavior prior to, during, and following each trial is often very informative. Qualitative factors such as general approach (haphazard vs. obsessive), speed of responding (impulsive vs. slow), repetition of errors (frequent vs. rare), response to failure (catastrophic vs. appropriate), and "holding" the correct idea throughout a sequence (loses idea vs. retains idea) are among the clinical data available from the Category Test.

In general, one can deduce the patient's typical approach to problem solving by analyzing the qualitative aspects of his/her performance. The patient's typical success at problem solving may be reflected in the total number of errors made.

The Category Test is sensitive to dysfunction throughout the brain. All things being equal, however, (i.e., if one can rule out visual problems, attentional deficits, or severe dyspraxia), patients with frontal lobe lesions tend to perform more poorly than those with more posterior lesions. Likewise, patients who perform very well on the Category Test are not apt to have acute, progressive or extensive cerebral dysfunction.

## CONCLUSION

In the preceding pages, I have attempted to present only an overview of the current status of brain-behavior relationships as they relate to cognitive rehabilitation. Certainly, one cannot expect to cover this area with much detail in a single book chapter. However, I hope that the clinician--whatever his/her field--has gained some insight into the highly complex nature of neuropsychologic assessment and, especially, how crucial such testing is to the identification of problems, prescription of treatments, and the determination of outcome for patients with brain disorders.

## REFERENCES

Benton, A. Revised visual retention test (4th ed.). New York: Psychological Corporation, 1974.

Costa, L., Vaughn, H., Levita, E., and Farber, N. Purdue Pegboard as a predictor of the presence and laterality of cerebral lesions. Journal of Consulting Psychology, 1963, 37, 133-137.

Dunn, L. Expanded manual for the Peabody Picture Vocabulary Test. Circle Pines (MN): American Guidance Services, 1965.

Dunn, L., and Markwardt, F. Peabody Individual Achievement Test Manual. Circle Pines (MN): American Guidance Services, 1970.

Folstein, M., Folstein, S., and McHugh, P. "Mini-Mental State" A practical method for grading the cognitive state of patients for the clinician. Journal of Psychiatric Research, 1975, 12, 189-198.

Golden, C. A standardized version of Luria's neuropsychological tests: a quantitative and qualitative approach to neuropsychological evaluation. In S. Filskov and T. Boll (Eds.) Handbook of clinical neuropsychology. New York: Wiley, 1981.

Goldman, R., Fristoe, M., and Woodcock, R. G-F-W auditory memory tests. Circle Pines (MN): American Guidance Services, 1974.

Halstead, W. Brain and intelligence. Chicago: University of Chicago Press, 1947.

Jastak, J., and Jastak, S. The Wide Range Achievement Test manual of instructions (Rev. ed.). Wilmington: Jastak Associates, 1978.

Levin, H., O'Donnell, V., and Grossman, R. The Galveston Orientation and Amnesia Test: a practical scale to assess cognition after head injury. The Journal of Nervous and Mental Disease, 1979, 167, 675-684.

Luria, A. Neuropsychological analysis of focal brain lesions. In B. Wolman (Ed.) Handbook of clinical psychology. New York: McGraw-Hill, 1967.

Massey, J. WAIS test profile. Palo Alto (CA): Consulting Psychologists Press, 1968.

Matarazzo, J. *Wechsler's measurement and appraisal of adult intelligence* (5th ed.) Baltimore: Williams and Wilkins, 1972.

Milner, B., Branch, C., and Rasmussen, T. Evidence for bilateral speech representation in some non-right handers. *Transactions of American Neurological Association*, 1966, *91*, 306-308.

Osborne, D., and Davis, L. Standard norms for Wechsler Memory Scale subtests. *Journal of Clinical Psychology*, 1978, *34*, 115-116.

Pfeiffer, E. A short portable mental status questionnaire for the assessment of organic brain deficit in elderly patients. *Journal of the American Geriatrics Society*, 1975, *23*, 433-441.

Porch, B. *The Porch Index of Communicative Ability, Vol. I*. Palo Alto (CA): Consulting Psychologists Press, 1967.

Reitan, R. *The effects of brain lesions on adaptive abilities in human beings*. (Unpublished mimeo.) Indianapolis: Indiana University Medical Center Neuropsychology Laboratory, 1959.

Reitan, R. A research program on the psychological effects of brain lesions in human beings. In Norman R. Ellis (Ed.) *International review of research in mental retardation, Vol. I*. New York: Academic Press, 1966, pp. 153-218.

Russell, E. A multiple scoring method for the assessment of complex memory functions. *Journal of Consulting and Clinical Psychology*, 1975, *43*, 800-809.

Strub, R., and Black, F. *The mental status examination in neurology*. Philadelphia: F. A. Davis, 1977 (pp. 163-173).

Swiercinsky, D. Significance of crossed eye-hand dominance. *Journal of Nervous and Mental Disease*, 1977, *165*, 134-138.

Wechsler, D. A standardized memory scale for clinical use. *Journal of Psychology*, 1945, *19*, 87-95.

Wechsler, D. *Manual for the Wechsler Adult Intelligence Scale*. New York: Psychological Corporation, 1955.

Zimmerman, I., and Woo-Sam, J. *Clinical interpretation of the Wechsler Adult Intelligence Scale*. New York: Grune and Stratton, 1973.

# BEHAVIORAL AND COGNITIVE DEFICITS IN CEREBROVASCULAR ACCIDENT AND CLOSED HEAD INJURY: IMPLICATIONS FOR COGNITIVE REHABILITATION

James D. Thomas, M.S.

Department of Psychology
University of Houston
Houston, Texas

Lance E. Trexler, Ph.D.

Neuropsychology Service
Medical Psychology Department
Community Hospital of Indianapolis

## INTRODUCTION

A major development within the discipline of neuropsychology involves the increasing contribution of the neuropsychologist to the comprehensive rehabilitation of the brain injured patient. Recent reports in the literature (Brinkman, 1979; Diller, 1976; Diller and Gordon, 1981; Giantusos, 1980; Gudeman, Golden, and Craine, 1978) have noted the recent expansion of the role of the neuropsychologist beyond the traditional ones of diagnosing, documenting, and localizing neurological damage. The new role includes the added functions of (1) developing paradigms which are basically theoretical, (2) planning strategies that will serve to remediate the behavioral and cognitive deficits that arise as a consequence of brain injury; the applied implementation of theory. Both activities may be subsumed under the title of cognitive rehabilitation.

The relative recentness in the development and dissemination of this area has limited the amount of organized research into the efficacy of different cognitive rehabilitative techniques. Thus the evaluation of treatment strategies is incomplete though progressing as more institutions attempt to remediate cognitive dysfunction (Diller and Gordon, 1981). Unfortunately, there has been a corresponding limitation on the development of a solid theoretical basis that is needed to empirically devise treatment strategies. This is to say, that an impediment to the coherent development of effective treatment strategies lies in the relative lack of a good theoretical base concerning the nature of cognitive dysfunction associated with brain injury. This problem is well illustrated by the assumptions that neuropsychology has imported into the rehabilitation setting. It is the opinion of the present authors that a greater understanding of these assumptions is both necessary and overdue. We believe that the way in which we view neuropsychological deficit, and the testing that elucidates the deficit, has a direct effect on the goals and form of cognitive rehabilitation. This is underscored by the intimate relationships between test procedures and remediation techniques (Diller, 1976). A hypothetical example synthesized from the literature may serve to illustrate this relationship and the previously mentioned assumptions.

Suppose that an individual has been referred for a neuropsychological evaluation following an instance of probable brain injury. Immediately upon entering the testing situation this individual could have been noted to have significant trouble navigating the furniture and doorways of the office or laboratory. Additionally, the person may have been unable to construct copies of two-dimensional visual designs using three-dimensional, colored cubes, and to efficiently connect a random array of numeric symbols with a continuous pencil line. These three deficits may occur even though there is a reasonable degree of visual acuity and the individual is able to manipulate the objects used in the test with a reasonable adroitness. This pattern of test performance is generally associated with deficits in visuo-spatial perception and is consistent with dysfunction of the non-dominant cerebral hemisphere (Golden, Osmon, Moses, and Berg, 1981; Lezak, 1977). One approach to the rehabilitation of such deficits involves the therapist's assumption that the best way to approach remediation is at a holistic, global level. Accordingly, the therapist may attempt to train the individual to more efficiently navigate unknown environments through behavioral modification. Thus the specific test-related deficits are not directly addressed during rehabilitation. Here the neuropsychological _syndrome_ is not seen as the appropriate level of intervention. A second approach to rehabilitation uses a treatment plan based on the specific tasks employed during the initial testing. In this case the therapist would drill the individual on these measures, while possibly ordering the task complexity in a hierarchical manner. In this instance, when a relatively lower level of task complexity had been mastered, relatively greater levels of complexity would be introduced until the trainee demonstrated a near normal performance. Here the therapist assumes that the most efficient way to remediate cognitive deficits is _test-specific_ and that rehabilitation aimed at this level of perceptual organization will carry over to the more naturalistic skills. A third approach is decidedly _reductionistic_, and seeks to 'decompose' complex skills into their component parts. Thus, visuo-spatial perception as assessed by a particular neuropsychological test can be reduced to a matrix of more unique and less integrated skills. The therapist may thus wish to concentrate on the remediation of visual scanning abilities with one remedial task and fine motor coordination with another separate remedial task. These tasks would then be different than the measures employed during assessment. Obviously efficacy of treatment is assumed by the therapist. More importantly the therapist is inferring that rehabilitation efforts directed at these component parts of higher order behaviors will have a beneficial effect on the more complex cognitive abilities. Diller and Gordon (1981) have referred to these three approaches as the behaviorist, psychometrist, and biologist models, respectively.

Several neuropsychology based assumptions may be garnered from this hypothetical case study. The most obvious of these is that assessment provides access to the content that cognitive rehabilitation should address, at any level of analysis. In that cognitive and behavioral assessment is the main strength of neuropsychology, this is somewhat of a moot issue, except when the psychometrist model is employed and a one to one convergence between testing and training exists. However, the common theme that runs throughout the three models is that the structure of the "normal" or intact hierarchy of cognitive abilities is essentially preserved (minus a specific deficit) when the central nervous system has been damaged. All three approaches to cognitive rehabilitation assume that neuropathology does not alter the basic structure of cognitive functioning, except to remove some relatively static function related to the location or the extent of the pathology. We do not know that this is absolutely not the case; however, it is ill advised to blindly accept this assumption as past neuropsychological research has been either statistically univariate or has violated the assumptions central to the more dynamic multivariate statistical procedures. Multivariate procedures address the complexity of the interrelatedness of brain functioning (or dysfunctioning) as measured by interrelated neuropsychological measures. Thus we propose a descriptive analysis based upon the pattern and hierarchy of deficits that result from central nervous system pathology. This is seen as a preliminary step in the process of defining the accurate content areas that cognitive rehabilitation should address. As such, this is basic research that is to be applied in the clinical setting as a preliminary step to the evaluation of specific treatment modalities. Thus it is intimately tied to data and subject samples available to the neuropsychologist working in the 'real world' rehabilitation setting.

We hypothesized that different types of central nervous system pathology should produce different patterns of neuropsychological deficits that should in turn provide some insight into the way that treatment protocols are designed. Instead of attempting to deal with the location and structural changes of neuropathology, which is to date an inexact science (Smith, 1981) we have concentrated on diagnostic categories derived from the medical histories of the patients seen in our neuropsychology laboratory. Additionally, we have limited ourselves to the two largest diagnostic categories seen in a rehabilitation setting, namely cerebrovascular accident (CVA) and closed head injury (CHI) patients. Based upon what is known of the biomechanics of these two it was hypothesized that they could be adequately discriminated by neuropsychological tests, and that they would produce different structural patternings. Although it was not central to the hypotheses tested in the present study, it was thought that the major differences between these categories would be related to the relative diffuse quality of CHI and the relatively greater focal damage associated with CVA. In order to avoid some of the problems associated with static univariate techniques, we decided to rely on an advised application of multivariate statistical techniques. The use of these methods was 'advised' because many of the neuropsychological studies in the literature that have used these techniques have unfortunately violated important statistical assumptions, thereby effectively invalidating any conclusions that could be drawn from these studies. The goals of the present study were realized through linear discriminant analysis (LDA) and factor analysis (FA). Before proceeding further, however, with details of our study, it seems important to clarify several points that are central to the assumptions of the present study. The first of these involves the biomechanics and natural histories of the CVA and CHI pathologies. The second involves the nature and statistical assumptions central to the multivariate statistics, while the third examines past applications of these techniques to neuropsychology.

## THE NATURAL HISTORY OF CEREBROVASCULAR ACCIDENT

It is in fact the case that stroke is a profoundly heterogeneous group of diseases of the vasculature of the central nervous system. Cerebral vascular accidents (CVA) can arise from a number of causes and there are two basic and general types of CVA's. Infarction refers to the death of neural tissue secondary to an insufficiency of blood and the oxygen and nutrients which it carries. The second major type of CVA is hemorrhage, although this particular type of CVA will not be further addressed in this chapter. We have concerned ourselves with infarctions which refer to insufficiency of blood reaching central nervous system tissue. Infarction can arise through a number of different pathophysiologic processes. One of the more common forms of infarction is atherothrombosis, where arteriosclerotic plaque forms inside an artery, thereby narrowing the vessel diameter. Atherothrombotic occlusions often occur in the carotid arteries and is an unilateral disease in approximately 95% of all cases in Gurdjian, Lindner, Hardy and Thomas (1961) and 50% in Castaingne, Lhermitte, Gautier, Escourolle, and Derouesne (1970). There exist no research which suggest that there is any predilection for either the left of the right internal carotid artery to become involved in an atherothrombotic occlusion. Two of the most common sights for atherothrombotic occlusion to occur is at the sight of bifurcation of the internal carotid artery and at the sight of the trifurcation of the middle cerebral artery. However, on some occasions it is common for pieces of this atherothrombotic lesion to break off and pass higher up into the central nervous system vasculature. These emboli are often referred to as athermomatous emboli and can potentially lodge in any of the cerebral arteries. Emboli can also, however, emanate from a number of sights, particularly the heart. Myocardial infarction (Hellerstein and Martin, 1974), bacterial endocarditis (Toone, 1941) and rheumatic valvular heart disease (Harris and Levin, 1941) has shown to cause cerebral embolism and subsequent stroke. Kane and Aronson (1970) demonstrated that mitral stenosis and mural thrombus of the left ventricle are clinically the most frequent causes of cerebral embolic infarction. The research indicates that a significant proportion, ranging from sixty to forty-nine percent of those patients with these types of cardiovascular disease have cerebral embolism compromising the central nervous system. In this case, the research reveals that a significant preponderance of cardiogenic cerebral infarcts involve the left cerebral hemisphere (Meyer, Charney, Rivera and Matthew, 1971). Further, Toole and Patel (1974) has suggested that the propensity for the left hemisphere to become infarcted secondary to cardiogenic cerebral embolism is due to the Vaso-anatomical structure of the aortocervical arteries and their hemodynamic characteristics. Blackwood, Hallpike, Kocen and Mair (1969) have shown that carotid atherothrombotic occlusions resulted in larger cerebral infarcts relative to infarctions secondary to emboli. However, in the case of cardiogenic cerebral emboli it cannot easily be assumed that the effects will be lateralized to one cerebral hemisphere or the other, particularly when a "shower" of emboli occur which may originate from the heart. In these cases, it is often likely that both hemispheres of the central nervous system will be involved.

With this brief discussion of the pathophysiology of cerebral vascular accidents, it becomes obvious that even within one category of CVA's that there is tremendous heterogenety between the disease processes themselves and the parts of the central nervous system which they may differentially effect. As a consequence, these different types of cerebrovascular accidents cannot be singly considered, as a group, when attempting to neuropsychologically assess the brain-behavior ramifications.

The lack of diagnostic specificity when neuropsychologically studying different types of CVA patients has fostered ambiguity regarding prototypical behavioral-cognitive impairment associated with neurovascular disease, as illustrated by Reitan and Fitzhugh (1971). Investigations by Goldstein, Kleinknecht and Gallo (1970) and by Perez and his collaborating investigators (Perez, Stump, Gay and Taylor, 1975; Perez, Gay, Taylor and Rivera, 1975; Perez, Gay and Hart, 1976) utilized subjects with more definitive neurovascular diagnoses which presumably represented some commonality in group pathophysiology. Further, Trexler (1979) has shown that four sub-types of cerebrovascular accident patients can be significantly statistically differentiated with multivariate analysis techniques and that the sub-types of cerebrovascular accidents result in specific (as opposed to general or global) neuropsychological impairment; those patients which evidenced the most global neuropsychological impairment were diagnosed with multi-infarct dementia.

In the present study, however, the focus of study is not particularly concerned with the differential diagnosis of these different cerebrovascular accident groups, but rather characteristic types of behavioral deficit. Further, in a clinical rehabilitative setting, it is not often possible to differentiate, diagnostically, these types of CVA patients. The natural selection of such patients to be involved in cognitive rehabilitative strategies is, therefore, of more significance in considering the present methodological design rather than differentiating between specific groups of CVA patients. All of this to say that while cerebrovascular accidents represent a very heterogeneous group diagnostically, the distinction is most likely somewhat artificial when considering the development of interventive efforts, and what becomes important is the delineation of the neuropsychological parameters by which these patients vary.

## THE NATURAL HISTORY OF CLOSED HEAD INJURY

In the general case, closed head injury (CHI) represents a class of craniocerebral injuries that result either from energy being imparted to the head in the form of momentum, or from the sudden withdrawl of momentum from the head where the skull remains reasonably intact and the contents of the cranial vault are contained. This classification is based upon the nature of the injury to the skull and as such does not aid in the prognosis and description of the individual who has sustained such an injury (Chusid, 1973). A more functional understanding of CHI may result from a multidimensional model that considers the mechanics of a traumatic injury. Such a model must consider (1) the forces that act on the skull at the time of trauma, (2) the resulting forces that act upon the contents of the skull at the time of injury, and (3) the situational or environmental factors that have an effect on the expression of the CHI. Such a model is diagramed in Figure 1. Gilroy and Meyer (1975) have summarized the mechanics of CHI by noting the physical forces that act on, or more specifically deform, the skull at the time of injury. These forces are acceleration, deceleration, and rotation. These may occur alone, in any simultaneous combination, or in any sequential combination. Acceleration, as the name implies, is the imparting of motion through space to the head. Deceleration is the cessation of movement, and rotation is the movement of the head on its rostral/caudal axis. To these three factors, Gurdijan (1975) adds the compression of the skull. This latter force is the result of the head being caught between the ground and heavy object,

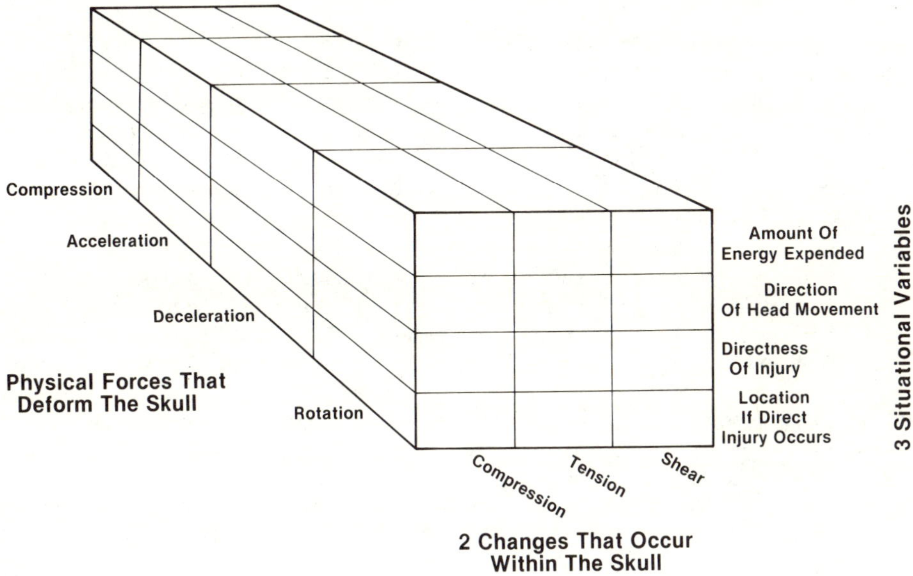


Figure 1. Model of the biomechanical factors in traumatic brain injury.

or between two blunt points moving closer together at a slow rate. This latter factor is the result of an object contacting the skull and is thus a direct or impact injury exclusively. However, Gurdijan also notes that the three previous factors may arise either through direct or indirect processes. In the case of direct injury, trauma may result from a relatively fast moving object striking the relatively slowly moving or stationary head (acceleration), or from the relatively fast moving head striking a relatively slower moving object (deceleration). Indirect injuries may result from the rapid movement of the head through space without physical contact with an object. In this case the sudden radical movement of the brain relative to the skull is the proximal cause of injury. The distinction of the directness of injury in actuality is a situational variable; however, its intimate relationship to the physical factors mandates its inclusion at this point.

The damage caused by the aforementioned forces actually occurs when there is a deformation in the normal shape of the skull which in turn alters the capacity of the cranial vault. The change in capacity introduces the second factor, which is involved with the physical changes that occur within the skull secondary to the physical forces. The decrease in the volume of the skull during deformation creates an increase in the normal pressure of the cerebral spinal fluid which may transverse the brain like a pressure wave distorting the substance of the brain. This distortion affects the brain through the processes of compression, tension, and shear. Gilroy and Meyer (1975) define compression as the forcing of tissue into close proximity; tension as the pulling apart of tissue; and shear as the sliding of one mass of tissue over another due to differences in tissue density. Additionally, the pressure wave may create a differential in the pressure of the cerebral spinal fluid where areas of negative (low) pressure and positive (high) serve to displace brain tissue.

The third factor in the model represents the situational variables that may affect the expression of a closed head injury. One of these variables has been mentioned. This involves the factor of the directness of injury. Direct injury has been found to produce greater injury than indirect injury partly as a direct blow to the head may fracture the skull (though not rupture it) and is associated with a greater amount of energy imparted to the skull. This is the second variable, where as a rule, the greater the amount of energy imparted to the skull, the greater the amount of resulting damage. This variable may be the result of several factors including the amount of time during which energy is imparted, the velocity of the head, and the relative mass and velocity of any contacting object. The third variable related to the situation involves the location of the energy imparted to the skull. When the initial injury is of the direct kind, and the energy is great enough, there is a high probability of laceration or tearing of the tissue below the site of injury (Gurdijan, 1975). The last situational variable involves the resulting direction of movement of the head regardless of the directness of indirectness of injury. Any rapid movement of the brain in an anteroposterior or an inferosuperior direction is likely to produce a bruising wherever the brain is near a bony prominence of the skull. Thus as Walsh (1975) notes, the frontal and temporal poles are susceptible to such injury because they rest against the base of the cranial vault. He reports that this type of injury is commonly seen in high speed, head-on automobile collisions and is termed the "exploded temporal pole syndrome". This type of event does not generally produce damage to the posterior, occipital portion of the brain as the shape of the skull in that area is rounded and featureless. The directional aspect of the model has a secondary importance due to the effects of the pressure wave that may be produced by a direct injury. The relative high and low areas of pressure may produce damage at the site contralateral to the site of the blow by this pressure gradiant. Such damage is termed a countre-coup injury. Thus a blow to the temporal hemisphere may cause damage to the brain directly at the site of the blow and also to the contralateral area of the temporal lobe.

The major purpose of this model is to provide a taxonomic or structural classification system that describes the location and amount of damage in terms of the context of the event causing the trauma. The model is not, however, designed to produce a series of diagnostic criteria. Instead it is an organizational system applied to the phenomena associated with CHI. The next step in this process is to delineate the immediate and proximal results of these three factors.

Two of the proximal effects of injury have already been reported. These are the pressure changes and the bruising that occur at the time of injury. This damage may cause the cerebral tissue to swell much as any body tissue can retain water following injury. This has the effect of forcing the cortex into close proximity with the interior surface of the skull and can subsequently inflict damage to the brain through compression of tissue. Pressure traveling through the brain can lacerate individual neural processes or more complex fiber tracts. These same processes may affect the supply of blood to the brain through the laceration of either deep or surface blood vessels. The resulting hemorrhage and hematoma can pose a medical complication that can turn a seemingly mild CHI into a life or death situation. As Jennett and Teasdale (1981) note, the proportion of head injury cases that produce hematoma is relatively small; however, hematoma of any type is the major cause of death in those cases where the patient was able to provide a verbal response after the injury. It is also worthy to note that many of the hematoma that result from CHI are the product of contusion and are often relatively diffuse. Disruption of the cerebrovascular system can also have the effect of producing areas of tissue damage secondary to hypoxia. This may in part be due to damage to the capillary beds supplying the brain tissue. It may also be due to metabolic damage following structural damage to individual neurons. Symonds (1974) reported that the acute effects of brain injury on individual neurons include (1) swelling of the cytoplasm, (2) enzymatic destruction of the neuron, and (3) destruction of the neuron's energy systems. If the damage to the neuron is severe enough it may degenerate as both the cell membrane and the glial tissue surrounding the cell 'dies'. These effects are not found immediately at the time of injury, and instead begin at

Table 1. A Summary of the Proximal Biomedical Effects of Closed Head Injury

1. General increase in cerebral spinal fluid pressure.
2. Bruising and Contusion of the cerebral surfaces.
3. Traveling pressure wave through the brain substance producing injury contralateral to site of injury.
4. Swelling or edema.
5. Laceration of neural processes or fiber tracts.
6. Laceration of cerebrovascular supply with resulting hemorrhage or hematoma.
7. Tearing of the brain at the site of injury.
8. Structural and metabolic damage in the individual neurons.
9. Unpredictable 'death' of individual neurons.

about fourteen hours post trauma. Much damage to individual neurons is reversible and a damaged cell does not necessarily 'die'. However, damaged cells may well develop an abnormal structure involving deformation of its structure and a generalized shrinkage. The variables that determine the potential death and recovery of neurons following trauma are presently unknown. Additionally, the relationship between neural transmission premorbidly and transmission following injury have not been sufficiently explored (Symonds, 1974).

Thus the range of effects following CHI are as complex as the forces that initially caused the injury. It should be noted that we have only considered the short term effects of trauma. For a more comprehensive treatment, the reader should consider other sources that deal more specifically with these matters in depth (Feirling, 1974; Gilroy and Meyer, 1975; Jennett and Teasdale, 1981; Lishman, 1978; Williams, 1979).

The review of the natural histories of cerebrovascular accident and closed head injury illustrate the pathophysiological and biomechanical differences characteristic of these two forms of brain insult. This review supports the contention that while cerebrovascular accidents may result in some generalized and diffuse cerebral compromise and closed head injury some focal neural tissue destruction, the most salient neuropathologic consequence of stroke involves relatively focal injury whereas closed head injury represents a more global and generalized form of brain insult, albeit great heterogeneity within each of these groups. It is because of this heterogeneity, and the multi-dimensional nature of brain-behavior relationships, that multivariate statistical approaches where utilized in examining our data.

## AN INTRODUCTION TO MULTIVARIATE STATISTICS

Although the mathematical bases of multivariate statistics are quite complex (and quite beyond the scope of the present chapter) they have an intuitive side that is understandable. At the most general level, multivariate statistics allow the experimenter to evaluate more than one dependent variable at a time by directly assessing the degree of interrelationship between them. In neuropsychology this is especially important because the domain of behaviors assessed is necessarily complex, and involves more than one measurement technique. If one attempts to use univariate statistical methods on a number of variables obtained from a single time sample (i.e., student's $t$ or the ANOVA $F$) in an attempt to determine which measures allow for the discrimination between diagnostic groups, there will be an increasing probability as each significance test is completed, that a significant difference found between two groups will be based on chance alone. In contrast, multivariate methods are able to consider and analyze a number of variables concurrently, as well as make statistical decisions based on the contribution of any one variable to the overall variance. Also, with multivariate methods, the responses of subjects are not artificially extracted from their behavioral context (McCall, 1970).

Although there are several techniques that fall within the domain of multivariate statistics the present study will only center on two of them. As mentioned previously, these are linear discriminant analysis (LDA) and factor analysis (FA).

In broad perspective, LDA is a method whereby a set of predictor variables (dependent) may be combined in a weighted linear composite which is termed a discriminant function. Two groups may be compared on this function using centroids. A centroid is analogous to a group mean in univariate parlance. If the group centroids are significantly differentiated then the groups may be said to differ significantly in terms of the set of dependent variables. With this method, groups may be established based upon some a-priori criteria and then subjected to a significance test that is not conceptually different from the null hypothesis test of traditional univariate methods. One difference, however, entails the use of probabilistic classification systems to see if the actual and predicted group memberships (based upon each subject's position along the discriminant function) is different from chance assignment (Sanathanan, 1973). Additionally, this technique allows the relative contribution of each dependent variable to the overall separation between groups to be assessed when an exploratory, stepwise procedure is used (Klecka, 1975). It must be stressed that this latter aspect of LDA is only exploratory. The actual ordering of variables in the analysis, to some extent, capitalizes on chance variation and tends to be unstable on replication. Additionally, this method is highly dependent on relatively high subject to variable ratios. If this latter assumption is violated, classification rates are prone to be overestimated and face a tremendous shrinkage on replication (Fletcher, Rice, and Ray, 1978). In context of the present study, the results of LDA may be seen to provide evidence of discriminant validity, or the ability of a set of neuropsychological measures to discriminate between different diagnostic groups.

Where LDA seeks to differentiate between subjects, FA ia a method used to determine the internal structure or relatedness in a set of dependent variables. Thus it has the ability to reduce a relatively large set of dependent variables into a smaller set of factors. Each factor in this case represents a cluster or related set of dependent variables based upon shared variance. Several varieties of factor analysis exist however all are based upon three related procedures. These include the preparation of a correlation matrix, the extraction of the factors (this is the step where data reduction actually occurs), and the rotation of these factors into a relatively stable and statistically unique configuration. Within each of these three procedures there are several statistical and conceptual variations that essentially make factor analysis such a complex entity. This technique is in no way unitary. The ultimate results of its application are dependent upon the preconceptions of the investigator, the goals of the analysis, the limitations of the statistical procedures, the nature of the data, and a relatively large number of related issues. Several complaints about the indeterminancy of factor analysis have been voiced; however, the technique is valuable when it is considered as one aspect of a larger research program (Howarth, 1972) and the various techniques are used with an eye to the manner in which they can affect the results and the interpretation of factor analytic studies (Guilford, 1952; Sternberg, 1977). Generally, the methodological applications involve the choice of factor extraction methods (components analysis or factor analytic methods), and the choice of rotational procedures (orthagonal rotation for independent factors and oblique rotation for correlated factors). These will be discussed in greater depth in terms of both previous studies and the present research.

## PAST APPLICATIONS OF MULTIVARIATE STATISTICS IN NEUROPSYCHOLOGY

The mathematical and procedural complexities that make multivariate statistics appropriate for the analysis of neuropsychological data, unfortunately also make these methods prone to misuse. Before attempting a new application of these methods it is obviously important to consider studies having serious statistical flaws, involving both LDA and factor analysis.

The four major published studies that form the cornerstone of multivariate discriminant validity in neuropsychology employ linear discriminant analysis (LDA) and unfortunately demonstrate five major violations of the assumptons that are integral to its proper use. All of these violations affect the accuracy and stability of the classifications. The first of these has already been briefly mentioned and refers to the subject to variables ratio seen in a particular analysis. In the case of uneven group sizes, this refers to the smaller of the groups included in the analysis. Other problems include, (2) the a-priori assignment of subjects to the particular groups before analysis; (3) the use of multiple LDA procedures within the context of a single study with a single sample (this has the same fault as using multiple univariate procedures); (4) the inclusion of heterogenous dependent variables that fail to sample an adequate domain or include a number of variables measuring a single domain of interest; and (5) the use of variables measured in differing metrics or units that may produce spurious correlations when the naturally occuring relationships between the dependent variables are assessed. The four "cornerstones" mentioned are Wheeler, Burke, and Reitan (1963); Wheeler and Reitan (1963); Goldstein and Shelly (1972); and Goldstein and Shelly (1973). These studies produced subject to variable ratios (in the best of many group comparisons) of 1.7 to 1; 4.9 to 1; 6.2 to 1; and 1.3 to 1, respectively.

All but one of these fall below the optimal values noted by Fletcher, Rice, and Ray (1978) of five subjects to every variable and thus are likely to produce lower rates of correct classification when replicated. In fact with their best subject to variable ratio, Wheeler, Burke, and Reitain (1963) obtained a correct discrimination rate of 90.7 percent which was reduced between 10 and 20 percent when additional subjects were included in the sample and a replication was conducted by Wheeler and Reitan (1963). This rate of shrinkage is consistent with Fletcher, Rice, and Ray (1978). The accuracy of these studies is questionable in that the control groups contain both normals and psychiatric patients (drug effects apparently were not controlled), while the brain damaged subjects were culled from patients having numerous pathological processes (ranging from evolving tumors to resolving lesions). Additionally, these groups with mixed pathologies were divided into groups reflecting the presence-absence of brain damage, and the laterality of damage based on neurological testing that is, at least to some degree, subjective. This has the problem of creating group classifications that may not be real. For LDA to function properly, the a-priori groups must reflect a real distinction (Pimentel and Frey, 1978). These studies also may be faulted in that they use the previously mentioned classification criteria to run multiple LDA's that may have the function of providing significant differences between groups by chance alone. They include a variety of dependent variables that have different numeric bases (for instance: age measured in years, time to complete a particular task, and the difference between two psychometric test scores) which has already been explained as a methodological flaw (Nunnally, 1978). Finally, these studies have the added problem of sampling dependent variables that share so much common variance that they cause distortions when the discriminant functions are computed. The inclusion of as many variables as can be collected from a group of subjects is no alternative to the analysis of a limited set of variables that accurately discriminates between the groups in question (Tatsuoka, 1976). These same problems, as noted earlier are found in the Shelly and Goldstein (1972, 1973) and in the more recent research of Swiercinsky and Warnock (1977) and Golden (1977). The "best" subject to variable ratios of these latter two studies were 3.1 to 1, and 1.3 to 1, respectively.

The shrinkage issue can be addressed, if not solved, in two ways. Fletcher, Rice, and Ray (1978) report that planned cross validations (especially when stepwise LDA's are used) with statistically derived shrinkage rates based on "Monte Carlo" methods allow the use of slightly less than optimal ratios. Thus a researcher may use a 2 to 1 ratio, if an implicit reference is made to the 30 percent shrinkage that is likely to occur when a replication is completed. Stuss and Trites (1977) suggest that a relatively large set of dependent variables may be reduced with factor analysis (as opposed to gathering more subjects) to provide a more favorable ratio. These latter two studies provide the best analysis of discriminant validity for neuropsychological tests, although they also suffer, to differing degrees, from the other methodological problems.

Previous research employing factor analysis also suffers from subject to variable ratio, subject classification, and dependent variable selection problems. Additionally, factor analysis is subject to the previously mentioned problems related to the many procedural options available to the researcher. However, it must be noted that there is a substantial amount of controversy related to the adequacy of factor analytic applications and thus the correctness of any particular study is much more difficult to assess. Generally, any aspect of a factor analysis that introduces random error into the statistical operations, or that causes the stability of the analysis to be reduced is to be avoided. Thus, idiosyncratic selections of either subjects, or dependent variables should be avoided (Comrey, 1978) in order to maintain the generalizability of the study. This does not mean that a selected population of either subjects or variables may not be analyzed. Instead, both should be collected in such a way as to adequately address the research goal to which the factor analysis is directed. Four general, and relatively more specific and important, procedural points should be considered. The first of these relates to the subject to variable ratio. Generally, the more subjects that are included in a factor analysis, the better (Bentler, 1976); however the absolute minimum ratio ranges between 4 to 1 (Rummel, 1970), and 5 to 1 (Bentler, 1976). It is also the case that the ratios generally hold for the number of factors that may reliably extracted from a subject sample (subject to factor ratio). The second point is related to the type of measurement that is used with the selected dependent variables. It is better to have the dependent variables in a similar metric or unit of measurement, for the same reasons as noted earlier in relation to LDA. One solution is to normalize the distribution of sampled data through the use of data transformations (Nunnally, 1978). A related point here is that dichotomous data should be rejected in favor of data measured on at least interval scales (Comrey, 1978). Thus the presence of absence of pathognomic neurological signs are not appropriate for factor analysis. The next major point is related to the relative independence of the dependent variables used in a factor analysis. As much as possible, the interrelationships in a data set should reflect the underlying structure of the domain that is being studied. It is thus important to not artificially introduce correlations between the dependent variables in a factor analysis. Accordingly, it would be inappropriate to use the scales of the Minnesota Multiphasic Personality Inventory (MMPI) because most of the scales are derived from item responses that are assigned to more than one of the scales. Thus a single response by a subject may be reflected in the scale score of more than one dependent variable. For similar reasons, it would be inappropriate to include the individual subtasks of the Wechsler Adult Intelligence Scale (WAIS) while also analyzing the three possible global (sic.) measures of intelligence (i.e., Full Scale IQ). The last point to be made here is related to the type of factor extraction process and is more complex. As noted previously, there are two main methods that may be used to actually extract factors from the correlation matrix. These are commonly referred to as principle factors analysis and common factor analysis. Without going into this in too much depth, it should be noted that the common method used in principle components analysis may be subject to severe distortions that render it unsuitable for many applications (Lee and Comrey, 1979). Thus the more exploratory common factor analysis, or one of the communality estimate methods related to common factor analysis should likely be preferred. For a more comprehensive list of the important issues related to the technical side of factor analysis, the reader is referred to Rummel (1970), and Sternberg (1977).

The application of factor analysis to neuropsychological data can be generally characterized in two ways, related to the number and complexity of the dependent variables included in the statistical analysis. Generally, the more variables that are analyzed in a factor analysis study, the greater the number of factors that will be extracted. However the more important aspect of this is the complexity of variables in the analysis. Here, complexity refers to the interrelatedness of the dependent variables. If a hypothetical study has fifty variables that are practically unrelated, the resulting number of factors that are extracted will approach fifty. Basically, this is to say that the number and type of dependent variables can radically influence the results of factor analysis. Royce (1967) notes that there are different levels of factor structure that are dependent upon this dependent variable complexity. Fifty dependent variables with some degree of relatedness may be termed first order factors. The resulting factors from a factor analysis would be fewer in number and thus represent second order factors. If in turn, these second order factors are subjected to another factor analysis, third order factors would result. There would be fewer third order factors than there were second order factors included in the second analysis.

An example of a factor analysis that resulted in a first order solution was conducted by Coppinger, Bortner, and Saucer (1963). They utilized 42 dependent measures with a sample of 88 subjects with mixed or no pathology. The resulting solution produced nine factors, of which five appear to be related to the MMPI and personality functions. These factors are difficult to interpret. Likewise, Blackwood and Long (unpublished manuscript) used 44 dependent variables with a large sample of 323 subjects (thus avoiding the low subject to variable ratio of the previous study) and generated 15 different factors. This study omitted the personality variables in favor of task-related and performance-related variables. The factors that were generated appear nearly all interpretable and appear relative task-related. Theoretically, if these factors were themselves factor analyzed, a second order structure would result. This two step process was accomplished by Royce, Yeudal, and Bock (1976) employing 49 dependent measures and a mixed pathology sample of 176 subjects. The first analysis yielded 13 factors, of which the authors deemed three uninterpretable. The ten "good" factors, as in the previous study, seemed related to specific types of cognitive and behavioral capacities. These included factors that the authors were able to label with rather specific abilities. Some of these included, perceptual-motor speed, pattern recognition, verbal comprehension, memory, etc. These are all relatively specific skills that could theoretically be individually assessed by the subtests of the WAIS. When these factors were in turn factor analyzed, only three factors were extracted. The authors labeled these (1) perceptual organization, (2) verbal memory, and (3) visualization. The absolute meaning of these is not actually important here. What should be noted is that the higher order or second order factors are more abstract and tend to be related to a greater number of underlying task-specific abilities. This distinction between the levels of analysis should appear similar to the earlier arguments related to the optimum "level" of intervention in cognitive rehabilitation. The first order factors represent the more reductionistic approach, while the second and third order factors tend to be much more holistic.

Several studies have produced factor structures that were much closer to the third order level without having to go through a preliminary stage of analysis. The first factor analytic approach to neuropsychological variables was done by Halstead (1947). Here, only thirteen dependent measures, taken from a sample of 237 subjects (normals, lobectomies, and brain injured) were analyzed. This resulted in four factors that were labeled (1) Central integrative field factor (dominant hemisphere and abstract reasoning); (2) Abstraction factor (non-verbal reasoning); (3) Power factor (attentional); and (4) Sensory modality directionality (residual perceptual factor). This structure is obviously more holistic than the first order factor structures noted earlier, in that each factor individually accounts for a greater number of test specific abilities. This same higher order structuring of ability (and thus possible dysfunction) is found in the factor analyses of Russell (1973) which is essentially a reanalyses of the original Halstead data, and of Goldstein and Shelly (1973).

The reader is urged to make the comparison between these "levels" of complexity or ordering of ability and the three models (approaches) to cognitive rehabilitation presented at the beginning of this section. If indeed some empirical evidence may be presented through factor analysis as to the "natural" ordering of cognitive and behavioral abilities, then the question becomes: where best can an intervention be made to address the rehabilitation of the brain injured individual? Unfortunately, this issue is partially obscurred because of the combination of pathologies in all of these factor analytic studies. Every one of them has based their analysis on a sample that touches a large number of cerebral pathologies. Thus as noted earlier, the individual factor structures are tremendously confounded. All of these factor analyses make the assumption that the pattern of dysfunction is unitary and follows the simple subtractive approach noted earlier. The question remains at the theoretical level: is it really possible to say that the structure of cognitive abilities following different types of brain injury remains essentially the same as before the injury, except that possibly one or more skills has been eliminated? It may well be the case that a particular form of cerebral pathology will produce a reordering of cognitive abilities, that is not only quite different from the "normal" individual; but also, different from individuals with other forms of pathology. Unfortunately, currently available studies of the structuring of cerebral dysfunction with factor analyses are difficult to compare because not only are different methods of factor analysis employed, on different sets of dependent variables; also, the sample studied in these studies have been combinations of different pathological processes.

### Goals of the Present Study

In the present study, we wish to attempt to compare the patterns of deficit that follow two distinctly different forms of cerebral pathology. It has been noted that the causal processes that underlie cerebrovascular accident (CVA) and closed head injury (CHI) are quite distinct, which leads us to suspect that the pattern of deficits for these forms of pathology may be distinctly different. If this is indeed the case, a methodologically correct application of linear discriminant analysis (LDA) should allow for a reasonably adequate discrimination between the two pathologies. This then provides a rational reason to submit each of the subpopulations to a separate factor analysis, in order to rationally compare the structure of deficits (or remaining ability) associated with each pathology. The LDA has the added benefit of supporting previous, less rational, LDA studies that have supported the discriminant validity of various neuropsychological tests.

## METHODS

### Subjects

The subjects included in the present study were culled from the files of the Neuropsychology Service, Department of Medical Psychology, Community Hospital of Indianapolis. Subjects were selected on the basis of documentable history of brain insult due either to cerebrovascular accident (CVA) or closed head injury (CHI). The CHI classification was made if the patient had experienced a known instance of major trauma to the head, resulting in a minimum of one day of unconsciousness, resulting from a documentable accident. The CVA classification was based upon a combination of historical information and medical diagnoses derived from neurologic examination procedures (E.E.G., CT scan, etc.). Patients with multiple neurologic diagnoses were excluded from the study. Selection of subjects was also dependent upon completeness of the neuropsychological evaluation. All subjects included had at least 85 percent of the neuropsychological measures herein utilized. Relevant demographic variables were recorded but were not used as selection criteria (sex, age at injury, age at test, and educational level). These sampling procedures resulted in 112 CHI and 57 CVA subjects being identified for inclusion in the present study.

## Tests Employed

A total of eight psychological tests were given to all subjects which yielded a total of twelve scores. The Wechsler Adult Intelligence Scale (WAIS) and the Wechsler Memory Scale (WMS) were two of these eight and were administered and scored according to the procedures described in their original publication (Wechsler, 1955 and Wechsler, 1945, respectively). All other tests, with exception of the Grooved Pegboard Test, were administered and scored in accordance with the suggestions of Reitan (undated). Further, the reader is urged to refer to Chapter 2 of the present volume for a thorough description of these neuropsychological tests.

Wechsler Adult Intelligence Scale (WAIS). The verbal Intelligence Quotient (VIQ) and the Performance Intelligence Quotient (PIQ) of the WAIS were included for analysis. The VIQ is a composite score of six subtests generally measuring a variety of language-related abilities. The PIQ reflects five subtests which require visuospatial, perceptual organization and perceptual-motor integration skills. The Full Scale Intelligence Quotient (FSIQ) was not included as the correlation between the FSIQ and the VIQ or PIQ would confound the results of the factor analytic statistics.

Wechsler Memory Scale (WMS). Only the Memory Quotient of the WMS was utilized in the present study. This composite score summarizes the scores yielded from seven subtests. These subtests measure such abilities as repertoire of geographically local information, orientation to present environment, ability to cognitively manipulate over-learned sequences (such as alphabet), immediate recall of auditorially presented paragraphs, immediate recall of complex visual patterns and ability to recall newly acquired verbal paired associates.

Seashore Rhythm Test (RHY). This test requires the subject to auditorially attend to paired non-verbal rhythmic patterns so as to determine if the patterns are similar or different.

The Trail Making Test (TR-A and TR-B). This test has two parts which were scored and analyzed separately. Part A of the TMT requires the subject to visually search a page and connect, by drawing a line, spatially random circles containing numbers. This task of visual scanning and search, sequencing, and visuo-motor integration was scored in terms of seconds to complete the task. The second component of the TMT (Part B) is identical to Part A, except the subject is required to sequentially alternate between letters and numbers when connecting the circles. Part B, therefore, involves the added requirement of cognitively sequencing alphanumeric symbols, simultaneously.

Speech Sounds Perception Test (SPCH). This measure of auditory acuity for consonants, attention and visual recognition of speech sounds is administered by having the subject listen to a tape recording which presents such sounds as "theeks" and "zeeks." The subject is then required to visually identify, given four typed choices, the auditory stimulus.

The Categories Test (CATS). The Categories Test is a measure of visual problem-solving, abstracting and ability to modify response set as a function of immediate reinforcement.

Finger Tapping Test (TP-D and TP-N). This task is merely a measure of motor speed of finger oscillation and is obtained for both the dominant (TP-D) and non-dominant (TP-N) upper extremities. This measure is obtained with the use of a keyboard with a key and counter, where the subject is asked to tap as quickly as possible for five ten second trials for each hand. This task is scored by averaging over the five trials for each hand.

Grooved Pegboard Test (PG-D and PG-N). The Grooved Pegboard Test requires the subject, utilizing only one hand at a time, to place small keyed pegs into a board as quickly as possible, first with the dominant and then the non-dominant hand. As such, it is a measure of motor dexterity and speed as well as of sensory-motor integration. This task is then scored for the amount of time required to place all of the pegs for each hand.

## Statistical Analyses

Both the stepwise linear discriminant analyses and the common factor analyses were performed on the DEC-10 computer at Indiana University-Purdue University at Indianapolis, using the Statistical Package for the Social Sciences or SPSS (Nie, Hull, Jenkins, Steinbrenner, and Bent, 1975). The method used in the LDA was Rao's *V*, a generalized distance measure between groups,where a dependent variable was accepted into the computation of the linear equation as long as it (in conjunction with previously included variables) offered any separation between the two group centroids. Both the initial step to test variable inclusion and the final step to test for the removal of a variable were based on a partial multivariate *F* with a minimum criterion of $F = 1.0$ ($p$ assumed to be 0.5). If a variable was thus found to contribute no significant separation between groups after each new measure was included into the analysis, it could be excluded. Thus redundant variables could be excluded from the analysis. These inclusion and exclusion criteria were relatively low, so that any variable with discriminatory power would be included in the linear equation. This produced an "optimal" set of variables, though not an exclusive one.

The factor analysis was based on the principle factors method (option PA2) with iteration of the communality estimates placed on the diagonal. The original communality estimates were derived from the squared multiple correlation estimates. This method determines the number of factors to be extracted essentially by the discontinuity of variance accounted for by the inclusion of each successive factor (Rummel, 1970). Because of the large amount of shared variance among these neuropsychological measures, no assumptions could be made concerning the independence or orthagonally of the factors resulting from this analysis. Thus on a-priori grounds an oblique rotational solution was employed. In SPSS this is equivalent to a direct oblimin procedure. In the present analysis, the controlling parameter for the degree of intercorrelation between the factors was set at zero.

In that the sample sizes were unequal, prior probabilities for the LDA were set proportional to the amount of the sample of each diagnostic category. In that a minor proportion of the data was missing from each of the analyses, data analysis programs were adjusted to account for this by including mean values for the respective missing elements.

## RESULTS

Demographic summary statistics denoting the level of educational attainment, age at injury, and age at the time of testing are presented in Table 2 for both the CVA and CHI subsamples. Additionally, although it was not central to the analysis or the conclusions drawn by the present study, a breakdown of the laterality of damage for each of the two samples is presented in Table 3.

Descriptive statistics for sex of the subjects demonstrated a male to female ratio of 1.85 to 1 for the CVA group and 4.33 to 1 for the CHI group. Table 4 presents frequency, mean, and standard deviation data for the 12 variables assessed with these neuropsychological tests for the CVA sample, the CHI sample and the total combined sample. All values are presented after transformation to $\underline{T}$ scores with a mean of 50 and a standard deviation of 10, except for the Wechsler Memory Scale which is presented in terms of an age adjusted memory quotient.

Table 2. Demographic Data for CHI and CVA Groups.

| Trait | Closed head injury (n = 112) | | |
|---|---|---|---|
| | $\overline{X}$ | sd | Range |
| Education | 11.8 | 2.3 | 6.0—19.0 |
| Age at injury | 26.2 | 12.7 | 5.0—68.0 |
| Age at test | 27.1 | 12.2 | 15.0—68.0 |
| **Trait** | **Cerebrovascular accident (n = 57)** | | |
| | $\overline{X}$ | sd | Range |
| Education | 13.2 | 3.2 | 3.0—19.0 |
| Age at injury | 46.4 | 14.4 | 15.0—74.0 |
| Age at test | 47.8 | 15.0 | 15.0—79.0 |

Additionally, correlation matrices for the twelve neuropsychological measures for the CVA sample are presented in Table 5 and for the CHI sample in Table 6.

The results of the stepwise LDA are presented in Table 7, demonstrating the stepwise ordering of variables into the analysis. It should be noted that only eleven of the test measures were included in the analysis, and that the final variable performance on the Grooved Pegboard for the nondominant hand was not included. Thus it may be assumed that this variable did not even minimally

Table 3. Laterality of Injury Ratings for CVA and CHI Groups.

| Type Lesion | CVA (n = 57) | | |
|---|---|---|---|
| | Frequency | Adj Percentage | Cumulative % |
| Right Hemisphere | 25 | 44 | 44 |
| Left Hemisphere | 12 | 21 | 65 |
| Bilateral/Diffuse | 16 | 28 | 93 |
| Unknown | 4 | 7 | 100 |
| | **CHI (n = 112)** | | |
| **Type Lesion** | **Frequency** | **Adj Percentage** | **Cumulative %** |
| Right Hemisphere | 5 | 5 | 5 |
| Left Hemisphere | 8 | 7 | 12 |
| Bilateral/Diffuse | 94 | 84 | 96 |
| Unknown | 5 | 4 | 100 |

Tabel 4. Descriptive Statistics for Neuropsychological Measures.

| | Cerebrovascular Accident (n = 57) | | | Closed Head Injury (n = 112) | | | Total Sample (n = 169) | | |
|---|---|---|---|---|---|---|---|---|---|
| | n | $\overline{x}$ | sd | n | $\overline{x}$ | sd | n | $\overline{x}$ | sd |
| VIQ | 55 | 44.38 | 12.88 | 110 | 37 .66 | 9.32 | 165 | 39.90 | 11.07 |
| PIQ | 55 | 34.42 | 16.31 | 110 | 33.30 | 12.85 | 165 | 33.67 | 14.05 |
| WMS | 37 | 105.14 | 21.66 | 57 | 82.56 | 18.90 | 94 | 91.45 | 22.80 |
| RHY | 48 | 33.04 | 19.04 | 111 | 38.01 | 16.73 | 159 | 36.51 | 17.55 |
| TR-A | 55 | 20.62 | 19.14 | 112 | 20.93 | 19.70 | 167 | 20.83 | 19.45 |
| TR-B | 55 | 22.78 | 18.80 | 112 | 15.64 | 17.78 | 167 | 17.99 | 18.38 |
| SPCH | 48 | 26.77 | 21.15 | 107 | 30.34 | 18.49 | 155 | 29.23 | 19.35 |
| CATS | 49 | 29.84 | 17.22 | 105 | 33.91 | 18.06 | 154 | 32.62 | 17.85 |
| TAP-D | 53 | 36.81 | 18.95 | 111 | 28.86 | 19.22 | 164 | 31.43 | 19.44 |
| TAP-N | 53 | 24.42 | 22.52 | 111 | 31.51 | 18.97 | 164 | 29.22 | 20.39 |
| PEG-D | 47 | 15.49 | 20.85 | 96 | 9.36 | 15.33 | 143 | 11.39 | 17.51 |
| PEG-N | 50 | 8.48 | 14.92 | 95 | 9.41 | 15.04 | 145 | 9.09 | 14.95 |

contribute to the overall separation of the two groups based on the change in Rao's V. It should also be noted that once variables were entered into the stepwise equation, none were excluded because of a major redundancy of information. However, the variables entered on the last three steps (numbers 9, 10, and 11) likely would not have been included if the criterion for inclusion had been slightly higher. This should have no effect on the overall classification rates as they are presented in Table 8.

These data indicate that the neuropsychological variables in this analysis did provide a relatively strong separation of the two

Table 5. Correlation Matrix for CVA Group.

| | VIQ | PIQ | WMS | RHY | TR-A | TR-B | SPCH | CATS | TP-D | TP-N | PG-D |
|---|---|---|---|---|---|---|---|---|---|---|---|
| **Cerebrovascular Accident** | | | | | | | | | | | |
| PIQ | .579 | | | | | | | | | | |
| WMS | .476 | .433 | | | | | | | | | |
| RHY | .216 | .475 | −.105 | | | | | | | | |
| TR-A | .190 | .676 | .203 | .478 | | | | | | | |
| TR-B | .486 | .690 | .317 | .478 | .646 | | | | | | |
| SPCH | .489 | .560 | .085 | .540 | .432 | .573 | | | | | |
| CATS | .346 | .656 | .170 | .420 | .435 | .488 | .360 | | | | |
| TP-D | .508 | .245 | .230 | .292 | .017 | .361 | .340 | .140 | | | |
| TP-N | .167 | .467 | .052 | .429 | .441 | .384 | .215 | .498 | .009 | | |
| PG-D | .255 | .333 | .312 | .223 | .444 | .614 | .385 | .141 | .535 | −.108 | |
| PG-N | .156 | .494 | .292 | .296 | .611 | .505 | .226 | .376 | .027 | .585 | .281 |

Table 6. Correlation Matrix for CHI Group.

| | VIQ | PIQ | WMS | RHY | TR-A | TR-B | SPCH | CATS | TP-D | TP-N | PG-D |
|---|---|---|---|---|---|---|---|---|---|---|---|
| **Closed Head Injury** | | | | | | | | | | | |
| PIQ | .543 | | | | | | | | | | |
| WMS | .300 | .143 | | | | | | | | | |
| RHY | .247 | .302 | −.035 | | | | | | | | |
| TR-A | .423 | .576 | .096 | .223 | | | | | | | |
| TR-B | .417 | .607 | −.080 | .385 | .722 | | | | | | |
| SPCH | .385 | .368 | .167 | .327 | .395 | .353 | | | | | |
| CATS | .425 | .498 | .043 | .336 | .213 | .306 | .113 | | | | |
| TP-D | −327 | .418 | −.049 | .125 | .244 | .340 | .102 | .150 | | | |
| TP-N | .301 | .485 | −.027 | .140 | .277 | .382 | .116 | .167 | .565 | | |
| PG-D | .280 | .534 | .298 | .253 | .476 | .509 | .122 | .413 | .447 | .372 | |
| PG-N | .233 | .436 | .200 | .244 | .419 | .470 | .064 | .369 | .249 | .378 | .690 |

forms of brain pathology (CVA and CHI). The overall rate of correct classification was 78.1 percent (Chi square = 53.402 with $\underline{p} < 0.001$). Also the size of the smaller of the two groups in relation to the number of variables in the analysis allowed a subject to variable ratio of 4.9 to 1 which although slightly outside the suggested ratio of 5 to 1 should create shrinkage rates of only about 10 percent on replication (Fletcher, Rice, and Ray, 1978). This result surpasses all but two of the "best" ratios in the literature and lends strong support to the discriminant validity of these neuropsychological measures for these diagnostic groups. More importantly, this analysis allows for a rational reason to factor analyze the two subsamples independently, thus allowing for a comparison of the two patterns of deficit. The relative positioning of the two group centroids relative to the single discriminant function needed to describe them is presented in Figure 2. This suggests

Table 7. Results of the Stepwise Linear Discriminant Analysis.

| Step | Variables | Standardized Discriminant Function Coefficients | F | df | Wilks Lambda | Sign | RAO's V | Change in RAO's V | Sign. |
|---|---|---|---|---|---|---|---|---|---|
| 1 | WMS | .310 | 11.691 | 1,167 | .935 | .001 | 11.691 | 11.691 | .001 |
| 2 | RHY | −.346 | 8.607 | 2,166 | .889 | .000 | 20.955 | 9.265 | .002 |
| 3 | TR-B | .847 | 10.913 | 3,165 | .833 | .000 | 33.387 | 12.431 | .000 |
| 4 | TAP-N | −.466 | 7.882 | 4,164 | .795 | .000 | 43.017 | 9.631 | .002 |
| 5 | SPCH | −.476 | 5.70 | 5,163 | .770 | 0 | 49.807 | 6.790 | .009 |
| 6 | VIQ | .402 | 4.795 | 6,162 | .748 | .000 | 56.223 | 6.417 | .01 |
| 7 | CATS | −.354 | 4.544 | 7,161 | .728 | 0 | 62.523 | 6.300 | .012 |
| 8 | TR-A | −.292 | 2.106 | 8,160 | .718 | .000 | 65.544 | 3.021 | .082 |
| 9 | TAP-D | .156 | 0.622 | 9,159 | .715 | 0 | 66.453 | .909 | .340 |
| 10 | PIQ | .090 | 0.121 | 10,158 | .715 | .000 | 66.632 | .179 | .673 |
| 11 | PEG-D | −.053 | 0.056 | 11,157 | .715 | 0 | 66.715 | .083 | .773 |

Table 8. Classification Matrix from the Stepwise Linear Discriminant Analysis

| Actual Group | Predicted CHI Group Membership | Predicted CVA Group Membership |
|---|---|---|
| Closed Head Injury (N = 112) | 102<br>91.1 Pct | 10<br>8.9 Pct |
| Cerebrovascular Accident (N = 57) | 27<br>47.4 Pct | 30<br>52.6 Pct |

78.1 Percent of all cases correctly classified
CHI-Square = 53.402
Significance = 000

that there were more individuals that had suffered a CVA by history, who presented a neuropsychological pattern of deficits more compatible with those individuals who had suffered a closed head injury (CHI).

This relatively higher rate of misclassification of CVA victims is also noted in Table 8, where 47.4 percent of the CVA sample were incorrectly classified as belonging to the CHI group. Inferrentially, based upon the previously biomechanics of these two pathologies, and this problem in classificaton, it may be suggested that the discriminant function represents a bipolar dimension dealing with the relative focalness or diffuseness of the injury. The left aspect of the function may represent non-focal dysfunction and the right aspect may represent relatively focal dysfunction.

The results of the common factor analyses are presented in Table 9 in terms of the two pattern matrices. These two matrices demonstrate the degree to which the 12 test measures are associated with the four factors that were condensed from the entire set of variables. These numerical values cannot be directly understood as correlations; however, the absolute magnitude of the values do represent the relative degree of association, where a relatively

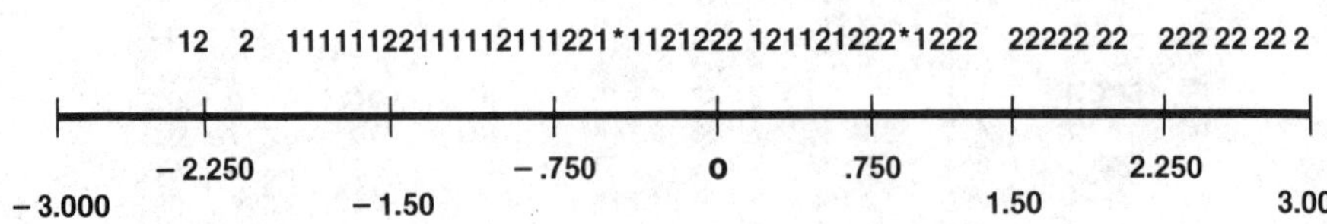


Figure 2. Discriminant Function with Centroids (*) for CHI (1) and CVA (2) Group.

Table 9. Common Factor Analysis Factor Loading Pattern Matrices After Oblique Rotations for Two Types of Brain Insult.

| | CEREBROVASCULAR ACCIDENT | | | | CLOSED HEAD INJURY | | | |
|---|---|---|---|---|---|---|---|---|
| | Factors | | | | Factors | | | |
| | I | II | III | IV | I | II | III | IV |
| VIQ | .326 | −.054 | .906 | .124 | .462 | .189 | .403 | .306 |
| PIQ | .653 | .028 | .440 | .030 | .500 | −.119 | .129 | .356 |
| WMS | .216 | .125 | .400 | .623 | −.066 | −.162 | .687 | −.100 |
| RHY | .373 | .091 | .159 | −.588 | .445 | −.076 | −.044 | −.019 |
| TR-A | .782 | .307 | −.146 | −.059 | .661 | −.197 | −.043 | .018 |
| TR-B | .521 | .392 | .257 | −.077 | .800 | .244 | −.313 | .073 |
| SPCH | .212 | .205 | .406 | −.356 | .608 | .219 | .140 | −.029 |
| CATS | .546 | −.114 | .274 | −.111 | .282 | −.209 | .140 | .091 |
| TAP-D | −.205 | .341 | .526 | −.117 | −.081 | .000 | −.045 | .819 |
| TAP-N | .728 | −.281 | .027 | −.123 | .006 | −.068 | −.066 | .700 |
| PEG-D | .058 | .986 | .013 | .036 | .081 | −.732 | .210 | .207 |
| PEG-N | .787 | .123 | −.139 | .152 | .131 | −.693 | .096 | .078 |

greater value represents a relatively higher amount of association. Underlined values in this table represent significant loadings of the test measures on each of the factors. There is no hard, fast rule for determining such thresholds, however, prior to the analysis a criterion of 0.350 was established. If the absolute loading of the test measure on the factor met or exceeded this level it was assigned to that factor. Because the factors may be correlated with the rotation method used in this study, a test measure may be associated with more than one factor. The interpretation of these factors will be considered below; however, it is interesting to note that the pattern of significant loadings is different for the

Table 10. Variance Accounted for by Each Factor.

**Cerebrovascular Accident**

| | Factors | | | |
|---|---|---|---|---|
| | I | II | III | IV |
| Adjusted % | 59.5 | 18.5 | 11.2 | 10.5 |
| Cumulative % | 59.9 | 78.3 | 89.5 | 100% |
| Eigen Values | 4.825 | 1.489 | 0.903 | 0.842 |

**Closed Head Injury**

| | Factors | | | |
|---|---|---|---|---|
| | I | II | III | IV |
| Adjusted % | 64.8 | 13.4 | 12.3 | 9.5 |
| Cumulative % | 64.8 | 78.2 | 90.5 | 100% |
| Eigen Values | 4.299 | 0.892 | 0.817 | 0.629 |

two types of pathology, suggesting a differential structure of cognitive and behavioral deficits between groups. Additionally, Table 10 illustrates the amount of variance for which each of the factors accounted for the CHI and CVA groups. Thus, this explains the amount of variation "explained" by each of the factors. This information is included because of the relatively greater amount of variation explained by the first factor in the CHI group as compared to the CVA group. This is not of major significance; however, it is parsimonious with the labels assigned to the factors in the present analysis.

## DISCUSSION

The results of the present study have indicated that the individuals that have suffered CVA can be discriminated from those individuals that have suffered CHI on the basis of neuropsychological test measures. This in turn suggests that there is a rational reason to study the pattern of deficits that arise from these two pathologies individually. Additionally, the results of the LDA suggest that CHI victims are more efficiently differentially from CVA victims. This latter finding may be the result of one of two possible factors. Demographic data has revealed that the age of the CVA victims is greater than that of the CHI victims and is likely due to the increased incidence of CVA later in individuals' life secondary to various forms of vascualr disease. Also this relatively older age of CVA victims may have unknowingly, introduced the possibility that a contaminating neuropathology in the form of a dementing process that would make individuals with a relatively focal CVA exhibit bilateral and diffuse neuropsychological patterns of deficit. Additionally, since the existence of vascular disease may allow for equal or bilateral infarcts in elderly people, again a relatively focal CVA that has been listed as the primary cause for referral for a neuropsychological evaluation can be found concurrently with bilateral infarct. The concept here is that in some percentage of cases, individuals diagnosed with CVA may present symptoms compatible with the deficits found in CHI. Thus, both diagnostic and cognitive rehabilitative efforts should be cognizant of this possibility. It also suggests that further research should consider the pattern of deficits seen within the entity that we have termed cerebrovascular disease.

The relatively noticable differences between the two subsamples in terms of the demographic variables of age (both at time of injury and at time of test) and sex may contaminate the conclusions we wish to draw concerning the neuropsychological measures. This is essentially a correlational study and ideally these variables should be somewhat better controlled (Parsons & Prigatano, 1978). It is however the case that all but one of the 12 test measures were normed on their appropriate age groups and this should serve to reduce the effects of age. Also, because the educational levels were so equal between the groups, a major source of contaminating error variance has been reduced. Thus, the CVA and CHI groups were more equated than they might initially appear. Tentatively, we are suggesting that the factor structures of these two groups may be compared with some confidence.

The labels that we have applied to the results of the factor analyses are noted in Table 11 for the CVA group, and Table 12 for the CHI group. It should immediately be noted that these are not immutable and represent only first approximations in a long term plan of study. We are applying these labels in order to try and explain the qualitative differences between the groups in order to generate hypotheses about the patterns of deficits secondary to each of them.

Before beginning a deeper analysis of these last two tables, the reader should note, that for the sake of theoretical clarity, we have labled the dominant-verbal hemisphere of the brain as the left hemisphere and the non-dominant, non-verbal hemisphere of the brain, as the right hemisphere in analysing the cognitive functions related to each factor. Obviously, the entirety of our samples were not left hemisphere dominant; however, the great majority were and, consequently, the labels are most likely minimally presumptious.

The factor analysis of the CVA group produced four factors that appear to represent relatively focal or lateralized functions. The first factor is comprised of test measures of a visual-perceptual nature. These range from simple motor functioning of the right (again, non-dominant) hemisphere, to more complex visual-motor tasks (Trails Making Test) to the more complex WAIS.

Table 11. Principle Neuropsychological Measures Comprising Each Factor for CVA Group.

| Factor 1 | Factor 2 | Factor 3 | Factor 4 |
|---|---|---|---|
| Pegs ND | Pegs D | WAIS VIQ | WMS |
| Trails A | Trails B | Tapping D | Rhythm (-) |
| Tapping ND | | Speech | Speech (-) |
| WAIS PIQ | | PIQ | |
| Categories | | WMS | |
| Trails B | | | |
| Rhythm | | | |
| Right Hemisphere Cognitive and Performance | Left Hemisphere Visual-Motor Performance | Left Hemisphere Verbal Comprehension and Motor Performance | Attention Memory |

Table 12. Principle Neuropsychological Measures Comprising Each Factor for CHI Group.

| Factor 1 | Factor 2 | Factor 3 | Factor 4 |
|---|---|---|---|
| Trails B | Pegs D (-) | WMS | Tapping D |
| Trails A | Pegs ND (-) | VIQ | Tapping ND |
| Speech | | | PIQ |
| WAIS PIQ | | | |
| WAIS VIQ | | | |
| Rhythm | | | |
| Global Cognitive | Bilateral Visual-Motor Performance | Memory | Bilateral Motor Speed |

Performance IQ. This factor is relatively easy to name and appears relatively pure. The second factor appears to be primarily a left hemisphere factor in that the variable with the highest loading involves fine motor control controlled by visual perception. This variable loads so strongly that the question of a distortion in the factor analysis should be considered (Comrey, 1978); however, in that Part B of the Trails Making Test also loads here, and is conceptually consistent with the functioning of the previously noted test, the possibility of distortion can essentially be ruled out. The third CVA factor appears to be primarily a left hemisphere factor in that the strongest loading tasks involve verbal skills (WAIS Verbal IQ and Speech Perception) along with a left hemisphere motor performance measuring motor speed with the dominant hand. It should be noted that a complex right hemisphere measure (PIQ) and a complex measure of global memory function (WMS) load here, although the association is at the bottom of the criterion of 0.350. Past research (c.f., Lezak, 1977; Thomas and Trexler, in preparation) has shown that parts of these measures are highly correlated with verbal functioning. Thus, even though this factor is not as "pure" as the previous two factors the contamination is likely due to statistical measurement of an existing relationship between the way in which the tests are presented to the subject and the degree of verbal mediation that even some nonverbal tests possess. In comparing the second and third factors it is interesting to note that left hemisphere functioning is seemingly divided into posterior-left and anterior-left functions respectively, while the right hemisphere functioning is reflective of all right hemisphere type tasks. The actual meaning of such a division of function is unclear but should be considered in localization research in the future. The fourth CVA factor is clearly a global memory factor dealing with the ability to maintain an attentional state. This attention may be referred to as focused arousal (Jasper, 1961). The weak attachment of a speech perception test here again is partially related to the verbal nature of many of the subtests integral to the WMS and to the arousal needed for performance of the measure. In summary, the CVA factor analysis has revealed a right hemisphere factor related to a broad range of visual perceptual and cognitive skills; a left hemisphere visual-motor factor; a left hemisphere language-motor factor; and an attentional-memory factor.

The CHI factor analysis produced four factors that seem to be related to bilateral brain functions. The first factor is comprised of test measures that represent higher level cognitive skills (i.e., both WAIS intelligence quotients) and accordingly, it has been named a global cognitive factor. The second factor appears to be a visual motor integrative factor, again representing both hemispheres of the brain simultaneously. The third factor appears to be a memory fact factor, although again, there is some residual relation to the verbal aspects of the Wechsler Memory Scale, with the relatively low association of the WAIS Verbal IQ measure. Additionally, it should be mentioned that one subtest of the Memory Scale and the WAIS VIQ is essentially duplicated in these two higher level measures, namely digit span. This helps to explain the intimate relationship found in both CVA and CHI analyses. The final CHI factor has been labeled bilateral motor speed because it is comprised of the performance of both hands on a test of simple motor speed, the Finger Tapping Test. This label has extra support in that the WAIS Performance IQ is also found to be herein associated. All but one of the five subtests that comprise this measure are dependent upon a patient's motor performance with an imposed time constraint, as is the case with the finger tapping. In any factor analysis, this kind of correspondence in the final factor extracted is encouraging in terms of the utility and stability of the factor structure, as it is often the case that theoretically unrelated measures are lumped together because of residual error variance alone. The final factor of the previous analysis had a similar theoretical basis in that both the rhythm and speech perception measures necessitate a moderate amount of focused arousal for adequate performance. The arousal and attention is needed for Seashore Rhythm because of the high rate of presentation, and is true for Speech Perception because of the relatively great length of the test. In summary, the CHI factor analysis produces four factors: a global or bilateral cognitive factor; a bilateral visual-motor performance factor; a verbal memory factor; and a bilateral motor speed factor.

An important consideration here is that to a great extent, the results of both factor analyses are quite consistent with the expectations made previously in noting the etiology of CVA and CHI pathology. CVA factors tend to be representative of localized, focal dysfunction, while CHI factors seem to be related to more diffuse, bilateral dysfunction. In support of this is the amount of variance that each of the initial factors "explains" or accounts for. The CHI initial factor accounts for slightly more variance than does the corresponding CVA factor, and this speaks for its designation as a global factor or "general factor: in the same vein of Spearman's general intelligence factor (Sternberg, 1977). As a minor caveat, it should be noted that we could not control the possibility that there were more patients with right hemisphere dysfunction included in the CVA group because of the base rates found in the population of subjects referred by various physicians for neuropsychological assessment, and because of the verbal nature of the tests used in our service, aphasics present more missing data than the statistical methods would allow. Thus, there is some chance that our CVA sample is biased regarding laterality; however, this is not seen as a major problem given the results of the factor analysis. Two left hemisphere factors were found. It is suggested however, that future research be attempted with laterality equated subsamples.

In considering the order or level at which the factor analysis is directed, it is obvious that the factors extracted are higher than the first order noted in previous studies; however, they are not representative of the higher order factors seen in previous research. They do not easily resolve down to single right, single left, and single attentional factors. It would seem that our factors are more consistent with an intermediate level of analysis, somewhere between the first and tertiary levels. This has implications for cognitive rehabilitation in addressing the content of the rehabilitative effort. These analyses provide general areas to which remediation tasks may be directed, although unfortunately, more exact areas of content were not found. Because of the relationship between the level or order of the measures that are included into the factor analysis and the resulting factor structure ordering, this lack of specificity was not unexpected. Future research can be directed to a lower level of analysis using the method that we have employed. It is much more important to simply note the difference in the structuring of the factor analyses for the two pathologies.

In essence, the subtractive ability approach to the conceptualizing of cognitive dysfunction has not been supported. Thus it appears incorrect to view the structure of cognitive abilities as essentially stable in its internal structure between normal and brain injured individuals, and between different types of pathologies. Thus it is suggested that these two types of pathology be treated as independent groups when planning treatment strategies. Again, although the present analysis cannot directly say what areas of content should be addressed in rehabilitation, two points are clarified. Namely that it may be appropriate to use more integrated or holistic, or third level tasks in the remediation of CHI while specific tasks may be more appropriate in the remediation of CVA. This may be supportive of the concept of inter-disciplinary collaboration in the treatment of CHI and potentially discourages a fragmented, deficit-specific approach to rehabilitation. This concern can be underscored by the fact that persons with CHI typically do not demonstrate generalization of learning. Rather, it appears to be the case that a diverse number of interrelated cognitive processing deficits are the most salient feature of CHI. These data may also be suggestive that the cognitive and behavioral compromise associated with CHI may relate to the complexity of the task, rather than to any specific brain-behavior deficit. Analysis of the tests which load into Factor 1 for the CHI group reveals that, with exception of the WMS, it contains those measures which have the greatest stimulus and response complexity. This may support the concept that CHI resluts in a general decline in information processing capacity, irrespective of the content of the task. Consequently, these data may suggest that cognitive rehabilitative efforts should focus on capacity and flexibility of information processing, at least with respect to CHI. Finally, because of the finding of a memory factor that is consistent with the dysfunction of both pathologies, it seems reasonable to suggest that both types of injury be offered either direct memory training or a more indirect training regarding the modulation of attention or arousal.

Moreover, we view the present research as the beginning in a series of projects into the nature of mental-cognitive abilities. We seek to go beyond this differential method into the underlying processes and components of human information processing (Sternberg, 1977; Sternberg, 1979). However, before we can elucidate the process, we need a clear and methodologically sound view of the content. This is merely the first tentative step in that greater goal.

## REFERENCES

Bentler, P.M. Factor Analysis. In P.M. Bentler, D.J. Lettieri, & G.A. Austin (Eds.), Data Analysis Strategies and Designs for Substance Abuse Research. Rockville, Maryland: National Institute on Drug Abuse, 1976.

Blackwood, D., & Long, C.J. Factor analytic investigation of Halstead Reitan Battery. Unpublished manuscript, Good Samaritan Hospital; Phoenix, Arizona, undated.

Blackwood, W., Hallpike, J., Kocen, R. & Mair, W. Atheromatous disease of the carotid arterial system and embolism from the heart in cerebral infarction: A morbid anatomical study. Brain, 1969, 92, 897-910.

Brinkman, S.D. Rehabilitation of the neurologically impaired patient: The contribution of the neuropsychologist. Clinical Neuropsychology, 1979, 1(2), 39-44.

Castaigne, P., Lhermitte, F., Gautier, J., Escourolle, R. & Derouesne, C. Internal carotid artery occlusion. Brain, 1970, 93, 231-258.

Chusid, J. Correlative Neuroanatomy and Functional Neurology (15th ed). Los Altos, CA: Lange Medical Publications, 1973.

Comrey, A.L. Common methodological problems in factor analytic studies. Journal of Consulting and Clinical Psychology, 1978, 46, 648-659.

Coppinger, N.W., Bortner, R.W. & Saucer, R.T. A factor analysis of psychological deficit. The Journal of Genetic Psychology, 1963, 103, 23-43.

Diller, L. A model for cognitive retraining in rehabilitation. The Clinical Psychologist, 1976, 29, 13-14.

Diller, L. & Gordon, W.A. Rehabilitation and clinical neuropsychology. In S.B. Fiscov & T.J. Boll (Eds.). Handbook of Clinical Neuropsychology, New York: John Wiley and Sons, 1981.

Feirling, E.H. Brock's Injuries of the Brain and Spinal Cord and Their Coverings (5th ed). New York: Springer Publishing Co., 1974.

Fletcher, J.M., Rice, W.J., & Ray, R.M. Linear discriminant function analysis in neuropsychological research: Some uses and abuses. Cortex, 1978, 14, 564-577.

Gianutsos, R. What is cognitive rehabilitation. Journal of Rehabilitation, 1980, 36-40.

Gilroy, J., & Meyer, J.S. Medical Neurology (2nd ed). New York: MacMillan Publishing Co., 1975.

Golden, C.J. Validity of the Halstead-Reitan neuropsychological battery in a mixed psychiatric and brain-injured population. Journal of Consulting and Clinical Psychology, 1977, 45, 1043-1051.

Golden, C.J., Osmon, D.C., Moses, J.A., & Berg, R.A. Interpretation of the Halstead-Reitan Neuropsychological Test Battery: A Casebook Approach. New York: Grune & Stratton, 1981.

Goldstein, G., & Shelly, C.H. Statistical and normative studies of the Halstead neuropsychological test battery relevant to a neuropsychiatric setting. Perceptual and Motor Skills, 1972, 34, 603-620.

Goldstein, G., & Shelly, C.H. Univariate v.s. multivariate analysis in neuropsychological test assessment of lateralized brain damage. Cortex, 1973, 9, 204-216.

Goldstein, S., Kleinknecht, R. and Gallo, A. Neuropsychological changes associated with carotid endarterectomy. Cortex, 1970, 6, 308-322.

Gudeman, H., Golden, C.J., & Craine, J. The role of the neuropsychological evaluation in the rehabilitation of the brain-injured patient: A program in neuroretraining. JSAS Catalog of Selected Documents in Psychology, 1978, 8, 44. (Ms. No. 1693)

Guilford, J.P. When not to factor analyze. In D.N. Jackson & S. Messick (Eds.), Problems in Human Assessment. New York: McGraw-Hill Book Co. 1967.

Gurdijan, E.S. Recent developments in biomechanics, management, and mitigation of head injuries. In T.N. Chase & D.B. Tower (Eds.), The Nervous System (Vol. 2): The Clinical Neurosciences. New York: Raven Press, 1975.

Gurdijan, E., Linder, D., Hardy, W., & Thomas, L. "Completed stroke" due to occlusive cerebrovascular disease. Neurology, 1961, 11, 724-733.

Halstead, W.C. Brain and Intelligence. Chicago: University of Chicago Press, 1947.
Harris, A. and Levin, S. Cerebral embolism in mitral stenosis. Annuals of Internal Medicine, 1941, 15, 637-643.
Hellerstein, H. and Martin, J. Incidence of thromboembolic lesions accompanying myocardial infarction. American Heart Journal, 1974 33, 443-452.
Howarth, E. Factor analysis has only just begun to fight - A reply to Lykken. Journal of Experimental Research in Personality, 1972, 6, 268-272.
Jasper, H.H. Thalamic reticular system. In Sheer, D.E. (Ed.) Electrical Stimulation of the Brain: An Interdisciplinary Survey of Neurobehavioral Systems. Austin, TX: University of Texas Press, 1961.
Jennett, B., & Teasdale, G. Management of Head Injuries. Philadelphia: F.A. Davis Co., 1981.
Kane, W. & Aronson, S. Cardiac disorders predisposing to embolic stroke. Stroke, 1970, 1, 164-172.
Klecka, W.R. Discriminant analysis. In N.H. Hie, C.H. Hull, J.C. Jenkins, K. Steinbrenner & D.H. Bent (Eds.) SPSS: Statistical Package for the Social Sciences (2nd ed.). New York: McGraw-Hill Book Co., 1975.
Lee, H.B. & Comrey, A.L. Distortions in a commonly used factor analytic procedure. Multivariate Behavioral Research, 1979, 14, 301-321.
Lezak, M.D. Neuropsychological Assessment. New York: Oxford University Press, 1977.
Lishman, W.A. Organic Psychiatry: The Psychological Consequences of Cerebral Disorder. Boston: Blackwell Scientific Publications, 1978.
McCall, R.B. Addendum: The use of multivariate procedures in developmental psychology. In P.H. Mussen (Ed.), Carmichael's Manual of Child Psychology (Vol.1), New York: John Wiley and Sons, 1970.
Meyer, J., Charney, J., Rivera, V. & Mathew, N. Cerebral embolism: Prospective clinical analysis of 42 cases. Stroke, 1971, 2, 541-554.
Nie, N.H., Hull, C.J., Jenkins, J.G., Steinbrenner, K., & Bent, D.H. SPSS: Statistical Package for the Social Sciences (2nd Ed.). New York: McGraw-Hill Book Co., 1975.
Nunnally, J.C. Psychometric Theory (2nd Ed.). New York: McGraw-Hill Book Co., 1978.
Parsons, O.A. & Prigatano, G.P. Methodological considerations in clinical neuropsychological research. Journal of Consulting and Clinical Psychology, 1978, 46, 608-619.
Perez, F., Gay, J. & Taylor R. WAIS performance of neurologically impaired aged. Psychological Reports, 1975, 37, 1043-1047.
Perez, F., Gay, J., Taylor, R. & Rivera, V. Patterns of memory performance in the neurologically impaired aged. The Canadian Journal of Neurological Sciences, 1975, 1, 347-355.

Perez, F., Stump, D., Gay, J. & Hart, V. Intellectual performance in multi-infarct dementia and Alzheimer's disease: A replication study. The Canadian Journal of Neurological Sciences, 1976, 3, 181-187.

Pimentel, R.A., & Frey, D.F. Multivariate analysis of variance and discriminant analysis. In P.W. Colgan (Ed.), Quantative Ethology. New York: John Wiley and Sons, 1978.

Reitan, R. and Fitzhugh, K. Behavioral deficits in groups with cerebral vascular lesions. Journal of Consulting and Clinical Psychology, 1971, 37, 215-223.

Reitan, R. Instructions and procedures for administrating the Neuropsychological Test Battery used at the Neuropsychology Laboratory, Indiana University Medical Center. Unpublished manuscript, undated.

Royce, J.R. Factors as theoretical constructs. In D.N. Jackson, & S. Messick (Eds.), Problems in Human Assessment. New York: McGraw-Hill Book Co., 1967.

Royce, J.R., Yeudall, L.T., & Bock, C. Factor analytic studies of human brain damage: I. First and second-order factors and their brain correlates. Multivariate Behavioral Research, 1976, 11, 381-419.

Rummel, R.J., Applied Factor Analysis. Evanston: Northwestern University Press, 1970.

Russell, E.W. Reanalysis of Halstead's biological intelligence factor matrix. Perceptual and Motor Skills, 1973, 37, 699-705.

Sanathanan, L.P. Discriminant analysis. In D.J. Amick & H.J. Walberg (Eds.), Introductory Multivariate Analysis for Educational, Psychological, and Social Research. Berkeley, CA: McCutchan Publishing Co., 1973.

Smith, A. Principles underlying human brain functions in neuropsychological sequelae of different neuropathological processes. In S.B. Fiscov & T.J. Boll (Eds.), Handbook of Clinical Neuropsychology. New York: John Wiley and Sons, 1981.

Sternberg, R.J. Intelligence, Information Processing and Analogical Reasoning: The Compenetial Analysis of Human Abilities. Hillsdale, NJ: Lawrence Erlbaum Associates, Publishers, 1977.

Sternberg, R.J. The nature of mental abilities. American Psychologist, 1979, 34, 214-230.

Stuss, D.T., & Trites, R.L. Classification of neurological status using multiple discriminant function analysis of neuropsychological test scores. Journal of Consulting and Clinical Psychology, 1977, 45, 145.

Swiercinsky, D.P., & Warnock, J.K. Comparison of the neuropsychological key and discriminant approaches in predicting cerebral damage and localization. Journal of Consulting and Clinical Psychology, 1977, 45, 808-814.

Symonds, C. Concussion and contusion of the brain and their sequelae. In E.H. Feirling (Ed.), Brock's Injuries of the Brain and Spinal Cord and Their Coverings (5th ed.). New York: Springer Publishing Co., 1974.

Tatsuoka, M.M. Discriminant analysis. In P.M. Bentler, D.J. Lettieri, & G.A. Austin (Eds.), Data Analysis Strategies and Designs for Substance Abuse Research. Rockville, Maryland: National Institute on Drug Abuse, 1976.

Thomas, J.D., & Trexler, L.E. On the stability of the factor structure of the WAIS and Wechsler Memory Scale: A comparative factor analytic approach. (Manuscript in preparation) Indianapolis, IN: Community Hospital.

Toole, J. and Patel, A. Cerebrovascular disorders, 2nd Edition. New York: McGraw-Hill, 1974.

Toone, E. Cerebral manifestations of bacterial endocarditis. Annuals of Internal Medicine, 1941, 14, 1551-1574.

Trexler, L. Behavioral deficit in vascular disease. Doctoral Dissertation, Purdue University, 1979.

Walsh, K.W. Neuropsychology: A Clinical Approach. New York: Churchill Livingston Publishers, 1978.

Wechsler, D. A standardized memory scale for clinical use. Journal of Psychology, 1945, 19, 87-95.

Wechsler, D. Wechsler Adult Intelligence Scale Manual. New York: Psychological Corporation, 1955.

Wheeler, L. & Reitan, R.M. Discriminant functions applied to the problem of predicting cerebral damage from behavioral tests: A cross validation study. Perceptual and Motor Skills, 1963, 16, 681-701.

Wheeler, L., Burke, C.J. & Reitan, R.M. An application of discriminant functions to the problem of predicting brain damage using behavioral variables. Perceptual and Motor Skills, 1963, 16, 417-440.

Williams, M. Brain Damage, Behavior and the Mind. New York: John Wiley and Sons, 1979.

# EMOTIONAL CONSEQUENCES OF BRAIN INJURY

William J. Lynch, Ph.D.

Director, Brain Injury Rehabilitation Unit
Veterans Administration Medical Center
Palo Alto, California

## INTRODUCTION

It should come as no surprise that there are significant emotional consequences to serious head injuries. Consider, for example, the extreme distress you yourself would experience if you were involved in a major automobile accident. As a result, you become unconscious for several days or weeks; you awaken half paralyzed in an eerie room full of strange sights and sounds, costing $500 per day. Because of the restraints, tubes, and catheters, you are unable to move your unaffected side. Your hemiparetic side both puzzles and frightens you. You are aware of a distressing memory loss for recently occurring events. Your ability to speak or to comprehend written or spoken language is disrupted.

Imagine 3 to 6 months of intense physical, speech, and occupational therapy. You must learn to ambulate with a cane or to maneuver a wheelchair. Getting in or out of a chair, bed, or bathtub becomes an exhausting and terrifying adventure. Basic motor skills such as dressing, grooming, or cooking must be re-learned.

Yet, even when all of this has begun to resolve itself, a new set of problems emerges. You become aware of drastic changes in your financial, occupational, and family status. Your spouse is forced to take out a second mortgage on your home since your disability insurance has proved to be inadequate. The savings account is rapidly dwindling. Your superiors at work are growing increasingly restless awaiting your return, and they are now broadly hinting that you should give serious consideration to an early retirement.

At home, your spouse seems somehow more distant and impatient with your slow progress. Your children seem to be more quick-tempered and disobedient. The ultimate indignity occurs when your family begins to talk about you among themselves while you are in the room.

What I have attempted to illustrate by the foregoing scenario is the fact that brain-injured persons have every reason to suffer emotionally at various stages of recovery and rehabilitation. In the following sections I will first discuss the common emotional sequelae of brain injury. I will then offer some suggestions for dealing with these problem behaviors.

## EMOTIONAL CONSEQUENCES OF HEAD INJURY

### Observations by the Family

In a recent survey (Mauss-Clum and Ryan, in press) of 30 families of brain-injured veterans, a number of interesting findings were noted. For example, 27 of the 30 families (90%) reported changes in the patient's personality after the injury. Table 1 shows a listing of the problems reported by at least half of the families.

Table 2 provides, for comparison, a partial listing of subjective reaction of family members to the stress of caring for the head-injured patient. It is noteworthy that both irritability and depression were observed with greater frequency in the wives (74% and 79% respectively) than in their brain-injured husbands (53% and 57% respectively).

Lezak (1978) has provided an excellent summary article on the impact of the head-injured patient upon the family. She stresses the importance of preparatory family education and counseling in the

Table 1. Changes in Head-Injured Patients Noted by Family Members (N=30)[a]

| Change Noted | Percentage Reporting |
| --- | --- |
| Decreased Memory | 87% |
| Dependency | 73% |
| Depression | 57% |
| Impatience | 57% |
| Decreased Ambition/Initiative | 53% |
| Irritability | 53% |
| Temper outbursts | 50% |

[a]From Mauss-Clum and Ryan (1981)in press

Table 2. Reactions of Family Members to Head-Injured Patients during Recovery[a]

| Reaction | Percentage Reporting | |
|---|---|---|
| | Mothers (N = 11) | Wives (N = 19) |
| Frustration | 100% | 84% |
| Irritability | 55% | 74% |
| Annoyance | 55% | 68% |
| Depression | 45% | 79% |
| Decreased Social Contacts | 27% | 74% |
| Anger | 45% | 63% |
| Decreased Time for Self | 36% | 58% |
| Financial Insecurity | 18% | 58% |

[a]From Mauss-Clum and Ryan (1981) in press.

process of adjusting to the return into the home of a characterologically impaired patient.

Bond (1975) has shown that families can accommodate much more readily to physical disability than to problems with personality or memory. Clearly, an understanding of the emotional consequences of brain injury is essential to any comprehensive rehabilitation program.

## Personality Determinants of the Head-Injured Patient

Kodimer and Styzens (1980) provide an excellent analysis of the personality of the head-injured adult. They stress the importance of pre-onset, primary and secondary factors.

Pre-Onset Factors. These include such factors as the physical state of the brain prior to injury, education level, occupational background, and overall socio-economic status. Certain personality features are worth noting in an attempt to re-create the patient's pre-onset personality. For example, his/her overall levels of assertiveness, tension, depression, hostility, insight, and resistance toward authority would be key variables. Simple factors such as use of leisure time may also be significant in that the clinician should not attempt to restore the patient to some "ideal" level of activity which bears little resemblance to the patient's "typical" premorbid level.

Primary Factors. These factors are felt to be more or less directly related to the injury, and are more likely to slowly resolve over time. An example of a primary factor would be the tendency to be selfish, insensitive, and generally focused upon the self, to the exclusion of other people. Another primary factor would be defective inhibition which results in poor judgment, impulsivity, and impaired self-control. Conversely, one frequently sees the opposite reaction, whereby the patient evidences diminished spontaneous activity, poor motivation, and poor tolerance for sustained activity. Some patients will exhibit a combination of cognitive rigidity and lack of insight into the true nature of their disability. Others will become emotionally unstable, with episodes of laughing or crying which bear little relation to ongoing events.

Occasionally, one sees a transient paranoid reaction which develops early in the recovery period and runs its course in two to three months. The syndrome includes delusions of reference, persecution, or unreality of the environment. For example, one patient in our program felt that he had been brought to earth by flying saucers and was in constant danger of being beaten or incarcerated, should he fail to cooperate with hospital rules. After two months of individual psychotherapy, the syndrome gradually faded to the point that he remained only mildly provocative and argumentative.

Depression is a common initial emotional response after head injury. Many patients who complain of problems concentrating or remembering are frustrated by their failure to improve appreciably in memory retraining. Not infrequently, the limiting factor is depression, and if left untreated, it can interfere with all phases of the rehabilitation process.

Secondary Factors. Kodimer and Styzens (1980) describe secondary factors as being those characteristics which develop during the course of recovery, often as a reaction to the situation in which the patient finds him/herself. They mention such responses as feelings of uncertainty, fear, lowered self-confidence, vulnerability or confusion. Commonly, these feelings will give way to defensive reactions such as belligerence and hostility. Typical defense mechanisms include denial, rationalization, compensation, flight into health and withdrawal (p. 55). Denial is often accompanied by rationalization and would be illustrated by the patient who denies his inability to read by rationalizing that it is not that he cannot read, but that he is simply not interested in what he is given to read. Another example would be the patient who refuses to accept a memory disorder, insisting, instead, that he did not forget his appointment but was never told about it in the first place.

Compensation may be seen in patients who become uncharacteristically abrasive, provocative, and demanding as a way of compensating for perceived weakness and disability. These patients will often become grandiose in terms of their future vocational and social plans, and will become bitter and vindictive toward staff members who seek to bring them down to earth in this regard. We have had patients who have serious math difficulties but insisted on seeking out work in the field of computer programming.

Still other patients may withdraw--i.e., become more silent, passive, and avoidant of interpersonal contacts. It becomes difficult to motivate these patients and to secure their participation in group activities. In extreme cases, the patient may develop schizoid adaptation which leads him to actively avoid friends and family.

## Emotional Consequences as Mental Disorders

In its most recent revision of the Diagnostic Manual of Mental Disorders (DSM-III), the American Psychiatric Association (1980) has recognized a number of organic mental disorders, four of which are relevant to this discussion:

| Code | Diagnosis |
|---|---|
| 293.81 | Organic Delusional Syndrome |
| 293.82 | Organic Hallucinosis |
| 293.83 | Organic Affective Syndrome |
| 310.10 | Organic Personality Syndrome |

The organic delusional syndrome includes suspiciousness, bizarre ideas, delusional jealousy, gradiosity, and bizarre beliefs. The term "organic hallucinosis" refers to recurrent or persistent hallucinations following the onset of a brain disorder. The organic affective syndrome may involve either depressive or hypomanic behavior, but in either case, the behavior must be related to a specific organic etiology. A patient who simply becomes depressed in response to events following a head injury may be more accurately diagnosed as "dysthymic disorder," (formerly, neurotic depression). Finally, there is the organic personality syndrome, which features a variety of changes such as emotional lability, impaired impulse control, apathy, indifference, suspicion, or paranoid ideation. Patients who evidence uncharacteristic outbursts of temper, poor social judgment, or exaggerated dependency are common examples of this syndrome.

In the hospital, as well as in the home, it is the irritable and/or paranoid patient who creates the greatest stress among staff and family members. Weddell, Oddy, and Jenkins (1980) observed that the most common change noted by relatives of severely head-injured patients was increased irritability. Kennie and Moore (1980) advise against attempting to deal with paranoid anger or suspicion by trying to outwit or argue logically with the patient. Generally, post-traumatic paranoia, which is not uncommon during the first few months of recovery, will clear spontaneously, providing the patient is placed in a supportive and non-threatening environment. This seems to be true with or without traditional psychotherapy. In certain degenerative conditions (such as Alzheimer's dementia), paranoia may persist and exacerbate despite efforts to treat it. These latter authors recommend medication for such stubborn cases (for example, Haldol or Mellaril).

Fauman (1978) points out that staff and family often become irritable with the patient for being irritable with them. As a result, physical and emotional distance between patient and staff is increased.

An unfortunate pattern often develops, whereby the patient's acting out is met by seclusion, restraints, or medication. All of this tends to exaggerate his/her panic, disorientation, and feelings of unreality. Eventually, this leads to further isolation, restriction, and rejection of the patient by staff and family alike.

There is a common tendency among staff or family to personalize what is essentially random acting-out behavior by the brain injured patient. This can develop into covert or overt attempts to retaliate. A further complication can be the development of guilt feelings in staff or family members in response to experiencing angry feelings toward the patient.

Sanford (1975) described the results of a survey in which he sought to determine the degree of tolerance (expressed as a "tolerance percentage") which family members expressed for various problems encountered with brain-injured patients. The survey indicated the following tolerance percentages: Urinary incontinence: 81%; inability to dress: 77%; personality conflicts: 54%; physically aggressive behavior: 44%. Interestingly, the least tolerated behavior patterns were: Sleep disturbance and night wandering: 16%; inability to get on or off the commode: 22 and 21%, respectively. Thus, it seems clear that families are quite sensitive to behavioral or personality changes, and are less concerned with physical inconveniences.

## SUGGESTIONS FOR TREATMENT

### The Agitated Patient

Booth, Doyle, and Malkmus (1980) describe three general objectives in dealing with the agitated patient: decrease the intensity, frequency, and duration of agitation. This can be accomplished, the authors feel, by first attempting to isolate factors in the environment (such as noise, unfamiliar surroundings, or sensory deprivation) which appear to be stimulating or prolonging the agitation, and then by modifying or removing them.

It is generally agreed that the staff or family should not yell at or "gang up" on an agitated patient unless circumstances require such desperate action. One should avoid using physical restraints, but if they are used, care must be taken to observe the patient frequently. Likewise, medication should be used sparingly, if at all.

In working with the agitated patient, the clinician should avoid introducing or insisting upon excessive structure in the treatment sessions. With regard to positive prescriptions, the clinician should attempt to reduce the amount of sensory-input and to remove all unnecessary or strictly-for-convenience medical paraphernalia such as I.V. tubes and urinary catheters. Should the patient begin to either raise his/her voice or to become behaviorally agitated, it is helpful if the clinician avoids becoming alarmed or panicky. Maintaining a sense of cool, confident self-control will often have the effect of calming the potentially agitated patient; whereas fear, threats, or raising of voice volume often exacerbate the problem. In some instances, simple distraction by diverting the conversation to a totally different topic can defuse a potentially explosive situation. If the patient tends to be disoriented, try to provide him/her with frequent reminders as to the date, time, and location.

Of course, one cannot stress enough the importance of becoming familiar with the patient so that his/her current and developing mood states can be quickly surmised by attending to subtle behavioral or verbal cues. During the critical times prior to an outburst, it may be helpful to try to provide reassurance by staying nearby and reassuring him/her by means of quiet words or touching.

Booth, Doyle and Malkmus (1980) make several useful suggestions for structuring treatment periods with the agitated patient. They suggest starting with relatively short work periods and frequent rest periods. The task content should begin with material that is elementary or overlearned, since this virtually assures early success for the patient. Since many brain disordered persons suffer from a lack of initiative, the therapist may have to begin responses for the patient. If the patient begins to fail, avoid prodding or "testing the limits." This tends to frustrate, anger, and alienate the patient. It is helpful to arrange to see the patient in an area where freedom of movement is encouraged. The clinician should not insist that the patient remain seated throughout the session. If friction between patient and clinician does develop, try first to alter the activity. Failing that, assign a different staff member to the patient. It is not effective to try to force harmony between an angry patient and staff member.

## The Depressed Patient

The development of depression is practically universal at some point during rehabilitation of the brain-injured person. Diller and Gordon (1981) point out that the patient who suddenly becomes aware of his/her deficit may become depressed as a result. They recommend certain strategies for establishing and maintaining motivation despite the presence of depression. The provision of prompt and meaningful reinforcers for performance is recommended. The clinician should seek to establish a supportive relationship with the depressed patient so that he/she will feel comfortable about expressing anger. Often, the therapist can ameliorate the patient's depression by seeking to identify specific short-term treatment goals and by taking pains to note and highlight the patient's successes.

It is generally fruitless to pursue a vigorous program of cognitive rehabilitation while the patient remains moderately-to-severely depressed. This caution applies especially to memory retraining, since poor concentration, fatigability, and pessimism are among the cardinal features of the depressive syndrome.

One should not presume the presence or absence of depression based upon casual observation or by simply asking the patient. Repeated observations in varying contexts, discussions with the family, and selected psychologic assessment are required to confirm the diagnosis. In certain cases of severe and apparently intractable depression, antidepressant medications may be helpful. However, pharmacotherapy alone should not be considered sufficient therapy for depression. Psychotherapy (individual, family, or group) should always be part of the treatment regime.

### The Apathetic or Inert Patient

Blumer and Benson (1975) note that apathy is one of the most common emotional alterations following brain injury. The patient appears listless, lacking in drive, and seemingly without spontaneous speech and activity. He/she may respond fairly promptly to specific requests for a response; yet, without external stimulation, there appears to be minimal inclination to act.

Some suggestions for dealing with this type of patient would include a general program of behavior modification in which apathy/inertia are not rewarded and spontaneous speech or behavior is promptly reinforced. The patient should be scheduled throughout the day so that long periods of inactivity between treatment sessions are avoided. It is helpful to require the patient to do something at all times (an exception would be an occasional scheduled nap for certain older, easily fatigued patients). Although he/she may watch television, read, or play cards, sleeping to while away the time should not be permitted in the clinic setting. Requiring the patient to eventually assume complete responsibility for getting to and from treatment sessions, lunch, and home will encourage more assertiveness and self-activation.

For certain patients who continually doze--even during therapy sessions--medication may be considered. Stimulants such as Ritalin or caffeine may prove effective when so indicated. The clinician should carefully assess the patient's sleep-waking cycle to be sure that the patient is not simply tired due to lack of sleep.

### The Paranoid Patient

Fauman (1978) notes that many brain disordered patients develop obstinacy, combativeness, and paranoia. In dealing with a patient who is excessively suspicious, critical, challenging, and negativistic, the clinician should follow the same basic guidelines which apply to psychiatric patients; for example, avoid crowding, suddenly touching, or surprising the paranoid patient. Although the patient may seem to take delight in arguing with staff and questioning their skill or integrity, avoid arguing with him/her. While you may offer alternative explanations or viewpoints, do not pursue your view too vigorously. This succeeds in little more than alienating the patient still further and may result in an escalation to violence.

It is always a good idea to seek to maintain maximum consistency in dealing with any patient, and this is certainly true in dealing with the paranoid patient. Be certain to forewarn the patient of changes in clinic routine or in his/her schedule well in advance of the day on which the change is scheduled to occur. Despite the difficulty in relating to the paranoid patient, the clinician should never permit staff to whisper or joke about him/her. In some instances, an impatient or disdainful facial expression may be quickly perceived by the paranoid patient as confirmation that you are not to be trusted.

## ASSESSMENT OF EMOTIONAL CONSEQUENCES OF BRAIN INJURY

While formal psychologic assessment is certainly not necessary in all situations, it is often helpful to have objective data to reinforce clinical impressions. The special problems of the brain-injured population require certain adjustments both in the selection of tests and in the ways in which tests are presented.

Generally, I have not found projective techniques such as the Rorschach or Thematic Apperception Test to be especially useful in this population. The visual-spatial and verbal expression requirements seem to be overwhelming to some patients. In addition, there is often a tendency to merely describe the cards or pictures without attempting to deal with them at an abstract or interpretive level. My experience indicates that simple and structured assessment techniques are apt to be more useful in the head-injured population.

### Assessment of Depression

Depression may be evaluated in a number of ways. The simplest assessment techniques are the scales developed by Zung (1965), and Beck and Beck (1972).

The Zung Self-Rating Depression Scale (SDS) is composed of 20 statements which relate to the depressive syndrome. Sample statements are "I get tired for no reason," and "My life is pretty full." The patient indicates his/her degree of agreement with each statement by placing a check under one of four columns ranging from "None or a little of the time" to "Most or all of the time." The clinician can assist disabled patients by reading the statements aloud and/or by marking the responses for the patient.

The Beck Depression Inventory consists of 13 sets of 4 statements dealing with various degrees of depression. The patient circles the statement(s) in each section which is most self-descriptive.

Both the Zung and Beck techniques yield numerical scores which can be interpreted by referring to tables provided with each test. Depression may also be assessed by utilizing some more complex scales or inventories; if the clinician is principally concerned with depression, a specialized measure designed for this purpose is recommended.

## More Comprehensive Assessment Techniques

Due to limitations in both time and staff, and considering the narrow attention span of most brain-injured patients, brief personality questionnaires or checklists are preferred over the more elegant--and lengthy--inventories available. The revised Symptom Checklist or SCL-90-R of Derogatis (1977) is a 90-item checklist on which the patient rates on a 5-point scale his/her current degree of distress along nine different dimensions or factors (such as Depression, Anxiety, and Hostility). An average distress level is calculated for each of the factors and these, along with three more global indices, are plotted on standard score (T-score) profiles. The SCL-90-R is designed for frequent administration (weekly or monthly) and is an excellent indicator of subjective distress in patients.

The Psychological Screening Inventory, or PSI (Lanyon, 1968) is a 130-item, true-false inventory composed of statements much like those contained in the more traditional Minnesota Multiphasic Personality Inventory (MMPI) which is discussed below. The PSI yields a standard score profile which contains the following scales: Alienation, Social Non-Conformity, Discomfort, Expression, and Defensiveness. As its name implies, the PSI is useful as a brief screening device which permits categorization of patients into broad types and levels of psychopathology. For this reason, refined interscale interpretations or lists of code types are not appropriate for the PSI. In the brain-injured population, the PSI is fairly easily administered in the standard fashion (patient reads the items and marks responses) or by either audio tape or oral administration of the items to the patient. The clinician may also choose to mark the patient's responses if it is felt that visual or motor deficits are too severe. The fact that the patient marks the responses directly onto the test form eliminates the possible confusion which can result from constantly switching attention between a separate test booklet and answer sheet (as in the MMPI). The significance of perseveration of "True" responses on the PSI has been investigated as a screening measure for organic brain dysfunction (Frankle, 1978, 1980), although such an application of a personality screening inventory should be regarded with caution.

The inventory which is most widely used in all clinical settings is the Minnesota Multiphasic Personality Inventory or MMPI (Hathaway and McKinley, 1943). Although the traditional formats of the MMPI (Group Form and Form R) have been widely used, in recent years more abbreviated versions have appeared. Those that relate most to the assessment of brain-injured patients are those based upon a 168-item format.

The MMPI-168 (Overall and Gomez-mont, 1974) consists of the first 168 items of the standard MMPI (either Group Form or Form R). Using the standard scoring templates, raw scores are obtained. These are transformed into extrapolated "Full" MMPI raw scores using regression equations provided by the authors. These extrapolated raw scores are then plotted directly on Standard MMPI profile sheets.

A related inventory entitled the OBD-168 (Sbordone and Caldwell, 1979) was designed specifically for the brain-impaired population. Each item has been reworded so that it assumes the form of a question, rather than a statement (as in the MMPI or MMPI-168). For example, "I like mechanics magazines" becomes: "Do you like mechanics magazines?"

The OBD-168 must be presented orally since the clinician must make occasional adjustments in market the standard MMPI answer sheet. Clearly, the OBD-168 is to be preferred for patients in whom there is any doubt concerning reading ability, alertness, or span of attention. The frequent confusion which brain-impaired and elderly patients experience with the standard MMPI statements is eliminated, to a large extent, by the OBD-168.

The MMPI profiles generated by these and other brief forms of the MMPI should not be treated as full MMPI profiles with regard to interpretation of code-types and minor inter-scale differences. Rather, the clinican should attend to general profile patterns and elevations which can suggest global categories of psychopathology. My experience with these brief forms of the MMPI has been generally favorable, although the reader is urged to consult the literature for a more thorough analysis of this area (see Graham, 1977; and Newark, Falk, and Finch, 1976).

Only a few of the many personality assessment techniques which are available have been reviewed. I would strongly urge that some objective assessment of personality be obtained both on admission and at intervals during rehabilitation. To ignore or inadequately assess the emotional status of a prospective patient is a serious oversight that will have repercussions throughout the treatment and follow-up process.

## CONCLUSIONS

In this presentation, I have attempted to provide an overview of the emotional consequences of brain injury from both the patient's and the family's standpoints. My emphasis was purposely upon what happens and how the clinician can cope with certain of these emotional changes. I did not explore the etiology--the why--of emotional changes because this is a very complex area which is fraught with uncertainty and speculation. Indeed, an entire volume could be devoted to the pathophysiologic and psychopathologic features of organic affective and personality syndromes.

As Lezak (1978) and others have pointed out so many times before, the professional must make every effort to understand the emotional status of both the patient and his/her family. Failure to do so makes treatment failure a virtual certainty. It is not an exaggeration to assert that the patient's emotional status is of equal importance to his/her neurophysical status in the process of acute and long-term rehabilitation. Too often, psychosocial factors are either de-emphasized or ignored entirely, while complete clinical attention is focused upon medical problems. Certainly, during the initial stages of critical care such a focus is justifiable. However, attention to the patient's and family's emotional needs should be initiated as soon as possible. Frequently, the tremendous stresses attending to long-term recovery from brain trauma can be anticipated, if not alleviated, by such early efforts.

## REFERENCES


American Psychiatric Association. Diagnostic and Statistical Manual: III. American Psychiatric Association, 1980, 115-120

Beck, A., and Beck, R. Screening depressed patients in family practice. Postgraduate Medicine, 1972, 52, 81-85.

Blumer, D., and Benson, D. Personality changes in frontal and temporal lobe lesions. In D. Benson and D. Blumer (Eds.) Psychiatric aspects of neurologic disease. New York: Grune and Stratton, 1975.

Bond, M. Assessment of the psychosocial outcome after severe head injury. In CIBA Foundation Symposium 34: Outcome of severe damage to the central nervous system. Amsterdam: Elsevier, 1975, 141-153.

Booth, P., Doyle, M., and Malkmus, D. Meeting the challenge of the agitated patient. In: Rehabilitation of the head injured adult: Comprehensive management. Downey, CA: Professional Staff of Rancho Los Amigos Hospital, Inc., 1980.

Derogatis, L. SCL-90 Administration, scoring and procedures manual - I for the revised edition. Baltimore: Johns Hopkins University School of Medicine, 1977.

Diller, L., and Gordon, W. Rehabilitation in clinical neuropsychology. In S. Filskov and T. Ball (Eds.) Handbook of clinical neuropsychology. New York: Wiley, 1981, pp. 702-733.

Fauman, M. Treatment of the agitated patient with an organic brain disorder. Journal of the American Medical Association, 1978, 240, 380-382.

Frankle, A. Sequential response shift rate: A correlate of human adaptivity measurable with existing personality inventories. Journal of Psychology, 1978, 98, 129-143.

Frankle, A. Perseverated yea-saying on a brief personality inventory (PSI) as a specific screening index for organic brain dysfunction. Paper presented to International Neuropsychological Society Meeting, San Francisco, CA Jan. 1980.

Graham, J. The MMPI: A practical guide. New York: Oxford University Press, 1977, pp. 219-224.

Hathaway, S., and McKinley, J. The Minnesota Multiphasic Personality Inventory. Minnesota: University of Minnesota Press, 1943.

Kennie, D., and Moore, J. Management of senile dementia. American Family Physician, 1980, 22, 105-110.

Kodimer, C., and Styzens, S. The psychology of the head-injured adult. In: Rehabilitation of the head-injured adult: Comprehensive management. Downey, CA: Professional Staff of Rancho Los Amigos Hospital, Inc. 1980.

Lanyon, R. The psychological screening inventory. Goshen, NY: Research Psychologists Press, 1968.

Lezak, M. Living with the characterologically altered brain injured patient. Journal of Clinical Psychiatry, 1978, 39, 592-598.

Mauss-Clum, N., and Ryan, M. Brain injury and the family. Journal of Neurosurgical Nursing, August 1981 (in press).

Newmark, C., Falk, R., and Finch, A. Interpretive accuracy of abbreviated MMPIs. Journal of Personality Assessment, 1976, 40, 266-268.

Overall, J., and Gomez-mont, F. The MMPI-168 for psychiatric screening. Educational and Psychological Measurement, 1974, 34, 315-319.

Sanford, J. Tolerance of debility in elderly dependents by supporters at home: Its significance for hospital practice. British Medical Journal, 1975, 3(#5981), 471-473.

Sbordone, R., and Caldwell, A. The "OBD-168": Assessing the emotional adjustment to cognitive impairment and organic brain damage. Clinical Neuropsychology, 1979, 1(4), 35-41.

Weddell, R., Oddy, M., and Jenkins, D. Social readjustment after rehabilitation: A two year follow-up of patients with severe head injury. Psychological Medicine, 1980, 10, 257-263.

Zung, W. A self-rating depression scale. Archives of General Psychiatry, 1965, 12, 63-70.

## CONCLUDING REMARKS

Lance E. Trexler, Ph.D.

Coordinator, Neuropsychology Service
Medical Psychology Department
Community Hospital of Indianapolis

The scope of issues addressed in the introductory section of the present volume reveals the inherent complexity of the consequences of dysfunction of the central nervous system (CNS) and their treatment. This scope included some preliminary examination of (1) the domain and conceptualization of what is herein referred to as cognitive rehabilitation, (2) a methodology for assessing the behavioral ramifications of cerebral dysfunction, (3) the patterning of behavioral impairment characteristic of closed head injury and cerebrovascular accident, and (4) the diversity and typology of emotional consequences of CNS dysfunction. These introductory considerations lay a foundation from which we can attempt to conceptualize what "cognitive dysfunction" is, for who, and what we should or should not do so as to facilitate its amelioration.

The conceptualization of cognitive rehabilitation as treatment efforts focused on (1) impairment of general information processing capability, (2) specific or circumscribed deficits, and the dynamic interaction of (1) and (2) mandates that rehabilitation therapies be highly integrated and cohesive. While most rehabilitation facilities are organized according to professional affiliation and consequently Departments of Occupational Therapy, Physical Therapy, Speech Pathology and Psychology often function relatively autonomously, each providing their own specific treatments for specific deficits, this conceptualization favors a team (not departmental) multidisciplinary approach to rehabilitation. A functional neglect of general information processing impairment, and its relatedness to specific deficits, and the relevance of information processing for learning may represent a serious threat to our expectations of the rehabilitation process. In other words, models of rehabilitation based upon departmental contributions (perhaps reflecting a compartmentalization of treatment efforts) may in fact fragment rehabilitative attempts to modify learning, be it motor, perceptual or linguistic learning. The herein proposed model of cognitive rehabilitation suggests that our professional contributions should be organized to address the nature of our patients, rather than reflective of our discipline territoriality.

The extent to which this conceptualization applies to all CNS injured patients is a matter of debate. The results of Thomas and Trexler suggest however that it may be more applicable to closed head injury (CHI) patients than victims of cerebrovascular accident (CVA). The factor analysis of neuropsychological data for the CHI group resulted in the finding that the factor which accounted for the greatest variance was composed of measures which were globally cognitive in nature, where neuropsychological tests of attention, cognitive set shifting or flexibility, speed of stimulus-response processing and overall language and non-language psychometric intelligence were selected. In contrast, factor loadings for the CVA group were neuropsychological measures sensitive to lateralized cerebral functions, suggestive therefore of a pattern of more deficit specificity, at least relative to CHI patients, in terms of CNS dysfunction. Further, the results of Thomas and Trexler argue against a subtractive conceptualization of viewing neuropsychological deficits in context of overall brain behavior relationships, in the case of either CHI or CVA. Rather, these data suggest that insult of CNS integrity eventuates in a reorganization of cerebral functions, as measured with behavioral tests, not specific to only the areas of dysfunction. Consequently, models of normal cognitive functioning may not resemble models of abnormal cognition. In this regard, empirical investigation of how people with CNS dysfunction learn is in its infancy. Further, the proposal that dysfunction of the CNS represents (1) compromise of information processing, (2) specific brain behavior deficits, and (3) an impairment of integrative and dynamic cerebral interrelatedness of (1) global information processing capabilities and (2) specific brain behavior functions requires considerable evaluation.

Lynch has described a neuropsychological repertoire for comprehensively assessing the functional status of brain behavior relationships. The diversity of test measures addressed in his chapter on neuropsychological assessment illuminates the multi-dimensional nature of brain behavior relationships. Historically, an awareness of the multi-dimensional nature of brain behavior relationships has not always existed and single, uni-dimensional tests for "brain damage" were utilized. Fortunately, rapid evolution of clinical neuropsychology has yielded testing procedures which are more diagnostic, descriptive and, with regard to planning strategies of rehabilitative or remedial intervention, informative, such as described by Lynch.

Inasmuch as emotions are integral to cognition in persons with intact cerebral functions are emotions in persons with dysfunctional cognition following injury to the CNS. Lynch has thoughtfully addressed the interrelatedness of patient, family and hospital staff emotional struggles and has included a discussion of the most prevelant emotional consequences of cerebral dysfunction with basic strategies and recommendations for assessment and intervention. The emotional consequences of brain injury are often terrifying for all concerned and there exists a phenomenal dearth of information about the behavioral and pharmacological treatment of the emotional consequences of cerebral dysfunction, particularly in the case of traumatic brain injury. As a consequence, many patients, and their families are left to their own coping resources, which are understandably fragile, to deal with an often bewildering and frightening pattern of behavior. The other alternative has historically been to place the patient in an excessively prolonged "chemical straight-jacket" with major tranquillizers, thereby even further decreasing the patient's capability for learning. It is very desireable that clinicians begin to invest much more clinical and research effort into this aspect of cerebral dysfunction.

# PART II: CONCEPTUALIZING COGNITIVE DYSFUNCTION

# PRINCIPLES OF COGNITIVE REHABILITATION

James F. Craine, Ph.D.

Neuropsychology Service
Hawaii State Hospital
Kaneohe, Hawaii

## INTRODUCTION

This present topic is seen as an attempt to bring some order and regularity into an extremely complex activity. So that we are in agreement as to the topic, it is suggested that we look more closely at the title, "Principles of Cognitive Rehabilitation". We can readily recognize rehabilitation as a program aimed at the restoration of functions and understand this to vary from general to specific in focus and from minimal to complete in terms of the amount of recovery achieved. The cognitive portion is not as clearly apparent, however, as it involves the entire process of knowing and understanding, which would include both awareness and judgment and which also comprises the decision-making process plus resultant actions. It is thus apparent that "cognitive" is a very broad term which will most probably include more than just the involvement of the neocortex of the human brain. Perhaps cognitive rehabilitation should be considered in the broader sense and pertain to the restoration of all higher level brain functions, which would also include subcortical brain functions as well. This is in agreement with Luria (1966) who states "It is obvious that the higher mental processes are functions of the brain as a whole and that the activity of the cerebral cortex can be examined only in conjunction with that of nervous structures at lower levels" (p. 1). Therefore, if we can formulate a broad and basic set of assumptions (principles) concerning the type of program that would seek to restore the higher level brain functions to a standard of usefulness, we would then comply with the title of this chapter, "Principles of Cognitive Rehabilitation".

There is no question but that the time has arrived for a greatly increased effort directed toward the rehabilitation of brain-damaged patients. In calling for a greater emphasis focused upon the retraining of these patients, Aaron Smith (1979) observes that "In attending numerous grand rounds in neurology, I have had the impression that many of them end where they should begin. Although we may now know that specific sensory, motor, and other neuropsychological deficits are due to a specific lesion, the cardinal question for the patient is what can be done about his persisting disabilities" (p. 237). Due to the widespread belief in the permanence and irreversible nature of brain damage, a great deal of pessimism has existed generally concerning the potential of environmentally based strategies for encouraging recovery following injury to the central nervous system. As a result, much of the rehabilitation efforts with these patients have been limited primarily to efforts to help the individual compensate for the effects of the injury and to adjust to the limitations imposed by his deficits. It is time to reverse the current conclusions involving the irreversible debilitating consequences of brain damage.

I represent a group of workers in Hawaii who have been involved in this specific kind of retraining process for a number of years. We were asked in 1972 to establish a neuropsychological laboratory for the purpose of testing and diagnosing clients who were suspected of having brain damage. We were not asked to establish a retraining program, however, because at that time it was not generally considered possible or feasible to retrain the behavioral consequences of human brain damage. Shortly after we commenced testing and were busily diagnosing various clients as having varying degrees of brain damage, it became apparent that we were only doing part of the job, just touching the tip of the iceberg. It seemed inadequate to recognize and diagnose brain damage and then leave it at that without any further recommendations and help as to what could be done. These people desperately needed help and were ready and willing to work long and arduous hours in order to make small improvements in their functioning.

When we asked ourselves the question, "Isn't there something we can do to help these people?", we were immediately hooked into a far greater challenge than was posed simply by the testing and diagnosis of brain damage. This took us directly into the retraining area and we searched the literature in order to find some clues as to how to proceed. Although this was only a few years ago, in 1972, we could find very little in the literature that seemed to be pertinent to our immediate application. We knew that work in speech pathology provided therapeutic intervention for people with brain damage, insofar as attempting to regain speech functions. Physical therapy also used a number of techniques for regaining use of motor functions subsequent to various types of cerebral insults. We also recognized that there were many behavior modification techniques which perhaps could be applied in these instances. We determined to use any and all of these techniques plus any useful principles derived from learning theory in order to put something together to aid the retraining process for brain-damaged patients. This work has proved to be a tremendous challenge because everyone we work with is a unique puzzle and life has been very fascinating for me every since. The challenge has been to unravel the puzzle and to provide therapeutic intervention strategies which maximize the patient's functional capacity.

During our work with our patients over the years, we have been able to formulate some treatment methods that appear to be of value. We have also been able to discard other methods that were not of value and have been free to make mistakes and to eliminate these from our procedures. Being somewhat isolated from the normal flow of ideas, in the middle of the Pacific Ocean, was both a blessing and a handicap. We have learned as we have gained experience in working with brain-damaged patients and as we have proceeded we have made attempts from time to time to try to make more sense and order out of what we were doing. It was apparent that a number of activities in which we were involved were successful and we wanted to describe our approach to others who were recruited to help us in the retraining process. We proceeded to boil down the essence of our training activities into a set of eight principles (Gudeman and Craine, 1976) which are proposed as a guide for structuring training activities for patients with central nervous system dysfunction. I want to present the results of our assumptions in the form of "principles" with the recognition that there will be extensive room for argument and for disagreement with the way these are formulated. We think of these as "working principles" because they have arisen directly from our involvement in the retraining activities. I want to present them in order to encourage others to become more active in this rewarding and intriguing process involving the retraining of those unfortunate individuals with brain damage.

The staff of the Neuropsychology Service at Hawaii State Hospital proceeded to systematize a training procedure to remedy the deficits of brain damage and applied the name "neurotraining" to this process. It is our contention that neurotraining is the systematic application of psychological and neurological principles for the purpose of enabling individuals to overcome or compensate for deficits that result from central nervous system dysfunction. A workbook describing neurotraining with examples and numerous training techniques, is now available (Craine and Gudeman, 1981). The procedures and knowledge that made it possible for us to structure neurotraining programs have emerged primarily in the last three decades. It was in an attempt to describe the neurological and psychological theory that underlies the practice of neurotraining and to provide the rationale for these structured training activities that we developed the eight distinct principles which I would like to present now for your consideration.

## PRINCIPLES OF NEUROTRAINING

### Principle One

The first principle establishes the basis for a training program by specifying that recovery of function following cortical damage is possible. We consider this to be the cornerstone principle because if recovery were not possible, there would be no necessity for a training program. Stated in greater detail, principle one says: "The plasticity of function within the central nervous system provides the basis for structuring neurotraining activities to promote and enhance recovery from brain damage" (Gudeman and Craine, 1976, p. 2).

It has long been noted that varying amounts of recovery take place subsequent to brain damage. As a result of these observations, numerous different theories have arisen to attempt to account for this phenomenon. One possible explanation for the improvement in behavioral deficits with the passage of time is the hierarchical explanation as described by Jackson (1869). This explanation takes notice of the fact that any given function within the central nervous system is represented at several different layers of the brain stem through a neural redundancy. In this theory, a given function appears to be represented at different levels and if a higher level is damaged, a disinhibition of a lower level of the brain will still allow that function to continue. We recognize that as a species climbs the phylogenetic scale the brain structures become increasingly complex. Humans, for example, retain a number of subcortical structures that at some point in our history were the primary cortex. This was later superseded by still higher levels. At the present time the neocortex is the most recent and highest functioning brain structure. If part of the neocortex is impaired, however, by some lesion, it is possible that a lower brain system can take over at least some of the function. This then represents one possible explanation for an apparent recovery from brain damage.

Another theory to account for recovery would involve the substitution explanation. This theory simply says that other areas of the brain have the capacity to take over the functions of the damaged portion. We recognize that the two hemispheres are almost mirror images of each other so that if the damage is in one area of one hemisphere, then it is perhaps possible that the corresponding area of the other hemisphere has the ability to take over the functions when this becomes necessary. The difficulty with this explanation involves the accounting for what happens to the functions that were the primary responsibility of the area that is substituting for the damaged portion. Perhaps the area is capable of carrying on many tasks at the same time. Another possibility in the substitution theory involves areas of the brain that may be held somewhat in reserve and therefore are capable of assuming a variety of alternative-type functions.

An explanation which is quite similar to the substitution concept involves multiple control. The concept of multiple control has been discussed by Rosner (1970). Briefly stated, this would note that any specific function is conceived as being controlled by more than one center within the brain; thus a destruction of one specific area would still leave several others still functioning and able to carry on the specific behavior required. Some of the excellent radioactive isotope studies of the brain would tend to substantiate this theory of multiple control of function (Lassen, Ingvar and Skinhoj, 1978).

Another theory that has risen to account for recovery of function after brain damage is von Monakow's diaschisis theory (1914) which suggests a temporary traumatic disruption of neural organization and integration. This would then tend to take the form of a "functional shock" in that the tissue involved is otherwise intact but is not functioning, or perhaps only partially functioning. This theory would indicate that although a certain area of the brain has been damaged or destroyed, some of the nearby areas may not have actually sustained physical damage but because of the shock reaction may act as if they are destroyed or completely non-functional and then later seem to revive and become functional once again. The name diaschisis was given to this type of reaction. Usually it is the adjacent areas to the main lesion site that are seen to sustain this kind of a shock reaction but sometimes corresponding areas in the opposite hemisphere have been found to have this same shock reaction and later recovery of function. It would appear that after shock dissipates, over a varying period of time, that the effected cells begin to function again. This theory suggests that these cells function abnormally, but after an indefinite period of time, they resume a more normal functioning. This return of cellular function would then give the appearance of a recovery from damage. Diaschisis is thus a very useful term for explaining this apparent recovery of function after brain injury.

Still another theory developed to account for recovery of function after brain damage involves dynamic reorganization through retraining. This theory was presented by Luria (1963) and has been reviewed extensively by Luria, Naydin, Tsvetkova and Vinarskaya (1969), at which point they make an important statement to the effect that recovery of higher cortical functions will not occur in the absence of specific rehabilitative therapy. In other words, Luria, who originally included various other theories in explanation of recovery of brain functions, finally reached the point where he felt that the cerebral cortex as a whole must be reorganized through a training program. He states this clearly as follows: "The cerebral cortex does not consist of separate, isolated centers...the recovery of the function must not be attributed to transfer of the function to a new, vicarious center but rather, to a structural reorganization into a new, dynamic system widely disbursed in the cerebral cortex and lower formations" (Luria, 1966, p. 29).

It is possible that all of the foregoing explanations for recovery of function are possible. They do not preclude one another and each may apply in different degrees or different situations so that they could be equally valid in explaining how recovery of function occurs. Certainly it is a fact that spontaneous recovery, particularly following cerebral vascular accidents, is a commonly observed phenomena. There is also a general agreement that spontaneous recovery occurs during the first 12 to 18 months post trauma. We take special notice in the first principle, therefore, that recovery is possible and include the various possible explanations as an aid to understanding this recovery. In addition, it is our opinion that whatever recovery would occur spontaneously or naturally can be considerably enhanced by a properly organized training program.

## Principle Two

The second principle refers to the neurological organization of the cerebral cortex as an "open system" that is highly maleable and adaptive. As you may recall, the human brain has been called the adaptive organ because it is through the brain that we are able to adapt to environmental changes. The organism adapts to its environment by means of the learning process which is controlled by the brain. Principle two is stated more completely as follows: "The cerebral cortex is a dynamic process of neurological organization that can be completely halted or slowed by injury or by environmental deprivation or it can be greatly increased or heightened by carefully planned environmental stimulation" (Gudeman and Craine, 1976, p. 4). This principle was adapted from Lewinn (1965) and refers to the learning capacity of the central nervous system.

In order to evoke adaptation, as controlled by the brain, we need heightened stimulation. The training program becomes the means by which we will provide the precise kinds of stimulation needed. One will tend to lose functions and abilities through lack of use or because of restriction of stimulation and conversely can gain or regain functions and abilities with the aid of properly administered stimulation. Because it becomes a learning process, it is possible to structure our training activities in such a way as to promote recovery of function. As we perceive the function of neurotraining, we must stimulate in the direction we want the learning or relearning to occur. Because the brain is the adaptive organ, the individual will be capable of making changes in his behavior in response to changes in the environment. The sensory stimuli are conveyed to the brain by afferent tract leading from the receptor organs to the specific projection areas of the brain. Stimulation through these afferent tracts represents the sole avenue by which learning takes place and allows the processes and organization of the brain to become modified. It is essential, however, that the stimulation be carefully planned and as specific and precise as possible.

It is apparent that our environment acts to stimulate us constantly and continually. This stimulation, however, is generally not planned stimulation and may indeed be quite haphazard. Kephart (1968) has noted that it is the task of the brain to enable the organism to adapt to its environment. It is thus apparent that if we are able to intervene in such a manner as to control environmental presentations, we are in a position to provide a special kind of training called "programmed stimulation". As the environment impinges upon the individual, accordingly does the brain proceed to develop. The central nervous system, even with a brain in a pathological condition, is not a closed system but is continuously reacting to external influences and continues to be affected by external events. Theoretically, if the individual is able to perceive stimulation, it would follow that he is also susceptible to changes in his behavior as a consequence of the changes in his environment. On this basis, it is possible to structure neurotraining activities in order to promote recovery of function.

Principle Three

This principle concerns the environmental influences which bring about an altered process or reorganization of cortical functions. At this point, the training program itself becomes the primary environmental influence affecting the impaired brain functions. Stated in more detail, principle three is as follows: "The organization of learning within the cerebral cortex results from the repeated activity on the part of the individual and becomes organized into functional systems of behavior" (Gudeman and Craine, 1976, p. 5).

As we review learning theory we note that initial learning or, as in our situation, the relearning as it pertains to the rehabilitation of our patients, occurs through repeated practice at specific tasks. As is necessary for the learning of all complex skills and especially so in relearning activities which have been decimated by cerebral lesions, it would appear that the practice must be repeated beyond the point of habituation. In other words, it is necessary to practice and practice and then practice some more. Actually, the relearning is quite similar to the initial learning of each of the skills or behavioral activities except that in some instances progress can be much more rapid. As in learning any new skill, at first a patient may be very halting and unsure in the activity. The more it is repeated and practiced, however, the more it is possible to produce an even and easy behavior almost without having to think about it. The relearning is the same as the original learning for any complex activity. You may recall learning a complex task such as driving a car or writing fluently on a piece of paper; at first it is an extremely difficult task and requires a great deal of concentration and effort. The innumerable practice sessions finally result in an ability to drive and talk and look at the scenery all at the same time. The complex act of writing with a pencil or pen on a piece of paper is improved in the same way. We practice and practice our penmanship until we reach the point where we can write and listen at the same time and perhaps also even carry on a conversation with someone else while taking notes. The ability to perform these complex activities in conjunction with other things at the same time cannot result unless we have practiced extensively on the task. The more we practice, the easier the task becomes and this exact same requirement applies to our brain-damaged patients as well.

It is at this point that I would like to interject a word of caution in terms of the tasks we are presenting to our patients for practice purposes. It is essential to commence the training for any particular task at exactly the right level of difficulty. This is a particularly crucial point in the training because if the task is too easy for the individual, little or no learning will be experienced. If, on the other hand, the task is too difficult, again no learning will occur and our patients may become discouraged. Ideally, performance should initially be hesitant and may contain many errors but the patient will be able to complete the task successfully with considerable effort. At that point, learning can take place as he works and works to improve his performance. Thus it is extremely crucial in presenting our tasks for practice purposes that we start at exactly the right level and recognize that this starting point will vary for every individual. If we start at exactly the right level, however, and then slowly increase the difficulty of the task as our patient gains proficiency, progress will be apparent.

At this point there may well be a question as to how to know exactly which is the right level to start an activity. This is not a difficult matter to resolve but it is extremely essential. For the purpose of establishing the right level to begin training in each of the activities, it is necessary to run base rates on every one of the exercises to be used for each patient. The base rates are established by beginning each of the tasks at a very simple level and quickly increasing the difficulty in ordered steps to a point well beyond the ability of the patient to succeed. As we review the data from these base rates, we note the point where difficulty began to be experienced. That is seen as the correct point to begin training for that particular activity.

As mentioned previously, this treatment methodology calls for slowly increasing the difficulty of the task as proficiency is gained. Just as it is essential to start at the right level, it is also essential to progressively increase the difficulty of the task as progress is made. In every instance, a criteria of success for the task is set and as soon as that criteria is reached for a sufficient number of trials or days or whatever is established, then a new

Criteria of increased difficulty is specified so that t
will have to continue to work and improve in order to c
ing the new criteria that are established.

Another essential point which should be mentioned at this
is the necessity of putting some numbers to all of the training activities. We have established a requirement to quantify each of our activities in order that we can keep track of the progress. It is in this manner that we are also able to know when each of the criteria has been completed. Quantification can be a score in terms of number of seconds to complete the task or the number of blocks piled or the number of items remembered or whatever else the criteria might happen to be. The essential point is that numbers are applied to the tasks so a score can be kept. Our patients may complain that is does them no good to reach a criteria point because as soon as they succeed, we make the task more difficult for them. They are correct in that we will increase the level of our expectations but it is by this method that they will continue to improve and make progress. Frequently our patients will not realize the progress they have made over time until we point to the level they were able to achieve six months earlier and they can recognize the amount of progress they have made since that time by looking at the graphs.

Principle Four

Principle four refers to the hierarchical nature of human development. In this instance hierarchy refers to a graded or ranked series of development. The full principle is stated as: "The activities of training must recapitulate the developmental stages involved in the individual's original acquisition of the learning or skill that is being trained" (Gudeman and Craine, 1976, p. 6). This is a relatively general statement and would appear to be fairly consistent with normal development. The hierarchical nature of human learning and development has been described by various authors in a variety of different ways (Kephart, 1968; Piaget, 1954; and Johnson and Myklebust, 1967). The idea is simply that the completion of the development of one stage is essential and is a prerequisite to the development of the next stage. In other words, first things come first. You must learn to crawl before you walk and you must learn to walk before you can run. The implications of this assumption includes the tenet that if an inadequate performance at an earlier level is not corrected, there may well be some implications for all later phases or more complex levels of learning. An adequate foundation should be laid in order to build a proper structure upon it.

In the training situation we recognize the importance of the hierarchical aspect of learning, both in describing and specifying a patient's deficits and in structuring the goals of the training activities. As a matter of course, developmentally earlier tasks are trained first and these in turn are used to structure later more complex kinds of activities. In this way the stages of neurotraining attempt to recapitulate the stages of normal development that are followed in the growth of an individual or in the normal acquisition of skilled behavior. It is even possible that a mature patient who has had abilities severely hampered in one particular area may well have to start training at a level that a four-year-old child would find appropriate. We will frequently receive objections from patients as to the level at which they will have to work, even though it may be ridiculous for a grown man to be practicing a task that a four-year-old child can do. However, it may be essential for this to be completed before he is able to progress to more difficult tasks. One consolation is that he will be able to progress much faster than the child at that same task. The importance of levels of training, however, cannot be minimized because we find that if the mastery of a prior level is not complete before we present the next level to the individual, he will have some difficulty with this next level and with all succeeding levels, simply because there is something missing in his repertoire.

As we observe our children at play we can note that they are continually doing something in their games that will prepare them for the next kind of activity that they are going to be doing next week or next month or next year. In the final analysis, all of these activities prepare them for life as an adult and it appears to be a natural progression. So once again we want to keep this in mind with our brain-damaged patients so as to provide them the proper kinds of activities in order to lay a solid foundation. It is also possible in referring to this particular area, the developmental sequence of learning, that neglect in this particular area may be why there have been so many failures in the past in attempting to retrain brain-damaged patients. Failure to initially meet a patient at a level well within his grasp and then failure to progressively carry him through more complex stages of development in the proper sequence may have made it difficult or impossible for the brain-damaged patient to re-establish a functional system.

## Principle Five

The fifth principle focuses attention on the complex integration of multi-modal processes. We can recognize that our window on the world depends completely upon our sensory reception. It is only through our senses that we perceive the world around us. If our window happens to be cloudy or distorted, we are at a distinct disadvantage when compared with others. Stated at greater length, principle five says; "Complex higher cortical functions represent an integration of multiple sensory modalities which supplement each other in the acquisition of learning" (Gudeman and Craine, 1976, p. 7).

The input channels to our brain arrive through the courtesy of our sensory receptors. Each sensory modality is equipped to handle specific types of data and all modalities are essential to the fully functioning intact individual. For humans, the visual system represents the preferred sensory modality with audition being a close second. The haptic senses, predominantly touch, are third in preference and taste and sm ll are of less importance and rank as a more distant fourth and fifth. It is extremely essential in the testing process to determine the status of all sensory systems; they represent the individual's window on the world. Whenever we discover impaired sensory modalities due to brain damage, we must pay special attention to our training program in order to rectify some of the imbalance. As noted in the order of importance, most of our training is performed in the visual and auditory modes.

It has been our experience that in most brain-damaged patients all modalities are not equally damaged but instead, some remain more intact and functional than others. This is fortunate because we are then able, by means of a technique called pairing, to use the relatively more intact sensory modalities to help retrain or re-develop the less intact or handicapped modalities. If, for example, audition is impaired and giving erroneous data to an individual patient but his visual input is intact, we can present various training exercises in such a way that the visual data is paired with the auditory data simultaneously, thus enabling his stronger sense to help in the learning process. By means of considerable repetition of the two sensory modalities in various exercises, the impaired modality begins to improve and we can gradually diminish the pairing of visual with the auditory information for this individual and continue to provide training primarily through auditory channels. Until we can reach the point where auditory information alone can provide the necessary data, however, the technique of pairing is used to enable a more intact sense to help train the impaired sensory modality.

Another form of pairing, but with a slightly different emphasis, is called "bridging" which was introduced by Luria (1963). We have been able to employ this technique in a number of different situations. Following Luria's example, we put together an apparatus for bridging between an intact visual modality and a severely impaired tactile modality. In this instance, if you have a patient who has finger agnosia (excessive difficulty recognizing fingers by touch), you can retrain the tactile sense by pairing with the intact visual sense through this bridging technique. The apparatus I mentioned uses five lights which represent the five fingers and these lights can be individually turned on or off and dimmed or brightened as we desire. At the beginning of the training, the patient is informed that when a finger is touched the light corresponding to that finger will be dimmed in comparison with the other lights. Obviously, as he watches the apparatus he can tell which finger is touched simply by whichever light is dimmed and he can then designate the finger touched even though his fingers are obscured from his sight. As the training proceeds, however, adjustments to the controls gradually makes the difference between the dim light and the brighter lights less and less so that he is required to obtain additional information from the sensation of touch because the visual is providing less and less information to enable differentiation. Over a considerable period of time some surprising results can be obtained with this technique of bridging from an intact to an impaired modality.

An additional problem has been noted which pertains to principle five and this is that although for an individual patient the reception and acuity of sensory stimulation may be intact, the patient may fail to effectively integrate the stimulation amongst the various modalities. This means then that at the cortical level the individual is getting ambiguous and undifferentiated sensory information. This provides an extremely interesting challenge in the training situation because it then becomes necessary to design exercises in such a way that the patient can practice to sort out the messages he is receiving and eventually to properly integrate incoming sensory information.

## Principle Six

The sixth principle refers to the "dynamic" or "process" aspects of neurotraining. In a sense, neurotraining is seen as a process through which a brain-damaged patient learns how to learn. It is almost as if he has forgotten how to learn and does not know how to start. Thus we think of the process as one designed to teach him how to learn. The complete principle is as follows: "The primary objective of neurotraining is to promote and develop the processes underlying learning and is concerned with the dynamics of learning rather than the specific content of any area" (Gudeman and Craine, 1976, p. 8).

The emphasis and procedures of neurotraining focus upon the learning process itself rather than upon any specific content area. For example, many of our patients are referred to us from Department of Vocational Rehabilitation or from the Department of Education and in each case they have not been able to teach the patient specific job information on the one hand or educational material on the other. These brain-damaged patients appear to lack the capacity to benefit from some of these specific training programs simply because they are unable to assimilate the training as it is presented to them. Because we are extremely careful to start each client at a level where he can succeed in whatever the task might be and only gradually increase the difficulty of the task, he begins to realize, over time, that he is capable of learning. In many cases we like to think of the kind of training we are doing as laying the groundwork so that the individual will be able to proceed from that point with more specific training, perhaps at school or in a vocation. We can think of neurotraining as preparing the patient to learn from these educational or vocational efforts by providing him with the basic cognitive skills necessary to learn.

Principle Seven

The seventh principle states simply that training should be deficit-specific. This means that we are working directly with the most impaired areas for each patient. In other words, we are purposely training in the area where the person is the most significantly impaired and are of greatest handicap. Stated at greater length, principle seven says: "The effectiveness of neurotraining activities is dependent upon and relative to the degree to which the deficits can be specified for each individual patient" (Gudeman and Craine, 1976, p. 9).

The more specifically the individual deficits can be articulated in behavioral terms the easier it is to structure effective training programs. As the assessment techniques are able to successfully differentiate and specify particular deficits, the training activities and procedures will begin to emerge. In addition, the training activities themselves may often serve to provide additional assessment data that can also be used to further develop or refine the training procedure.

We believe that the reason traditional rehabilitation programs have tended to become rather pessimistic about working with brain-damaged patients, and have not been more successful in their endeavors, stems partly from their failure to specify in detail the deficits of their patients, plus their failure to structure their rehabilitative activities to be deficit-specific. If the training activities have not been tailor-made to the unique needs of each patient, it is quite possible that the activities will serve instead to overwhelm him rather than to help him regain impaired abilities. This means that the diagnostic program has vital importance to the retraining program and serves to supply critical information. The backbone of our testing is the Halstead-Reitan Neuropsychological Test Battery (Reitan & Davison, 1974) but in our opinion this does not provide sufficient information in order to properly structure the training program. Further, the Luria-Nebraska Battery (Golden, Purisch, and Hammeke, 1980) has similar limitations. We find it necessary to supplement the Halstead-Reitan Battery with many, many other tests in order to provide more precise information regarding the status of current functioning.

I should perhaps digress briefly at this point to emphasize that the specificity of deficit is not synonymous with localization of the lesion in the assessment of brain dysfunction. For training purposes, we are primarily concerned with the gap in the performance, the behavioral deficits, rather than with the location of specific lesions of the brain. Although there is a definite relationship between the status of the brain and the performance of the individual, neurotraining intends to deal with the performance of the individual and to make use of the brain model only as it has further meaning in terms of the performance of the individual patient.

The importance of the assessment program becomes apparent when an attempt is made to write a training plan for the brain-damaged patient as individual strengths and weaknesses should be completely described. The neurotraining plan should include a long-term goal and a detailed description of the patient's deficits. Each deficit or constellation of deficits in turn will have short-term goals or objectives which must be attained if the deficits are to be eliminated. Finally, the training plan will contain a list of activities or training techniques to be pursued in order to attain the short-term goals or objectives. As the various activities are completed, the patient will successfully achieve the short-term goals; satisfactory completion of all short-term goals in turn should result in achievement of the long-term goal. At this point the training can be considered completed successfully.

If careful attention is paid in the determination of the specific deficits for each patient and if the training activities are carefully structured on the basis of these deficits, it is possible to promote considerable recovery within the brain-damaged population. An additional aid in training can also be derived from the assessment program through enumeration of strengths that the individual may possess. A training plan will frequently utilize a patient's strength paired with a weakness in order to help improve the weakness and gradually phase out the strength as the weakness improves. No matter which way it is achieved, however, the emphasis is always upon the deficits and their remediation.

## Principle Eight

The eighth and last principle states that consistent and systematic feedback is needed. In our program we provide training on a one-to-one basis which means one trainer per patient. The decision to proceed in this manner was made quite early in the program and makes it especially easy to comply with this eighth principle in terms of supplying the feedback to the patient. Stated in its full form, principle eight says: "Consistent and direct feedback to the patients about their performance is a crucial aspect of neurotraining." (Gudeman and Craine, 1976, p. 11).

Not only does the graphing of the daily training results, thus producing learning curves, provide the best means for monitoring performance but also these learning curves can provide information to our patients as to their progress. The immediate criteria for success on each training activity is frequently discussed and the progress or the lack of progress in each area examined. We find they are extremely interested in their learning curves because through these means they can tell immediately how they are performing in relation to the previous work they have done.

The additional importance of feedback is stressed because the patient needs to know how to modify his response in order to bring it closer to his expectation. The growth and learning of our patients appears to be maximized by having specific objectives clearly in mind and a direct system of feedback constantly in use, thus insuring that they are able to monitor their activities and performances. Without consistent feedback and without continuous reinforcement, the brain-damaged patient seems to be overwhelmed by the environment and by his limitations. The importance of precise and frequent feedback is also stressed by Luria et al. (1969) and they define the feedback broadly so as to include any and all means of reporting back to the patient the results of his actions. By having one trainer for each patient, we are able to provide appropriate and timely feedback and want to emphasize that this is of utmost importance.

## CONCLUSIONS

The greatly expanded interest in programs directed toward treatment and rehabilitation of patients with brain lesions is attested to by the interest and attendance at the symposium on which the present volume is based. In Hawaii, we have attempted to formulate a basic set of assumptions to be used in a structured program aimed at remediation of cognitive deficits resulting from brain insults. We call these "principles" but they can more correctly be called "working principles" as they were derived primarily from clinical practice, observation and considerable trial-and-error effort. There is no question but that extensive gains can be made by these patients suffering from impairment of cognitive functioning providing environmentally based strategies designed to encourage recovery are properly administered. Significant recovery from cortical dysfunction requires considerable time, however, involving years rather than months, and many helping hands. We no longer have to contend with arguments specifying the "irreversibility" of the effects of the cortical lesions and, in addition, our experience with neurotraining suggests that considerably more recovery is attainable than has ever before been thought possible.

## REFERENCES

Craine, J.F. and Gudeman, H.E. _The rehabilitation of brain functions--Principles, procedures, and techniques of neurotraining._ Springfield, Illinois: Charles C. Thomas, 1981.

Golden, C.J., Purisch, A.D., and Hammeke, T.A. _The Luria-Nebraska neuropsychological battery: A manual for clinical and experimental uses._ Los Angeles: Western Psychological Services, 1980.

Gudeman, H.E. and Craine, J.F. _Principles and techniques of neurotraining._ Privately published manuscript, Hawaii State Hospital, 1976.

Jackson, J.H. _Selected writings, Vol. 2._ New York: Basic Books, 1869.

Johnson, D.J. and Myklebust, H.R. Learning disabilities, educational principles and practices. New York: Grune and Stratton, 1967.

Kephart, N.C. Learning disability: An educational adventure. West Lafayette, Indiana: Kappa Delta Pi Press, 1968.

Lassen, N.A., Ingvar, D.H., and Skinhoj, E. Brain function and blood flow. Scientific American, 1978, 239, 62-71.

Lewinn, E.B. Neurological organization: The basis for learning. In Hellmuth (Ed.) , Learning Disorders, Vol. 2. Seattle: Special Child Publication, 1965.

Luria, A.R. Restoration of function after brain injury. New York: MacMillan, 1963.

Luria, A.R. Higher cortical functions in man. New York: Basic Books, 1966.

Luria, A.R., Naydin, V.L., Tsvetkova, L.S., and Vinarskaya, E.N. Restoration of higher cortical function following local brain damage. In R.S. Vinken and G.W. Bruyn (Eds.), Handbook of clinical neurology, Vol. 3. Amsterdam: North-Holland, 1969.

Monakow, C. von. Die lokalisation in grosshirnrinde und der abbau der funktion durch korticale herde. Wiesbaden: J.F. Bergmann, 1914.

Piaget, J. The construction of reality in the child. New York: Basic Books, 1954.

Reitan, R.M. and Davison, L.A. Clinical neuropsychology: Current status and applications. New York: Winston/Wiley, 1974.

Rosner, B.S. Brain functions. Annual Review of Psychology, 1970, 21, 555-594.

Smith, A. Practices and principles of clinical neuropsychology: "Focusing on the hole rather than the donut". International Journal of Neuroscience, 1979, 9, 233-238.

# A CONCEPTUAL FRAMEWORK FOR INTERVENTIVE COGNITIVE NEUROPSYCHOLOGY

Yigal Gross, Ph.D.

Psychology Department, and the Unit for Neuropsychological Treatment and Rehabilitation
Bar Ilan University, Ramat Gan, Givatayim, Israel

Clinical neuropsychology puts a heavy emphasis on diagnostics, i.e., the detailed differential labelling of sets of functional deficits as they correlate with given sets of physiological disturbances. Such terms as "frontal syndrome" result from these diagnostic operations.

The basic goal of any diagnostic approach is twofold. First, a diagnosis enables one to predict behavioral dimensions not directly observed on the basis of tested behaviors, e.g., if we observe a deficient score on verbal components of the Wechsler Memory Scale in a left temporal lesioned patient, we can expect a low performance on other verbal memory tasks. We cannot however predict the patient's ability to perform in real life situations complex tasks which depend on spatial memory. In this way the differential status label of verbal memory impairment is meaningful.

The other purpose for which diagnosis is used is to provide predictions about patient's <u>future</u> performance on the basis of a present diagnostic label provided by medical data, test results, and behavioral observations.

Thus, knowing that a patient has lost, due to surgical intervention, the best part of his frontal lobe, and knowing the extent to which this loss has affected the flexibility of his thinking, one can predict what jobs the patient can hold and even the types of marital difficulties he may confront. An assumption can be made that beyond the point of physiological recuperation, the <u>pattern</u> of behavioral and cognitive deficiencies will remain stable, although the impairment may increase in degree.

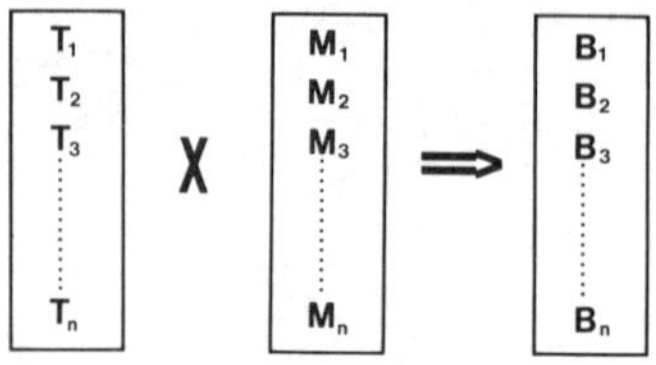


Figure 1. Model of utilizing psychometric test (T) and medical (M) data to predict behavior (B).

It is the purpose of this chapter, however, to address another, non-diagnostic, aspect of clinical neuropsychology. We are shifting our attention to the ways in which we can, and should, intervene in the usual course of events following brain injury. We are here to examine the various interactions between initial diagnosis of the patients and rehabilitative treatment, and to produce abilities and behavioral repertoire not predictable on the basis of the initial diagnosis alone. The focus of this chapter is to make the term rehabilitative or interventive neuropsychology meaningful.

Initially, let us examine whether the variables currently used in clinical diagnostic neuropsychology, whilst being effective, are sufficient, when we are dealing with an interventive model. Two paradigms should be contrasted: one in which clinically complex data are used as independent variables to predict current or future untested behaviors, these being considered the dependent variables (see Figure 1); the second considers the interactions between two sets of independent variables which are qualitatively different, namely the interaction between neuropsychological and medical data and clinical interventions variables, which are supposed to bring about future behavior (see Figure 2).

The first model is static and descriptive inasmuch as it deals with fundamentally concurrent data. The second is dynamic and manipulative inasmuch as it deals with the ways in which organismic variables interact with environmental treatment variables. Since a

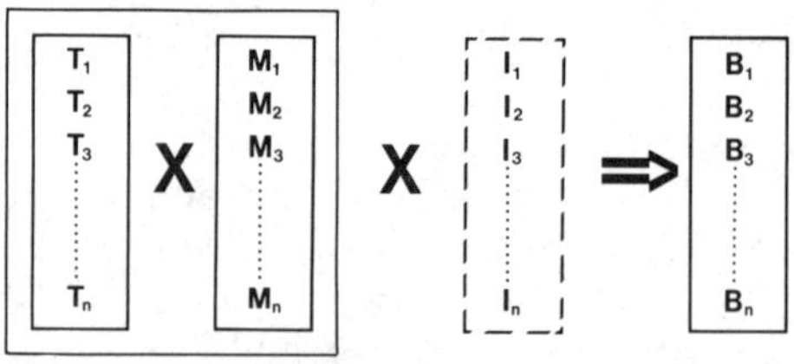


Figure 2. Model of the interaction between psychometric test (T) and medical (M) data and clinical intervention (I).

variable is defined in terms of other ones with which it is functionally related, it is clear that test data which have been of great significance using the first paradigm do not necessarily have the same role according to the second. In other words, once rehabilitative intervention is allowed to take place, it is possible that we have to look for test data of a different kind. How different, and in what way the new test data should differ from the old data should at the moment be left an open question. We hope that the following discussion will provide some guidelines.

The transition from descriptive clinical neuropsychology to interventive clinical neuropsychology came about as a correlate of two other transitions in our thinking. First, greater emphasis is now put on the concept of recovery of functions and the variables which determine this process. The widely held notion that recovery of function is strictly limited to a relatively short period is now being put to question. The new perspective emphasizes the dynamic dimension of brain activity. The influence of this transition on our thinking as neuropsychologists, and the amount and kind of hope we can give our patients can not be exaggerated. Only through the recognition that the recovery of the brain injured individual is not affected only by the tissue response to trauma have we come to pursue methods which take advantage of and guide this conceptual transition.

The other change in our thinking is a growing de-emphasis on the analytic aspect of the research into the working of the brain. Neuropsychological research and conceptualization followed the localizationist tradition in one way or another. The limitations of this tradition in explaining many newly discovered facts are becoming more and more apparent. As a result, models which attempt to describe the function of the brain in intergrative and synthetic rather than in discrete and analytic terms become more influential (e.g., Lashley, 1950; Sperry, Gazzaniga, Bogen, 1969; John, 1967; Pribram, 1971).

Two concepts which emphasize the synthetic aspect are the "organic syndrome" of which we address in relation to intelligence testing, and the concretic personality syndrome which was conceived by Goldstein and Scheerer (1941) and collectively describe the cluster of symptoms displayed by brain damaged individuals who suffer a variety of lesions to their brains. The implications of these two related concepts, the "organic syndrome" and the "concretic personality" are vast. They point to the fact that in addition to discrete detrimental effects of localized lesions, and without denying the existence of these discrete effects, there are also global deficits. These are not particularly related to a circumscribed location of a lesion. Rather, they are related to a diffuse disturbance in the operation of the brain as an integrated, synthetic system. I suggest that analyzing the discrete symptoms which make up the organic syndrome, and the individual characteristics of the concretic personality should lead us to the unveiling of some communality among them which may point to basic features of the synthetic aspect of the way the brain functions.

First, let us be reminded of some of the symptoms which make up the organic syndrome and which portray the concretic personality. Among them we find disturbances in judgement, abstraction and paradoxical combinations of impulsivity - with lack of initiative, outburst with flat emotional tone, and memory disturbances with perservation.

Since these symptoms tend to be correlated, let us investigate the suggestion that to some extent they are different reflections of a single basic malfunction of the brain system. The brain as a system deals with many units of information which are represented in it, by active processes, sometimes referred to as complicated reverberating circuits or cell assemblies (Hebb, 1972). The research in the area of attention has supplied proofs that those processes which represent aspects of behavior not overtly expressed are in fact active at a subliminal level. [Compare for example Broadbent's original theory (Broadbent, 1958) with that proposed by Treisman (1969)]. The modulation of the level of activity of different brain processes is accomplished through their interactions both in terms of facilitation and inhibition. The phenomenon of lateral inhibition (Kuffler, 1953) is an example of how brain processes interact with one another.

What happens when the brain can allow fewer processes to interact than in normal situations? The result may be reflected in concretic behavior. As an example let us examine the vulnerability of brain damaged patient's memory traces to the effect of interference. It is easy to see that this syndrome could be explained on the basis of the damaged brain's inability to accomodate a number of active, separate brain processes at the same time. Hence the few processes which are active fade as soon as an input imposes on the brain a certain new pattern of activity. As an example of the way a brain damaged patient is effected by interference, I always think of a patient who told the present author that whenever he boils water to prepare a cup of coffee, he has to stay in the kitchen holding the handle of the kettle until the water boils. If he were to move from the kitchen anything may catch his attention and he would never remember to turn off the flame and proceed with his original plan to prepare a cup of coffee.

Internal modulation of activity is dependent on the interaction between the brain process which is currently above threshold activity - the process which is relatively more structured - and the other processes which are currently active in the subthreshold level but nevertheless constitute modulatory effects as contextual effects. Without them the response to a given situation is stereotyped, unidimensional and lacking in depth. In terms of actual behavior we may be speaking about behavior which lacks the judgemental dimension, which is stimulus bound and impulsive. For example, the present author has a young patient whom, for reasons which are not quite clear to me, has a need to call me a day or two before our weekly meeting. Our phone conversation goes something like this: "Hello". "Hello". "How are you and how is your health?" "Fine, fine." "How are the kids and how is the family?" "Fine, fine." After all this social politeness ritual, he would continue to deal with his business of confirming our meeting or cancelling it. At least two types of contextual effects are lacking in this patient's behavior. First, being polite to a member of the family or a friend may require, according to our social conventions, to ask all these ritualistic questions. But talking to your psychologist requires a different social code. For this particular patient the context of the identity of the person to whom he was talking did not matter. The other missing aspect of contextual effects is that the purpose of the phone call, what he was about to say immediately after he finished the social ritual, also did not effect that ritual. In summary, if one were to listen to the opening sentences, one could not guess with whom he was talking nor the purpose of the conversation.

A limited capacity system in which only few processes can be active at a given moment and where modulation of activity is impaired, is a competitive system in which the various processes tend to act according to an all or none principle. Hence, the paradoxical appearance of continuous unaltered activity which is expressed in rigidity and perseveration with, concommitently, extreme changes in the processes which are active (impulsivity) becomes explainable.

In summary, clinical neuropsychology is concerned more than ever before with the problem of the integrated operation of the brain. Analysis of the concretic personality syndrome suggests the possibility that the various symptoms which make up this syndrome share a common origin. Further analysis of the interactions between brain processes which are simultaneously active suggests that a healthy efficient brain has a broad capacity and can accommodate many active processes at the same time, each modulating and being modulated by others. The interrelationships between various brain processes are seen as a most important quality of the active brain. We further contrasted the efficient, broad capacity brain with the one which has only a limited capacity in which different processes compete rather than interact in many different ways. We finally proposed that the broad capacity brain can serve as a model for understanding the way a healthy brain functions. A limited capacity brain can serve as a model for understanding the way a damaged brain produces the behavior of the concretic personality.

Let us now analyze the other concept which reflects an emphasis

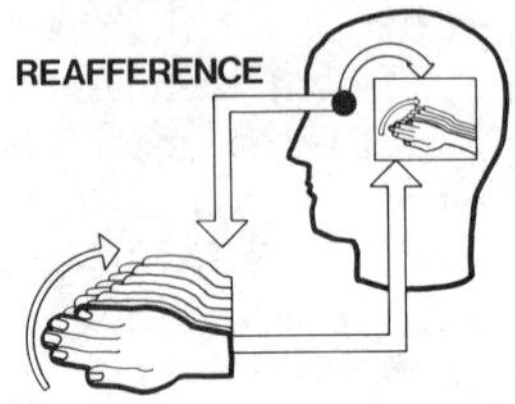


Figure 3. Schematic of Reafferent Processes.

on the integrated aspect of the activity of the brain, the concept of "function" as defined by Luria (1973). Luria defines a function as a complex relationship between "a constant (invariant) task performed by variable mechanisms bringing the process to a constant result" (Luria, 1973, p. 28). The complex functional systems cannot be localized in narrow zones of the cortex or in isolated cell groups, but must be organized in concertedly working zones ... which may be located in completely different and often far distant areas of the brain" (Luria, 1973, p. 31).

A neuropsychological function is a part of the integrated activity which is "represented" so to speak in many different cortical and subcortical areas. We have to restate that a function is defined in terms of its "goal" or the equivalent in brain processes of, what we call in motivation, consumatory behavior. A function is therefore a system which defines the relationship between an initiating process and its reafferent brain processes.

Reafference is the input which reaches a system and which is highly correlated with that system's output. Think, for example, of the fact that when you move your eyes in the normal fashion from right to left, the scenery seems to be stationary. However, when a similar movement of the eye is produced not through occulomotor output but by pressing on the eyeball, the external world seems to be moving. In the first case we have an input (movement of the image on the retina) which is correlated with the system's output. This input is called reafference. In the second case we have input which is not correlated with the system's output, and is termed exafference.

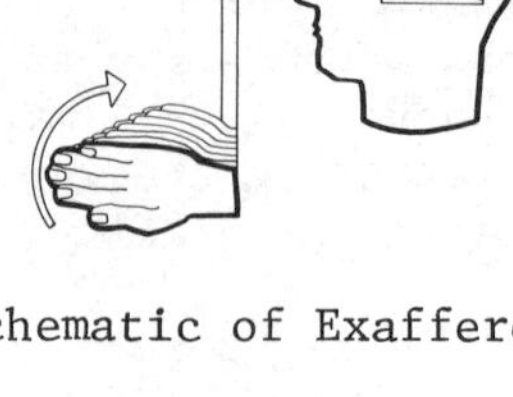


Figure 4. Schematic of Exafferent Processes.

The basic feature of reafference is that it is expected before it actually happens. (See Van Holst and Mittelstaedt, 1950; Held & Hein, 1963.)

When we look on a function as the relationship between an initiating process and its reafferant process, we have a two dimensional circular element of the integrated activity of the brain. Once a process has been initiated, the reafferent activity of the brain tends to be highly predictable and to have a one to one relationship with the initiating process. Is there anything else besides that two dimensional circular element be it as complicated and as evolved (i.e., have many stages) as it may?

At this point I would like to draw our attention to the analogy between the one-to-one direct convergent relationship between the initiating and the reafferent processes, and the one-to-one direct convergent relationship between stimulus or impulse and response displayed by so many of our patients. Here again an example which will be familiar to many of us can serve as an illustration. A brain damaged war veteran in Israel needed to get a refrigerator. The reader should know that due to the economic conditions in Israel, buying a refrigerator is a major operation involving the investment of significant capital. At one point during his treatment he related to the following story: "I was strolling with some friends in the town near the village where I live. I saw a store with electrical appliances and I went in to get a refrigerator. I asked the store keeper to give me that refrigerator and I asked him for the price. He told me the price and I put my hand into my pocket to fetch my check book." The impulsivity of the patient and the fact that his behavior was controlled to a large extent by external stimuli was obvious. This example illustrates the lack of depth characteristic of the brain injured in reasoning and the extent to which this particular patient's behavior was totally convergent with the input (the presence of the refrigerator). The patient's reaching for his check book was a reafferent process, synchronizing his own behavior with the input information, without judgement or benefit from contextual information.

Several factors may interfere with the one-to-one relationship between the initiating process and the reafferent one. Factors such as motivation and the degree to which the correspondence between initiation and reafference is over learned or repeated excessively and opponence. The concept of opponence was first derived by Solomon and Corbit (1974). However, these authors treated this concept only with regard to motivation, whereas it appears to be a viable concept in understanding brain processes as well. The basic thesis of Solomon and Corbit is that once a (motivational) process has been repeatedly initiated, or activated for prolonged periods of time, the organism supresses it by producing its inverse process. Solomon and Corbit use an example of a woman who notices a lump in her breast. I'd like to give my own description of such a case. At first the woman becomes distressed and her behavior is significantly disturbed. For a few days she might even stop functioning as a mother or a housewife, spending much of her time crying. As time passes her apparent distress subsides giving way to what looks to be her normal behavior. Then she goes to her doctor and finds out that she definitely did not develop breast cancer. Her apparent behavior now changes. Her behavior might be again disorganized but this time in a completely different way. She may go out of the office with a broad smile. Then she might be singing in the street, she may buy herself a new expensive dress which she wanted for some time but knew she could not afford, or do all kinds of "crazy" things. Again her normal routine as a mother and a housewife is disturbed and it may take a few days until she exhibits her more typical behavior. Solomon and Corbit point to the contrast between the seemingly relaxed "normal" mood the woman is in before going to the doctor, and the mood with which she leaves the office. Apparently she was "worried" in some sense, even when it did not effect her immediate overt behavior. The opponent process theory assumes that the processes which were activated by perceiving the lump in her breast got inhibited by other processes and that the observed behavior is the net outcome of interaction between the two. Once the distress is removed by the doctor's diagnosis, the "distress" processes are not activated any longer but their opponents remain. The net behavioral result being the opposite of worry and distress emerge. The generalization which Solomon and Corbit make is that any motivational process tends, when activated, to produce its opponent. It may be the case that initiating processes tend to produce an opponent which is reafferent in nature. The correspondence between the initiating process and the reafferent process, both in terms of spatial and temporal organization,

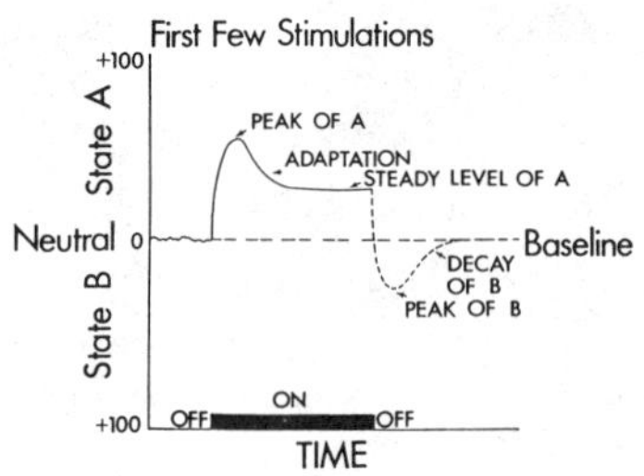


Figure 5. The manifest temporal dynamics generated by the opponent-process system during the first few stimulations. (The five features of the affective response are labeled.) Note. From "An opponent-process theory of motivation: I. Temporal dynamics of affect" by R. L. Solomon and J.D. Corbit, Psychological Review, 1974, 81, 119-145. Copyright 1974 by American Psychological Association. Reprinted by permission.

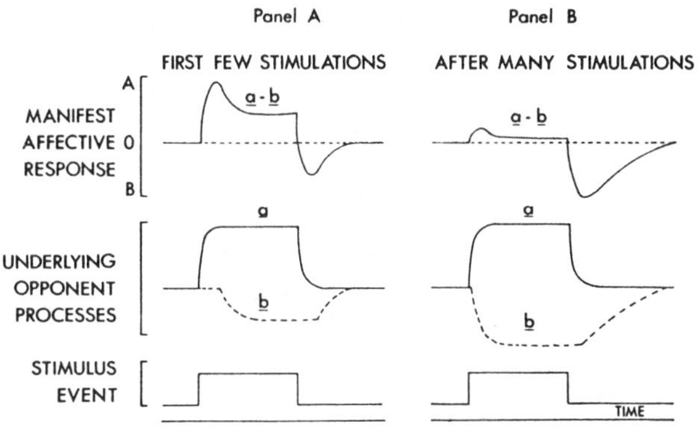


Figure 6. Panel A: The operation of the summing device for the first few stimulations. (The summation of the underlying opponent processes, A and B yields the manifest affective response.) Panel B: The operation of the summing device after many repeated stimulations. Note. From "An opponent-process theory of motivation: I. Temporal dynamics of affect" by R.L. Solomon and J.D. Corbit, Psychological Review, 1974, 81, 119-145. Copyright 1974 by American Psychological Association. Reprinted by permission.

increases as a function of several factors. The first is, of course, learning, i.e., repeated exposure to the same signal which is followed by the response (and its supression). The second is whether the initiating process does involve motivational systems. Solomon and Corbit argue that non-motivational initiating processes do not produce the inverse, reafferent processes. The apparent analogy between the opponent response and the negative after image in perception is discarded by them, because the negative after image disappears after a short interval, whereas the opponent process is a long lasting one. They have overlooked at least two cases in which the sensory after-effect takes a long period of time. One is the McCulloch (1965) effect in which case the brain is habituated to horizontal lines of one of two complementary colors (e.g., green), and vertical lines of the other color (e.g., red), and a negative differential effect is produced for both horizontal and vertical lines simultaneously. This after-effect can take place for quite a long time. The other case in which we have opponent, long lasting, phenomena in perception is the effect of an anchoring stimulus on the adaptation level, and the adaptation level itself.

I remember, for example, my first experience in New York. I live in Israel in a relatively small community. Coming to New York I was startled by the enormous noise, the number of people, the size of the buildings, et cetera. Having been there several times over the years, and getting somewhat accustomed to the city, I still perceive it with the eyes of a countryman. The opposite experience happens to my firends from the big cities who come to stay with us and find what is for me, a relaxed atmosphere, distressing. The point that I wanted to make is that opponence is a general principle of brain function, a principle which is related not only to motivational processes. There seem to be situations and stimuli in which the opponence is more pronounced and creates long lasting after-effects and others in which the opponence is less pronounced and creates after effects which subside relatively soon after the stimulus which produced the initial process disappears. Rather than dividing processes into two groups, as suggested by Solomon and Corbit, one which creates opponents and one which does not, I suggest to see the continuity between these two groups. The obvious question is therefore, what are the variables which effect the ability of an initial process to produce a long lasting reafferent opponent process.

It is the tenent of the present paper that the relevant dimension is the degree to which the initiating process is a tightly structured one. Namely the degree to which the elements of this process are interdependent. Repeated occurences strengthen the structure of a process to the point of automaticity. Take for example the performance of a learned skill after it has been initiated. Heredity is another factor which creates highly structured process and the fixed complexity of instinctive behavior. Motivational processes are therefore one class of processes in which there is a high correspondence between the initiating process and the reafferent one. Here the opponence is clear and obvious, and we have what we have called before, a circular two dimensional state brought about. The obvious answer is that this happens whenever the conditions which create a close correspondence between the initiating and the reafferent processes do not exist.

When a situation arises in which a very loosely structured set of processes are activated, the brain produces, according to the opponents principle, supression of those processes. Now since the initiating process is to some extent amorphous, it is highly unlikely that an opponent, reafferent process be created which is synchronized

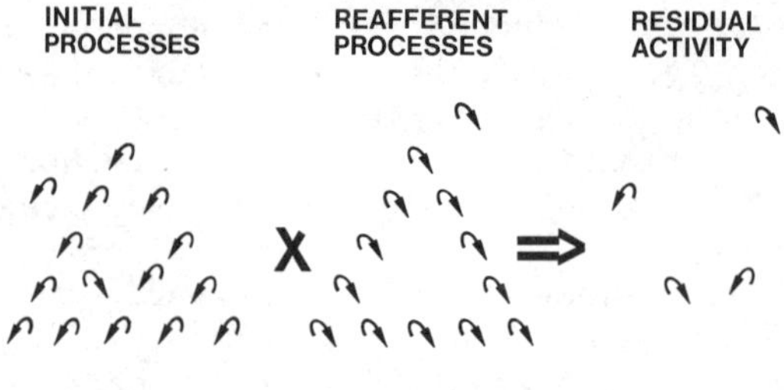


Figure 7. Schematic of a relatively structured initiating process with highly corresponding reafferent process, resulting in a minimum of residual activity.

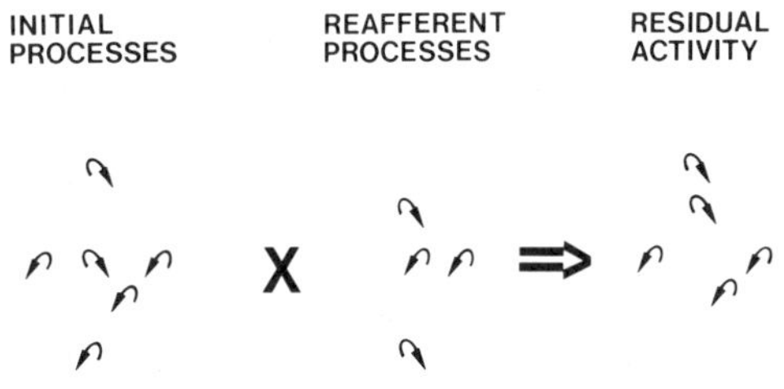


Figure 8. Schematic of quite unstructured initial processes with, concomitantly, an amorphous reafferent, resulting in a significant residual sustaining arousal and poorly directed orienting response.

in time and space with the initiating process. Speculating this way, we can further assume that only part of the activity of the initiating process is suppressed and inhibited. Taking the most simple minded approach we may propose that some residual activity remains as a result of an interaction between an initiating process and a reafferent process which does not fully correspond. Sustained arousal is one of the components of orienting response. This sustained arousal is the result of the lack of correspondence between the initial process aroused by the novel, unexpected stimulus and its oppenent process. In the case of the orienting response the lack of correspondence results from the fact that the initial process itself is not structured and therefore no opponent can be formed which corresponds in temporal and spatial organization to the initial process.

A different type of residual activity is formed, when, due to factors like specific attitude, detailed analysis of the situation is carried out so that minute details of the situation get to be represented in the initiating process. In the latter case every situation is a new one.

We have all experienced orienting responses, and have also experienced cases in which we perceive time and again the same stimulus always discovering new aspects. Take, for example, the attitude an art lover has towards a piece of art, always discovering its hidden layers. The constant process of discovering new facts of the situation produces initial processes which do not have already prepared and structured opponents. The result is lack of habituation and sustained arousal produced by the piece of art.

Residual activity can be a new initiating process to which the brain is responding by again trying to inhibit it. This can provide a model for activity which never ceases, which perpetuates itself endlessly. The description of self-perpetuating, though ever changing activity, stands in sharp contrast to the two dimensional closed circular element which we have described before.

If we may shift between the physiological speculative level and actual behaviors, this distinction is reminiscent of the distinction between habituation and perceptual learning phenomena. Perceptual learning is defined as "an increase in sensitivity to existing but initially undetected or poorly detected variables of stimulation. The process whereby perceptual learning occurs is assumed to be one of differentiation, that is, of the tendency to see more and more what is present in stimulation by progressive analysis, rather than by synthesis of stimulation" (Tighe & Tighe, 1966). Isn't the above a description of what happens to our art lover? On the other hand, habituation occurs as a result of the repeated presentation of the same stimulus to which the observer develops a leveling attitude. Perceptual learning would occur in those cases in which the observer has a sharpening attitude.

In habituation we have a gradual decrease in the organism's responsiveness to a stimulus. To put it in our words, we have an increase in the complementarity between the initiating and the reafferent processes. In perceptual learning on the other hand, we have an initial partial complimentarity between the initial and reafferent processes which decreases with repeated presentations. Another behavioral analogue would be the distinction between latent inhibition and sensitization effects of pre-exposure to potentially anxiety provoking stimuli.

In addition to the question of the quantity of the residual processes, i.e., the degree of complementarity between the initiating and reafferent processes, we have to mention another aspect of the residual activity, this time a qualitative dimension. This is related to the degree to which the residual activity forms a structured as opposed to amorphic activity. This dimension is related to the difference between the amorphic orienting response, and response which is directed and differentiated. To sum up, continuous inte-

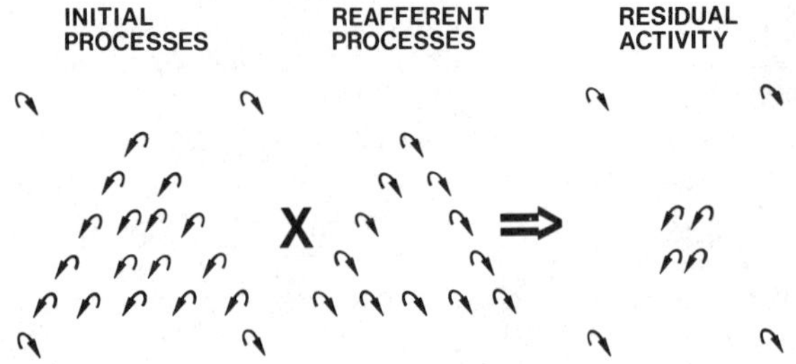


Figure 9. Schematic of process which result in a highly structured residual and consequently, a directed and differentiated response.

grated behavior depends on partial complementarity between initiating and reafferent processes, and interrelatedness between parts of the residual activity.

In review, it has been suggested that the deficiency shared by different brain damaged patients is an inability to deal simultaneously with many different processes. Luria's concept of "function" has been expanded such that it defines the relationship between initiating and reafferent processes. However, this concept of "function" lacks in that it looks on a unit of behavior which is isolated from the constant flow of activity. The concept of reafferent and opponent processing were related such that the continuity and integration of behavior are dependent on the residual brain activity which remains after initial processes have been partially neutralized by opponent processes. We said further that the amount and interrelatedness of the elements of the residual activity are related to the degree to which contextual information is processed.

We can plausably consider that brain damage produces (in addition to specific deficits) a disruption in the continuity and integration of the activity in one of two ways; either through reactivity similar to the amorphic orienting response, or reactivity of the habituation type. Seen in this way, the purpose of cognitive interventive neuropsychology is to enable the patient to develop <u>significant</u> residual activity. "Significance" is related to both quantitative and the qualitative dimensions. At this point, it is clear that interventive cognitive neuropsychology should aim at directing patient's attention and perception to the context within which the external stimulus or internal process are embedded. Residual activity is a function of the patient's ability to notice many aspects of the context of a stimulus, namely the degree to which an event (occurrence of a given figure on a given background) is psychologically unique. Then the degree to which the context is analyzed and coded in medium and long term memory systems rather than just registered in the short term memory system determines the interrelatedness of the processes which represent that background or context.

Having returned from the realm of theory into the world of practice we can state in operative terms the goals of interventive neuropsychology. Basically, the goal is to allow the patient to divert his attention from the figure in his experimental field to its ground, and back again. The assumption is made that a healthy brain is able to shift its attention from figure to ground and back in a dynamic way. Furthermore, a healthy brain does this dynamic shift habitually. Can we train a damaged brain to change the way its attentional mechanism is functioning? This question should be dealt with from two different aspects. First, a word should be devoted to the very basic assumption of interventive neuropsychology regarding the modifiability of the functioning mode of the brain.

Secondly, the problem of generalization of training with brain injured patients should also be discussed.

Many attempts illustrate the ability of the brain to change the way it functions when changes arc forced on it. Recovery of function which cannot be explained by restoration of physiological balance in the damaged brain is often mentioned in this context. In fact, the brain changes its mode of functioning constantly in response to experiences, as well as in response to the daily loss of thousands of neurons. It is only logical to assume that these spontaneous changes could be channeled in a "right" direction through intervention, provided we know what this "right" direction is, and provided we know how to develop an effective training procedure.

The problem of generalizability should be dealt with in some detail because we all agree that for a training program to be effective, it has to bring about a desired change in behavior which was not specifically trained, and in situations which are new for the trainee. These requirements are very problematic when one deals with brain damaged patients. We know that one of the ways in which their concretic personality is reflected is through a limited ability to transfer training from one task performed in a given situation to another task or another situation. Can this problem be overcome or at least circumvented? It seems to us that indeed it can, if the whole problem of generalization and transfer of training can be avoided altogether.

Generalization occurs as a result of dual evaluative process: one which deals with the comparability between two processes, the other with the differentiation between them. Two contrasting operations are therefore involved, and their combination allows one to estimate the degree of similarity between two situations. The brain damaged patient tends to have difficulties in engaging in two contrasting mental operations and in working with abstract concepts such as degree of similarity. He prefers to paint his world as either consisting of repeated events or of events which are completely irrelevent to one another. This is one of the facets of his concretic attitude. If only we had a principle which the patient could apply equally to all situations and all tasks of his concretic attitude might even be an asset, since once he has learned to apply that rule indiscriminately, he will do so automatically and continuously. It seems to me that the model which we have described above leads to the formation of such a rule. That rule would be: "Always pay attention to the context of that which you are dealing with but make sure that you keep in your mind the distinction between figure and ground".

Like so many other rules this general instruction is not only easier said than done, but also easier said than explained. We cannot expect our patients to be psychologists and to understand our professional concepts and jargon.

Even if they do understand the jargon, what meaning does the sentence 'pay attention to contextual information' convey in terms of actual new behavioral strategies the patient has to adopt? The question that we raise here is related to the desired methodology which will enable the patient to comprehend what it is we are meaning when we say contextual information, and what he can do to attend to contextual information. Some training methods which we have used in Israel in the last few years and which we believe are helpful to patients will be described in Chapter 11 of the present volume.

## REFERENCES

Broadbent, D.D. *Perception and communication*. London: Pergamon Press, 1958.

Goldstein, K. and Scheerer, M. Abstract and concrete behavior. *Psychological Monographs*, 1941, *53*.

Hebb, D.O. *A textbook of psychology*. Philadelphia: Saunders, 1972.

Held, R. and Hein, A. Movement produced stimulation in the development of visually-guided behavior. *Journal of Comparative and Physiological Psychology*, 1963, *56*, 872-876.

John, E.R. *Mechanisms of memory*. New York: Academic Press, 1967.

Kahneman, D. *Attention and effort*. Englewood Cliffs: Prentice-Hall, 1973.

Kuffler, S.W. Discharge patterns and functional organization of mammilian retina. *Journal of Neurophysiology*, 1953, *16*, 37-68.

Lashley, K. In search of the engram. *Symposium of the Society for Experimental Biology*, *Volume 4*, p. 454-482.

Luria, A.R. *The working brain: An introduction to neuropsychology*. Hardmondsworth: Penguin Books, 1973.

McCollough, C. Color adaptation of edge detectors in the human visual system. *Science*, 1965, *149*, 1115-1116.

Pribram, K.H. *Languages of the brain*. Englewood Cliffs: Prentice-Hall, 1971.

Solomon, R.L. and Corbit, J.D. An opponent-process theory of motivation: I. Temporal dynamics of affect. *Psychological Review*, 1974, *81*, 119-145.

Sperry, R.W., Gazzaniga, M.S., and Bogen, J.E. Interhemispheric relationships: The neocortical commisures: Syndromes of hemispheric disconnection. In P.J. Zenken and Fruyn (Ed.), *Handbook of Clinical Neurology*, *Volume 4*. Amsterdam: North-Holland, 1969.

Stein, D.G., Rosen, J.J. and Butters, N. (Eds.), *Plasticity and recovery of function in the central nervous system*. New York: Academic Press, 1974.

Tighe, H.S. and Tighe, T.J. Discrimination learning: Two views in historical perspective. *Psychological Bulletin*, 1966, *66*, 353-370.

Treisman, A.M. Strategies and models of selective attention. Psychological Review, 1969, 76, 282-299.

Von Holst, E. and Mittelstaedt, H. Das Reafferenz-Prinzip. Die Naturwissenschaften, 1950, 20, 464-467.

# THE RELEVANCE OF BRAIN-BEHAVIOR RELATIONSHIPS FOR REHABILITATION[1]

Eugene B. Piasetsky, Ph.D.

Department of Behavioral Sciences
Institute of Rehabilitation Medicine
New York University Medical Center
New York, New York

In order to assess the implications of brain-behavior relationships for rehabilitation, two separate yet related issues will be considered:

(1) How can recovery be understood in terms of the capacity of the central nervous system to respond to injury? Specifically, what mechanisms have been proposed to account for recovery?; and,

(2) To what extend may a role for environmental influence in the recovery process be defended?

Having considered these issues, the relevance of brain-behavior relationships to rehabilitation will further be explored in terms of dynamics which are common to both the principles underlying the organization of functions and those underlying cognition.

The context for this discussion is the manner in which complex behaviors are understood to be achieved by the normal non-damaged brain. Early theorists argued this issue from one of two basic perspectives: That which depicted the brain as a conglomeration of discrete functional centers, each exerting control over one or another class of behaviors (localizationism); and, that which depicted the brain as functionally unitary with no absolute sub-differentiation of control over complex behaviors (mass actionism). While each of these drew basic support from observations on the post-injury state (localizationism reflecting the consistency in relationship between damage to certain structural regions and primary deficits; and, mass actionism reflecting the persistence of recovery in the

[1]The preparation of this paper was supported in part by grants from NIH-NINNCDS (10236-08) and the Pew Memorial Trust.

face of structural damage), neither adequately accounted for both the specificity of acquired deficits following injury and the subsequent recovery therefrom. Current thinking has done much to reconcile the implications drawn from observations on the post-injury state. Complex behaviors are presently seen as arising through dynamic systems of regional cooperation. Basically, while different regions are seen as devoted to certain complex processing activities, it is only through the integration and coordination of these activities that complex behavior is achieved.

While a systems approach to brain function is generally accepted, individual researchers differ markedly with respect to the kinds of processing activities they ascribe to anatomically distinct regions (i.e., integrations, transformations, mental acts, behavioral units). These differences are reflected in differing interpretations as to what has been lost subsequent to injury, and what specific organizational properties might be available to support recovery.

## MECHANISMS OF RECOVERY

Within this context, there are three main principles from which mechanisms of recovery have been derived: Dis-inhibition; compensation by virtue of redundancy; and, functional re-organization. The first two are largely descriptive, reflecting those intrinsic organizational properties of the system which may predispose it to retain its functional integrity after injury. The third, functional reorganization, is dynamic, involving the active adaptation of the system to the effects of injury. Such adaptation implies an interaction with the environment and affords a potential application for intervention.

### Dis-inhibition (Recovery from Shock)

The behavioral consequences of injury processes reflect the influence of two underlying sources of disruption in neural activity: permanent cessation of activity in regions where no structural damage has been sustained. Dis-inhibition addresses recovery from deficits attributable to the latter.

Areas often far removed from the actual site of injury may become functionally inhibited secondary to shock. Von Monakow (1914) characterized this shock as being uniquely neurogenic ("diaschisis"), transmitted to distant regions along neural pathways. Luria (1963) ascribed the effects of shock to a combination of predominantly systemic (i.e., edema, vascular reactions, biochemical alterations), and occasionally psychogenic, factors. To the extent that these two formulations might be distinguished, systemic factors would effect an influence along geographic lines in relation to specific sites of injury, being most pronounced and longest lasting nearest those sites. Neurogenic factors would effect an influence along functional lines in relation to any area in which cessation of activity has occurred (involving projections to and from damaged regions and regions which have fallen under the influence of systemic factors). In most instances, these effects would be reversible.

Dis-inhibition refers to a return to normal activity in undamaged regions as the state of shock abates. As a rule, affected areas which are farthest from the sites of injury would be dis-inhibited earliest, with the final stages of dis-inhibition occurring in spared portions of damaged regions. Some distant effects may persist longer than others. For example: 1) Transmission along fiber pathways which traverse a site of injury may remain disrupted as long as there is edema present in and around that site. Such pathways may "connect" regions apart from and wholly unrelated to the damaged region. Normal communication along these pathways would not be restored until the final stages of dis-inhibition are achieved; or, 2) areas receiving projections from the damaged region, and thereby innervated by it, may remain inhibited unless and until there is a substantial return of neural activity in the damaged region. This would constitute a potential source of permanent referred inhibition where activity in the damaged region could not be restored (owing to extensive tissue destruction).

In the overall process of recovery, dis-inhibition accounts for the re-activation of spared processing activities upon which the organism must come to rely. Its influence would be most prominent early in the post-injury recovery period, affecting a wide range of behaviors, and is likely the basis for recovery often characterized as spontaneous. Yet, dis-inhibition does not directly address recovery from losses attributable to a permanent cessation of neural activity. To explain this, some compensatory action must be presumed.

## Compensation by Virtue of Redundancy

Compensation might be achieved without changing the underlying processing dynamics as they were constituted pre-morbidly. This would assume the existence of certain intrinsic organizational properties, specifically some degree of functional redundancy, by which the lost processing activity could effectively be duplicated. Redundancy would allow for the restoration of function within the confines of pre-morbid processing dynamics, and would either arise spontaneously upon dis-inhibition or, subsequent to dis-inhibition, be rapidly evidenced upon exposure to the environment.

Redundant Representation. One source of redundancy may reside in the local organization of cells within the damaged region. Rosner (1970) has proposed that a region's contribution to behavior may be sustained by some minimum number of cells within that region. This, he reasoned, would account for the results of laboratory studies in which cats retained the ability to perform tasks requiring complex visual discriminations despite massive lesioning of the optic tracts (Galambos, Norton & Frommer, 1967) or both, optic tracts and visual cortex (Chow, 1968). Yet, as other investigators have pointed out (Dawson, 1973; Laurence & Stein, 1978), interpreting the results of such studies is complicated by the availability of more rudimentary cues by which animals might complete the tasks.

Still, animals have consistently been found to be less impaired by partial damage to a region than by total damage. To the extent to which this may reflect redundant representation, it could be argued that some of a region's processing activities may be sufficiently unsophisticated so as to be accomplished through a minimal application of its organizational properties. Behaviors which might be accomplished through an application of these simpler activities would constitute the limits to which redundant representation accounts for recovery.

Multiple Representation. The argument of redundancy might be extended to include structures at different hierarchical levels within a system. During the course of development, earlier-developing structures may retain aspects of functioning which become incorporated into the activities of later-developing hierarchically adjacent ones. Structurally distinct regions may, then, be functionally concentric, so that the processing activities of any one might be partially represented in the activities of another. Following injury, those operations of a functional system which may be mediated by lower centers as readily as higher ones may be retained. Behaviors which may be supported by those operations would be spared the effects of injury.

## Functional Re-organization

Dis-inhibition and the presence of intrensic redundancy provide for the limits of recovery which might be mediated through pre-morbid processing dynamics. Further recovery would necessitate some change in the deployment of available processing activities so as to effect compensation for what has been lost. Yet, such re-deployment must occur within the context of a still enormously complex set of established organizational priorities. Intuitively, it would follow that even small changes in the way processing activities are utilized could be disruptive. The success or failure of a particular re-organizational effort rests, not simply in whether restoration is achieved, but, also, in how well the adaptive changes in utilization may be integrated into the ongoing operations of the brain as a whole.

Rosner (1970) suggests that re-organization may occur in instances where functions were pre-morbidly controlled through the activity of several regions. His concept of multiple control appears to embody two properties which might facilitate re-organization: 1) The presence of a degree of functional redundancy (referred to earlier as multiple representation) which serves to minimize the processing loss; and, 2) the existence, among functionally related regions, of common access to required processing centers. While this provides a structural basis for re-organization, Rosner offers no explanation for how this process occurs.

Luria (1963) considered functional re-organization to be an active learning process which may only be achieved after long periods of special training. The structural basis for re-organization, as provided for in his theory of dynamic localization, inheres in the complex neural processes which characterize association cortex. These processes give rise to a broad hierarchy of inter-related and progressively more complex associative integrations. The dynamic structure of this complex hierarchy derives from the differentiation of cortical regions into primary (projection), secondary and tertiary zones. During development, different locations within this complex hierarchy become established as "afferent fields," which serve as centers of automated control over individual functional behaviors. These fields are said to monitor the processing activities which comprise a particular functional system and ensure that those activities remain consistent with intended action. A functional system may involve the coordination of several afferent or efferent links (i.e., vision, audition), each of which may contain embedded subdivisions which permit numerous variations on a general functional theme.

In instances where damage has disrupted the operation of one link in a functional system, Luria proposed that function may be restored through an internal re-organization of spared components. In example of this, he describes a training regimen which was applied to a patient who could not discriminate between complex or phonetically similar speech sounds. The patient was trained to make a discrimination by referring each of two similar sounds back to words beginning with those sounds. On each training trial, the patient was provided with sufficient cues so as to understand which sound-word referent was being signified. This provided the patient with a means of internally validating the experience of each sound and, thereby, facilitate his finding a relevant dimension along which to make the discrimination. In this instance, a spared activity of the functional system (generating meaningful speech-sound combinations) was adopted to serve a more generalized purpose (modeling for individual speech-sounds). Training was required, initially to establish the adaptation and, finally to automatize it.

In instances where damage results in the total destruction of a link in a functional system, rendering the system inoperable, Luria proposed that restoration may be achieved through an inter-system compensation. With training, the role in behavior played by the destroyed link may be assumed by another which had not previously taken part in the behavior. Luria (1963; 1969) cites several examples of inter-system compensation. The substitution of visual guidance for a loss of proprioception in directing the movements of a limb; the use of kinesthetic-proprioceptive feedback (tracing) to facilitate recognition of visually presented symbols; the use of auditory or visual signals to pace sequencing of motor movements.

In reference to inter-system re-organization, Luria suggests that "... links which hitherto never participated in the deranged functional system, can now be made to do so" (1963, p. 77). Yet, it stands to reason that re-organization based upon genuinely novel relationships would necessitate considerable overall accommodation and be unlikely to achieve synchrony within the existing organizational framework. There would be a decided advantage to seeking re-organization which has at least some basis in pre-morbid inter-modal relationships. Where an inter-system re-organization is called for, one might seek instances from general behavior which establish a precedent for substitution. Many such instances may be found. In fact, between the diversity of human behavior and the complex changing nature of human development, it is improbable that the majority of purposeful inter-modal relationships which may be formed, have not already been so. Several sources may be explored:

(1) Less efficient organizational components, prominent during early stages in the development of a behavioral function, may be re-emphasized after injury. So, for example, the involvement of somesthetic mechanisms (haptic exploration) in early exploration and cataloguing provides a basis for the substitution of these mechanisms in instances where the more efficient visual substrate fails;

(2) Specialized applications of a behavioral function may provide a precedent for substitution. For example, within the context of a class of functional behaviors (such as those involving guidance of limb movements), a particular inter-modal relationship (such as visuo-motor) might be a variable component, evidenced in certain applications (throwing, kicking) but not others (lifting, walking). These specialized applications may potentially be generalized to serve a broader purpose in the accomplishment of a class of functional behaviors;

(3) Components which normally play a secondary role in the accomplishment of a functional behavior may be advanced to primacy through refinement and elaboration of their contribution. So, the involvement of auditory mechanisms in guidance and identification may be intensified in conjunction with a refinement of their capacity to discriminate relevant stimulus parameters.

Each of these sources would provide a basis for restoration of function, albeit not in the same way, nor likely as efficiently, as it was carried out premorbidly. While the examples provided involved overt behavioral acts, the principle is equally applicable to the restoration of psychological functions, as well. It is reasonable to assume that the organizational properties underlying brain function are sufficiently rich in complex inter-relationships so as to provide an ample basis for all forms of functional re-organization. These inter-relationships exist within a complex balanced organizational framework. Hence, selecting appropriate strategies by which to implement a re-organization, and, determining the best methods with which to engage those strategies, necessitates careful planning and remains a matter for continuing research.

## ENVIRONMENTAL INFLUENCE

A discussion of the potential role of environmental influence on recovery of function must inevitably lead to a consideration of what minimum assumptions are met concerning the structural basis of those functions. The observed tendency of functional properties to lateralize and localize cannot be simply discarded as arbitrary.

Whether one decides that brain mass is the determinant of function, or whether, from an evolutionary prospective, one considers that functional demands give rise to structural development, it may be presumed that the evidenced relationship between structure and function constitute a most effective utilization of brain mass. Given a reduction in the range of available structural layout (following injury), how much variation on the basic theme is possible without relinquishing the functional properties which define human cognition. For the present discussion, we will briefly examine the extent to which functional properties may be preserved in the absence of certain structural features.

Laboratory studies have often demonstrated that, when comparable damage is sustained by immature and adult animals, the immature ones exhibit less functional impairment (e.g., Benjamin and Thompson, 1959; Sharlock, Tucker and Strominger, 1963; Wetzel, Thompson, Horel and Meyer, 1965). Moreover, immature animals may retain a marked propensity to achieve adequate levels of functional development despite damage to critical (by adult standards) brain regions (Kennard, 1938). Comparable observations have been made in studies of early brain damage in children. Recovery from childhood aphasia is often complete or with relatively limited residual defects (Hecaen, 1976; Lenneberg, 1967). Moreover, in instances where damage is sustained very early in childhood (but after the onset of language development) no language impairment may be evidenced (Lenneberg, 1967). In contradistinction to inferences drawn from observations on the effects of localized damage in adults, studies of childhood brain injury argue in favor of considerable organizational plasticity during development. So much so, that even the removal of an entire hemisphere during infancy is often insufficient to prevent extensive functional development (Dennis & Whitaker, 1976; Smith & Sugar, 1975).

Functional plasticity is a generally accepted characteristic of the developing nervous system. It has been suggested that the degree of plasticity evidenced in cases of early damage may be dependent upon the maturational state of the system at the time damage is sustained, favoring periods where functional commitments are minimal (Goldman, 1974). Yet, there is some evidence that functional plasticity may also be characteristic of the adult, functionally committed, system. This evidence emerges from studies of the differential effects of serial versus single stage lesioning on animal behavior. It has been demonstrated that removing a given region (unilaterally or bilateral-symmetrically) in segments over time is associated with far less in the way of functional impairment than lesioning of the same area in a single operation (Stein, Rosen & Butters, 1974). It would be difficult to understand such an occurence in a system where particular structural entities are indespensable in the genesis of function. Hence, it might be said that the organizational dynamics which support function in both the immature and mature system inhere with a capacity to meet functional demands in more than one way.

It may be concluded, then, that: 1) Under normal conditions, there is a developmental course which may best suit the complex functional needs of the organism as a whole. This course is not, however, immutable. When blocked, another course may be undertaken; 2) Functional development following early brain damage, while less than ideal, is sufficiently adequate to suggest that few, if any, structures are truly indispensable in the overall functional scheme; and, 3) Established functional organization in the mature nervous system inheres with a decided potential for flexibility, revealed under certain conditions of structural loss.

## Environmental Influence In Development

The developing nervous system has often been found to exhibit susceptibility to environmental influences. Gross differences in early environmental experience have been associated with discernible differences in morphological development (see Greenough, 1976). Different rearing conditions have consistently been found to influence the functional physiology of the developing visual system (see Freeman, 1979). Directional selectivity of cortical visual receptors is substantially reduced or abolished in animals reared in total darkness. Monocular deprivation (suturing one eye closed) and artificially-induced monocular astigmatism selectively alter the number of directionally-specific receptors accessed through each eye. Yet, functional changes may be less dependent on either the innate properties of the system or the presence of environmental stimulation, than on an interaction of the two.

Kittens reared in total darkness have been found to exhibit a reduction in orientation selectivity of receptors in the visual cortex. They are said to behave as if blind upon initial exposure to a lighted environment, but recover normal functioning over time. Complete behavioral recovery has been demonstrated for deprivation lasting up to six months (Timney and Mitchell, 1979). Buisseret, Gary, Bobo and Imbert (see Imbert, 1979) found that reversing the effects of dark rearing in two month old kittens may depend upon both the presence of an appropriate environment and the manner of the animals' interaction with it: 1) Animals permitted to run free in a normal environment for six hours evidenced substantial recovery of orientation specificity; 2) animals exposed to a normal environment but restrained from free movement showed somewhat less recovery; and, 3) animals exposed to a normal environment under drug-induced paralysis (preventing even ocular motility) showed no recovery. It would appear, then, that some minimum environmental exposure is necessary to allow for the maintenance and further development of the functional properties of cortical visual receptors; but that this environment must be engaged actively in order to advantage its presence.

### Environmental Influence In Recovery

It was noted earlier that serial lesion studies provide evidence of organizational plasticity in the mature brain. It is particularly significant, then, that the advantage afforded serial-lesioned animals over single-stage lesioned ones may be dependent upon environmental factors. Petrinovich and Bliss (1966) compared the effects of serial versus single-stage lesioning of the visual cortex on retention of a learned visual discrimination task in rats. To the basic paradigm, they added the condition that their serial-lesioned animals were maintained in different visual environments between operations. One group remained in normal lighted conditions, while another was maintained in total darkness. Only the serial-lesioned animals, caged in a lighted environment, retained the ability to perform the previously-learned visual discrimination task. Those caged in darkness evidence no advantage over the single-stage lesioned animals. Petrinovich and Carew (1969) subsequently replicated these findings. Hence, while the mature nervous system retains a certain capacity to adapt to injury, this capacity may not be realized in the absence of appropriate environmental stimulation.

## THE DYNAMICS UNDERLYING FUNCTIONAL ORGANIZATION

Plasticity, with respect to functional organization, is more readily evidenced in the developing immature organism than in the developed mature one. Yet, certain dynamic mechanisms may be common to both. The primary distinction would seem to lie in the context

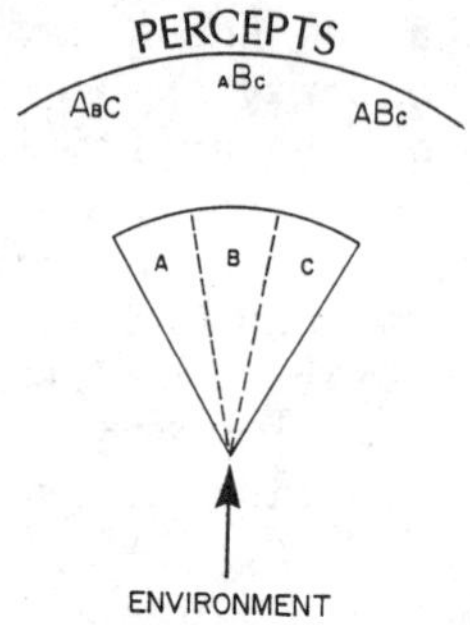


Figure 1. Schematic of a sensory system in early development.

within which these mechanisms must work. The immature system would demonstrate greater malleability and appear more readily receptive to dynamic alteration, owing to a lack of commitment to organizational priorities. Hence, the immature organism's central nervous system, by virtue of this lack of functional commitment, and inhering with the momentum of growth, readily accepts an organizational flow. The mature organism's central nervous system retains a capacity to demonstrate organizational plasticity, but must accomplish this within the context of an established and "phenomenologically balanced" set of functional priorities. Given this basic difference in internal environments, a single set of dynamic mechanisms may adequately describe the functional operations of both. To illustrate this, we might trace the course of functional development into maturity.

The first figure schematically depicts a sensory system (i.e., one definable pathway) at some point early in its development. It is, arbitrarily, afforded the capacity to discern three distinct characteristics of the environment. The extent of this system's contribution to a perception of the environment is defined by all the ways in which these characteristics may be converged. Through

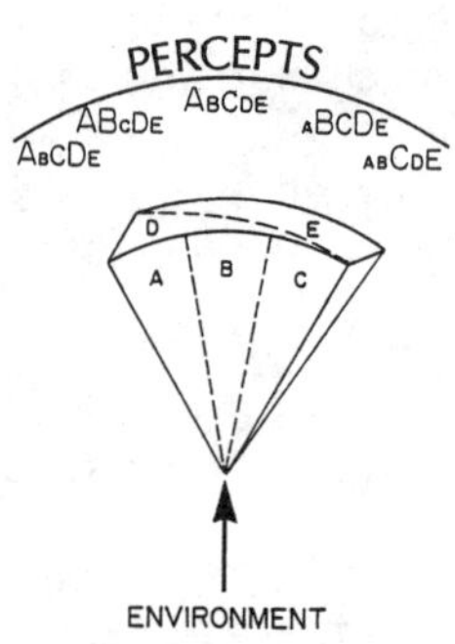


Figure 2. Differentiation, through maturation, of sensory system.

vertical development (maturation of a later developing component along the functional pathway), the system's capacity to represent the environment is enhanced through integration. This integration results in a more differentiated coding of sensory impulses and, thereby, provides for a more sophisticated contribution to general perception (see Figure 2). Yet, this is only a single component in the overall developing organizational network. That network includes numerous systems (subdivisions of primary sensory and motor modalities), each undergoing development and participating in the functioning of the organism. Figure 3 depicts this extended relationship at a particular moment in development, represented by two sensory systems and one motor system, each at different stages in their respective vertical development. The display has been limited to include only three basic systems, solely in the interests of simplification. More appropriately, one might imagine a multi-dimensional lattice, with numerous rungs intersecting at different stages in the development of individual systems. This would open the possibility for establishment of an inumerable variety of organizational arrangements with which to meet functional demands. At this moment in time, the functional life of the organism is defined by its utilization of these capacities and their various intersections.

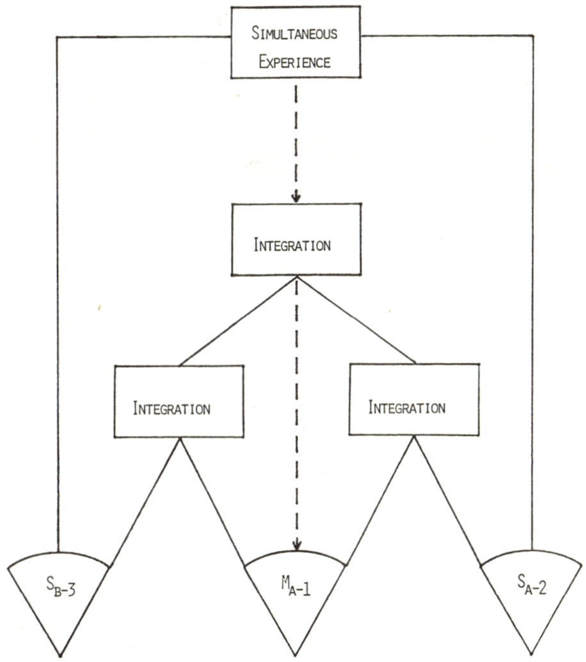


Figure 3. Inter-relatedness and integration of two sensory systems ($S_A$ and $S_B$) and one motor system ($M_A$).

Just as a single system does not develop in isolation, the organization underlying an individual functional behavior does not take form independently. Some patterns of utilization might serve one behavioral goal but be incompatible with the accomplishment of others. Hence, it is incumbent upon the organism to arrive at those processing arrangements which, weighted by behavioral demand, are mutually compatible and effective. Such arrangements become established as primary organizational schemes by their being engaged with greater regularity. Over the course of development, functional organization may be seen as an active process of schematization through which the deployment of available processing capacities is maximized. While this process is undoubtedly guided by innate structural imperatives, it is ultimately founded in functional relevance (as evidenced in studies of early brain damage).

The concept of functional relevance must be understood in terms of the organism's internal experience of contingencies. The ongoing operation of processing activities becomes schematized in recognition of a set of experienced results. At a very fundamental level, schematization is intent, conveyed through patterns of selective activation and inhibition. Figure 4 represents the network of

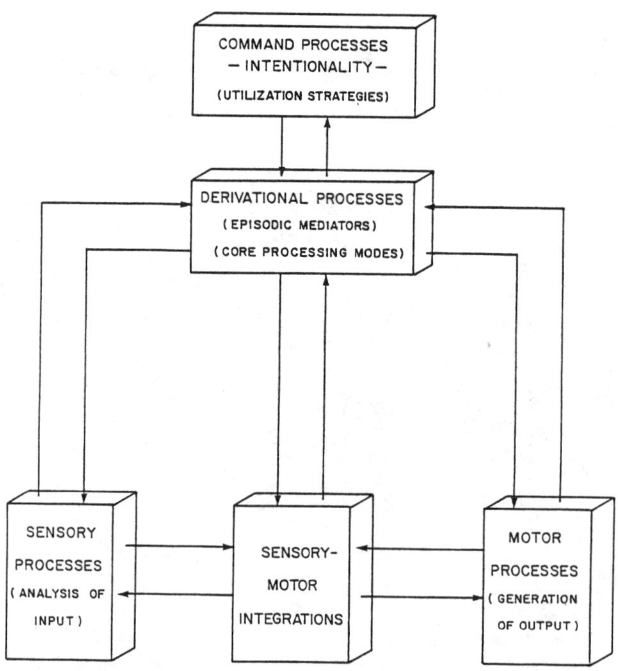


Figure 4. Schematic of inter-relatedness between command processes of intentionality and sensory, motor and sensory-motor integrative hierarchies, as mediated by derivational processes.

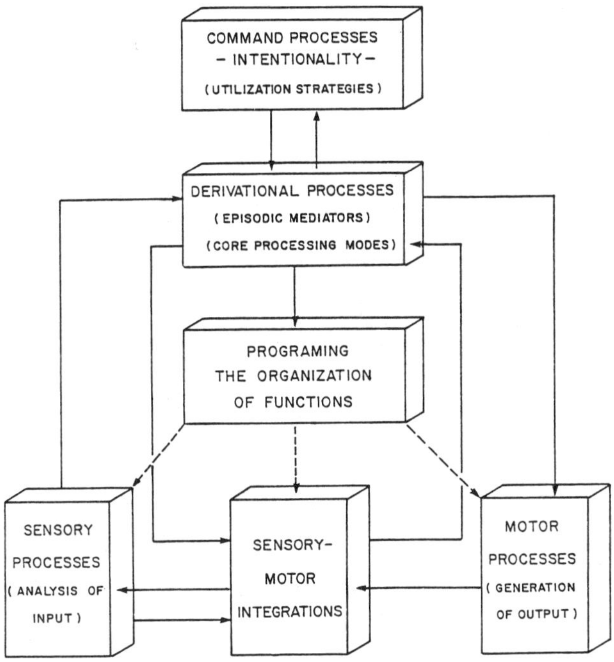


Figure 5. Schematic depicting the relationship of maturationally more sophisticated units of organized functions to command processes and integrative hierarchies.

developing systems in relation to the primary dynamics through which organization is effected. The complex inter-relationships represented in Figure 3 have been collapsed (for display purposes) into sensory, motor and sensory-motor integrative hierarchies. As development proceeds, schematized units of functional behavior begin to emerge (Figure 5). These units inhere with an hierarchical configuration reflecting a development progression from simpler and more general coordinations of activity through more complex and specific functional routines. Continued development leads, finally, to the emergence of more specialized routines (skills) which are applied during selected environmental interactions (Figure 6). It is in maturity that both the advantages and disadvantages of schematization may readily be evidenced. The availability of complex automated routines, applied with a minimum of segmented arousal, permit the highest levels of functional behavior to be accomplished without taxing the working limits of the organism. Yet, owing to their functionally unitary status, these routines might be particularly vulnerable to disruption (following damage) at a level not readily accessible to higher cortical supervision.

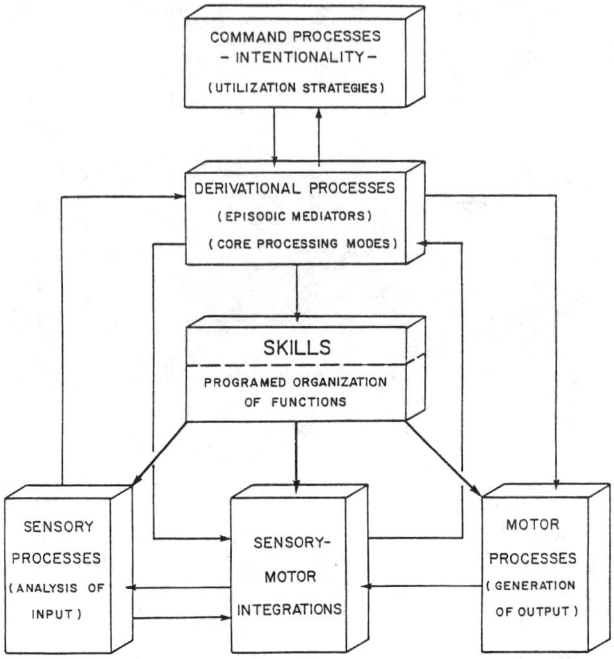


Figure 6. Schematic representation of the development of specialized skills in context of the hierarchial configuration.

Throughout development and into maturity, functional organization is effected by virtue of fundamental intent. In the immature organism, intent is expressed in the organization of processing activities into functional units. In the mature organism, it is expressed in the organization of established functional units into complex behavioral (psychological) activities. It follows, then, that if re-organization is to be effected, it is only through the organism's fundamental intent that this might be accomplished. Yet, intent is not embodied in the performance of a particular task nor is it necessarily reflected in verbal statements. It is, rather, the organism's experience of its processing in recognition of results. Hence, if change is to be achieved within a broad context, methods must be devised by which to ensure that the organism experiences that context and intends it. This, I suggest is the principle challenge facing us today.

REFERENCES

Benjamin, R.M. and Thompson, R.F. Differential effects of cortical lesions in infant and adult cats on roughness discrimination. Experimental Neurology, 1959, 1, 305-321.

Chow, K.L., Visual discriminations after extensive ablation of optic tract and visual cortex. Brain Research, 1968, 9, 363-366.
Dawson, R.G. Recovery of function: Implications for theories of brain function. Behavioral Biology, 1973, 8, 439-460.
Dennis, M. and Whitaker, H. Language acquisition following hemidecortication: Linguistic superiority of the left over the right hemisphere. Brain and language, 1976, 3, 404-433.
Freeman, R. (Ed.) Developmental neurobiology of vision. New York: Plenum Press, 1979.
Galambos, R., Norton, T.T. and Frommer, G. Optic tract lesions sparing pattern vision in cats. Experimental Neurology, 1967, 18, 8-25.
Goldman, P. An alternative to developmental plasticity: Heterology of CNS structures in infants and adults. In D.G. Stein, J.J. Rosen and N. Butters (Eds.), Plasticity and recovery of function in the central nervous system. New York: Academic Press, 149-174, 1979.
Greenough, W.T. Enduring brain effects of differential experience and training. In M.R. Rosenzweig and E.L. Bennett (Eds), Neural mechanisms of learning and memory. Cambridge Mass.: M.I.T. Press, 255-278, 1976.
Hecaen, H. Acquired aphasia in children and the ontogenesis of hemispheric functional specilization. Brain and Language, 1976, 3, 114-134.
Imbert, M. Maturation of visual cortex with and without visual experience. In R. Freeman (Ed.), Developmental neurobiology of vision. New York: Plenum Press, 43-49, 1979.
Kennard, M.A. Reorganization of motor function in the cerebral cortex of monkeys deprived of motor and pre-motor areas in infancy. Journal of Neurophysiology, 1, 477-496, 1938.
Laurence, S. and Stein, D.G. Recovery after brain damage and the concept of localization of function. In S. Finger (Ed.), Recovery from brain damage, New York: Plenum Press, 1978.
Lenneberg, E. Biological foundations of language. New York: Wiley, Chapter 8, 1967.
Luria, A.R. Restoration of function after brain injury. New York: Macmillan, 1963.
Luria, A.R., Naydin, V.L., Tsvetkova, L.S. and Vinarskaya. Restoration of higher cortical functions following localized brain damage. In P. Winken and G. Bruyen (Eds.), Handbook of Clinical Neurology, 3, Amsterdam: N. Holland Publishers, 1969.
Petrinovich, L. and Bliss, D. Retention of learned brightness discrimination following ablation of the occipital cortex in the rat. Journal of Comparative and Physiological Psychology, 1966, 61, 136-138.
Petrinovich, L. and Carew, T.J. Interaction of neo-cortical lesion size and interoperative experience in retention of learned brightness discrimination. Journal of Comparative and Physiological Psychology, 1969, 68, 451-454.
Rosner, B.S. Brain functions. Annual Review of Psychology, 1970, 21, 555-594.

Sharlock, D.P., Tucker, T.J. and Strominger, N.L. Auditory discrimination by the cat after neonatal ablation of the temporal cortex. Science, 1963, 141, 1197-1198.

Smith, A. and Sugar, O. Development of above normal language and intelligence 21 years after left hemispherectomy. Neurology, 1975, 25, 813-818.

Stein, D.G., Rosen, J.J. and Butters, N. (Eds.). Plasticity and recovery of function in the central nervous system. New York: Academic Press, 1974.

Timney, B. and Mitchell, D. Behavioral recovery from visual deprivation: Comments on the critical period. In R. Freeman (Ed.), Developmental neurobiology of vision. New York: Plenum Press, 1979.

Von Monakow, C. Diaschisis (1914). Excerpted in K.H. Pribram (Ed.), Mood, states and mind. London: Penguin Press, 27-37, 1969.

Wetzel, A.B., Thompson, V., Horel, J., and Meyer, P.M. Some consequences of perinatal lesions of the visual cortex in the cat. Psychonomic Science, 1965, 3, 381-382.

# LANGUAGE-COGNITIVE DISORGANIZATION FOLLOWING CLOSED HEAD INJURY: A CONCEPTUALIZATION

Chris Hagen, Ph.D.

Speech, Hearing and Neurosensory Center

San Diego, California

Closed head injury (CHI), defined here as a blow to the head which may or may not produce a skull fracture, does not cause tearing of the dura but does alter the individual's level of consciousness, frequently causes profound language and cognitive impairments that present the Speech-Language Pathologist with a diagnostic, prognostic and treatment challenge that is at once unique and complex. If the traditional language assessment instruments are applied one will obtain a diagnosis, prognosis and embark on a course of treatment only to find that all three aspects of patient management are inappropriate later that day, the following day or week. However, if one waits until the patient "stabilizes" they will find that not only have two to three months of valuable treatment time been lost but also that they are now confronted with a patient who has developed coping strategies that interfere with the effectiveness of treatment. Clearly, such patients cannot be successfully understood, diagnosed and treated within the framework of our traditional approach to language disorders.

The literature is not unanimous with respect to the nature and temporal course of post CHI language impairments. Early studies, (Arseni, 1970; Caveness, 1969; Fahy, 1967; Hooper, 1969; Lewin, 1966; Russell, 1932) which were directed primarily towards charting and identifying the natural course of general recovery from head trauma, reported that head injured patients experience an initial period of complete dissolution of language abilities but then gradually and spontaneously recapitulate the ontogoney of language with eventual attainment of "normal speech." The most frequent behavioral residuals reported were cognitive problems of impaired concentration and short term memory. In contrast, investigations that have studied post CHI language impairments present evidence that "speech" does not return to "normal" in the majority of patients.

In a series of 16 patients Glasser and Shafer (1932) reported one to have complete motor aphasia, four with mixed sensory-motor aphasia and ten as having partial motor aphasia. Smith (1974) found anomic errors to be a prominent characteristic of the majority of her subjects and of the 13 subjects studied by Heilman, Safrran and Geschwind (1971) nine were determined to have anomic aphasia and four were classified as Wernickes aphasia. Other investigators have found CHI patients to exhibit both specific language impairments and "confused" language. In general, confused language can be described as receptive/expressive language that is completely or predominantly intact phonologically, semantically and syntactically yet lacking in meaning either because the behavioral responses are completely irrelevant, confabulatory, circumlocutious or tangential in relation to a given topic and/or because of a lack of logico-sequential relationship between thoughts. The response of one of Weinstein's (1966) subjects is an example of this type of language dysfunction. When asked why he had come to the hospital he replied: "They sent me back, sir, on my one arm. I had one arm here in Korejit and this one here on for corgent. They took part of that on the way back in and my rove renetted up and we got a crane secker and thats where I got my injury in my head and my base. Both my eyes were blackened and this lady that brought me back took them out."

Levin's (1979) subjects presented with specific language disorders of paraphasic errors, jargon and auditory comprehension impairments as well as conversational language that was frequently fragmented, tangential and "often drifted to irrelevant topics." Thomsen (1975) found that 13 of his 26 subjects presented with symptoms of amnestic aphasia and verbal paraphasia four months post onset. However, impaired language organization was also a predominant symptom. His subjects had their greatest difficulty with verbal tasks that required them to formulate precise and conscise expressions. Groher (1977) found confused language to be the primary residual four months after onset. At the beginning of the study all subjects presented with anomia as well as other receptive and expressive language deficits. At the end of four months the anomia symptomatology had remitted but test scores were still indicative of reduced expressive and receptive language abilities but not to a degree that prohibited conversational interaction with others. Striking, however, was the finding that the majority of the subjects carried on conversations in which their "thought content was confused, seldom relevant to the discussion and inappropriate in length." Groher concluded that the major post CHI deficit is the discrepancy between the seemingly normal ability to communicate and impaired organizational and retention skills. Halpern, Darley and Brown (1973) also found confused language to be characteristic of CHI patients. They investigated the language characteristics of patients with various neurologic etiologies including head trauma. In addition to the typical areas of language testing the subjects were also measured with respect to "relevance of responses." While all patients in the confused language group manifested some degree of impairment in all areas measured, it was the category of "relevance" that clearly differentiated this group from the other three.

Cognitive impairments have also been found to be a major residual of CHI. Initially the most frequently reported problems were those of inability to sustain concentration and impaired memory (Brock, 1960; Walker, 1969; Hooper, 1969; Russell, 1932; Lewin, 1966; Jacobsen, 1963). The primary memory deficits were seen as retrograde and anterograde or post traumatic amnesia (Russell and Smith, 1961; Brock, 1960; Lewin, 1966). As early as 1932, Russell (1932) suggested that the memory impairment may be a factor underlying the language dysfunction. It appears, however, that the amnesic types of memory loss are not the only memory disturbances caused by CHI. Such patients also experience long term deficits in immediate and recent memory as well (Levin, 1979; Schilder, 1934; Smith, 1974; Jacobsen, 1963; Brooks, 1972).

CHI has also been found to produce other cognitive impairments. Levin's (1979) finding that his subjects were inefficient in filtering extraneous material is suggestive of possible selective attention problems. Miller (1970) interpreted his findings of slower reaction time in relation to task complexity as suggesting a reduced speed of information processing and decision making. Several investigators (Cronholm, 1972; Miller and Stern, 1965; Thomsen, 1975) have found abstract thought to be impaired. The findings of Schilder (1934), Mandleberg (1975) and Omar (1979) may suggest one of the bases of these patients difficulties with abstract thought processes. All found CHI subjects to have particular difficulty with the integration and synthesis of elemental parts of a whole perception.

Taken individually these studies would appear to conflict as to what are the residual language impairments of CHI. The various results would seem to indicate that the language impaired CHI patient is one who regains completely normal language, exhibits symptoms of oral-motor apraxia, has a specific language disorder of an anomic nature, experiences confused language, or retains cognitive deficits in the areas of attention, selective attention, retention span, immediate and long term memory and abstract thought processes. In part the variations in these findings may reflect the focus of each study. Quite possibly the earlier studies would have found residual language disturbances had they carried out specific testing in this area rather than relying solely on behavioral observations. Similarly, as Groher (1977) and Smith (1974) identified coexisting short term memory problems, it may be that a wider range of cognitive problems would have been identified by all investigators who studied the language sequelae of CHI had this been an area of focus of their investigations and, in a similar fashion, those studying cognitive deficits may have found linguistic impairments as well. However, taken as a whole, these various findings may also be indicative of the highly complex and varied neuropathological consequences of CHI. Clearly, CHI does not constitute a homogeneous population from the standpoint of neurophysiological sequelae. It is probable that the variability in both the nature and recovery course of the linguistic and cognitive impairments reported in the previous studies also reflects the neuropathological heterogenity of this population.

The force of a blow to the skull is distributed to all parts of the brain. Thus, all parts of the brain suffer to a greater or lesser degree (Brain, 1969). At the moment of impact the brain accelerates, rotates, compresses and expands within the skull. The dynamics of these motions produce pressure waves within the brain substance (Brain, 1969; Field, 1970; Walker, 1944). All of these factors function to damage cerebral tissue through the dynamics of compression, tension and shearing forces. (Brain, 1969; Greenfield and Russell, 1963; Tomlinson, 1964; Walker 1944) Compression causes the forcing together of tissue. Tension pulls it apart, and shearing, which produces contusions and lacerations, develops at the points where the brain impinges upon bony or ligamentous ridges within the cranial vault. Cerebral edema, which produces increased intracranial pressure, occurs shortly after this mechanical displacement and disruption of the brain substance. (Meyer and Denny-Brown, 1955) In view of the magnitude and multiplicity of these negative forces, Russell (1932) and Adam's (1968) description of the effects of CHI as being a "molecular commotion" would appear quite appropriate. The very molecular structure of the brain is disrupted, disorganized, bruised and/or lacerated. These gross neuropathological effects of CHI have been found to produce permanent microscopic alterations of both white and gray matter. Brain (1969) reports wide scattered punctate hemorrhages throughout the brain. Severe localized demyelination was found by Greenfield (1938) but others (Stritch, 1956; and 1961; Tomlinson, 1964) have reported wide spread white matter degeneration. Nerve cell damage has been reported both by Courville (1953) and Horowitz (1966). Other permanent neurological impairments result from the contusions and lacerations of cortical tissue (Brain, 1969; Courville, 1942).

The variety of the potential neuropathological consequences of CHI suggests that the initial generalized impairment of language/cognitive processes is a manifestation of the massive yet, to a degree, reversible disruption and disorganizaton of neurophysiological activity. The irreversible neurologic damage would, subsequently, produce a potentially wide variety of cognitive/language impairments that would not be expected to remit spontaneously. Typically during the initial phases of recovery most CHI patients not only present with symptoms of specific language impairments, confused language and cognitive disorganization but also the qualitative nature and severity of these sequelae fluctuate drastically and randomly across time. At certain times they may be completely unresponsive though not comatose and at other times one may observe an outpouring of a fluid stream of jargon with localization to sound being the highest level of intact auditory processing. On other occasions they may grasp bits and pieces of what they hear and express themselves in fragmented and disjointed sentences composed of a combination of jargon, neologistic, paraphasic and meaningful words with only portions being relevant to their environment or the specific focus of discussion. These early symptoms are occurring at a time when the neurophysiological activity of cerebral tissue has been temporarily interrupted and is beginning to function again. As the course of recovery continues, the patients may begin to comprehend the general meaning of what has been said and be able to express their thoughts in sentences that are semantically and syntactically complete. However, they fail to convey meaning because their expressions are either irrelevant to the topic, confabulatory, circumlocutious, tangential and/or lacking in a logico-sequential order of related thoughts. During this same time period, other patients may exhibit these characteristics of language disorganization as well as signs of specific deficits in auditory processing, word retrieval, grammatical structure, and/or praxis of speech. Simultaneously all of these oral language symptoms will be observed in the patients reading comprehension and graphic language expression abilities as well. This later phase of language/cognitive impairment represents the potential long term residuals that are secondary to the irreversible structural damage caused by the punctate hemorrhages, cell body changes, demyelination of white matter and localized contusions or lacerations of cortical tissue. While the severity of these impairments often decrease during the first three months of recovery their presence and impact on functional language abilities continues for a considerable length of time.

In a certain sense the initial generalized impairment of language/cognitive processes may be the consequences of disturbances in three very broad cognitive functions: (1) the ability to internally structure one's thought process; (2) the ability to fluidly and rapidly shift cognitive sets in relationship to either internal needs or demands of the external environment and (3) the ability to modify or dampen emotional reactions. Throughout the course of daily cognitive/communicative activities one is called upon to engage in one or any combination of these three general higher cognitive functions. While their implementation may not always require conscious thought, they are not wholly automatic either. It would seem that we must intend to focus these cognitive processes on our inner and external behavioral demands. It is through this intentional focusing that we bring internal order and structure to our rather random, fragmented and fleeting environment. Thus it may be that the cognitive/linguistic symptomatology observed during the initial recovery phases that is related to reversible neurophysiologic processes is related more to the inability to purposefully focus on and manipulate these three functions.

It has been our experience over the past eighteen years with more than 2,500 head trauma patients that three general groups ultimately emerge from the diffuse symptomatology of the initial post CHI phase: (1) those with disorganized language secondary to cognitive disorganization who may or may not have a coexisting specific language disorder; (2) those with the predominant feature of a specific language disorder and coexisting minimal cognitive impairment; and (3) those with attentional, retentional and recent memory impairments but without language dysfunction. The remainder of this paper will focus on the assessment and treatment of those patients who fall into the first category, those whose primary communication disorder is one of language disorganization.

Our approach to assessment is based on several postulates:

(1) In this group of patients, the CHI has permanently weakened or frankly impaired the non-modality specific cognitive processes of: attentional abilities (i.e. attention, attention span and selective attention), discrimination (discerning differences and/or similarities between simultaneously and/or sequentially arriving stimuli), maintaining temporal order of groups of stiumuli, memory abilities (i.e. retention span, immediate, recent and remote memory), categorization and association of stimuli on the basis of their intrinsic properties and part to whole or whole to part integration/synthesis of stiumuli;

(2) The majority of the patient's language impairment is a symptom of the dysfunction of these cognitive processes that support language processing;

(3) While the severity of the cognitive disorganization diminishes during the first several months of recovery, in the majority of cases some or all of these cognitive processes will remain permanently impaired to some degree and, consequently, the patient's receptive/integrative/expressive language abilities will also remain impaired to some degree.

(4) A portion of the cognitive linguistic dysfunction is caused by the impeding or blocking of cognitive/linguistic processes that arise from the inner tension created by the competition between one's innate expectation and desire that language can be processed and used at it always has and the need to consciously find new ways of processing language.

Because of the relationship between cognition and language, it is necessary to assess both the patient's language and cognitive processes. The assessment must also address four general problems that are common to this population. In the early phases of recovery the patients are confused, disoriented and unable to purposefully deal with internal and external stimuli. Consequently, the assessment approach should not be completely dependent upon the ability of a patient to volitionally cooperate in the more typical stimulus-response test taking procedures. Two other characteristics of this population are that they present with extremely diffuse (i.e. phonological, semantic, syntactic and cognitive) language/cognitive impairments and that these impairments fluctuate rapidly and randomly across time. It is not unusual to find that during the first four to eight weeks of recovery, a patient's communication disorder may result from the combined effects of the global temporary interruption of neural activity, the language/cognitive disorganization secondary to irreversible diffuse structural damage and, possibly, a specific language disorder. Predictably the typical language assessment approach that is based on the administration of tests designed to identify categorical areas of language impairment will result in an inconclusive, inaccurate, and/or inappropriate diagnosis, prognosis and treatment plan. As a consequence, the assessment approach should not only employ standardized tests but also provide a means of describing, categorizing and scaling the type and nature of language/cognitive behavior at very frequent intervals. During the later phases of recovery it is not unusual to find that a patient, who is clearly experiencing difficulty with receptive and expressive language in the natural environment, demonstrates minimal to no impairment on our standard aphasia testing instruments. This often occurs not because the patient has attained normal language abilities but because our tests do not directly assess the more subtle levels of language organization. It is entirely possible for a patient to have regained the parts of language (phonology, semantics and syntax) but have considerable difficulty organizing these parts into the whole of an ongoing flow of ideas. Most tests assess only the parts of language. Consequently the patient's ability to organize and use verbal language beyond the level of denoting objects, events, needs and wants must be understood. One must assess the verbal reasoning processes that lie behind the use of language to convey thoughts. In addition to an assessment of all levels of language utilization one will also need information relative to the patient's non-language cognitive abilities of attention, attention span, selective attention, discrimination, temporal ordering, retention span, immediate, recent and remote memory, categorization, associaton, integration and synthesis.

The assessment approach that we have found to be the most helpful consists of four evaluation methods. The categorization and scaling of the patient's spontaneous behavioral responses to randomly occurring environmental stimuli. Scaling their responses to non test stimuli that are purposefully presented and controlled by someone other than the patient (e.g. the daily nursing routine, the general but predictable routine of hospital living, the specific treatment tasks involved in rehabilitation). The administration of a standardized aphasia test battery and supplementing this battery with higher level cognitive and verbal integration, synthesis and reasoning tests. Depending upon the patient's level of functioning at the time of the initial contact, this approach may take the form of sequential assessment steps that parallel the longitudinal course of recovery or, when appropriate, combinations of all four methods are applied simultaneously.

We have found the Levels of Cognitive Functioning (Hagen and Malkmus, 1979) to be quite helpful in the categorizing and scaling of behavioral responses. It consists of eight levels of function with descriptions of general, cognitive and language behaviors that are characteristic of each level. The following is an abbreviated version of the scale.

I. No Response: Patient appears to be in a deep sleep and is completely unresponsive to any stimuli;

II. Generalized Response: Patient reacts inconsistently and non-purposefully to stimuli in a non-specific manner. Responses are limited and often the same regardless of stimulus presented. Responses may be physiological changes, gross body movements and/or vocalization;

III. Localized Response: Patient reacts specifically but inconsistently to stimuli. Responses are directly related to the type of a stimulus presented. May follow simple commands in an inconsistent, delayed manner, such as close eyes, squeeze hand;

IV. Confused-Agitated: Behavior is bizarre and non-purposeful relative to immediate environment. Does not discriminate among persons or objects, is unable to cooperate directly with treatment efforts, verbalizations frequently incoherrent and/or inappropriate to the environment, confabulation may be present. Gross attention to environment is very short and selective attention is often nonexistent. Patient lacks short term recall;

V. Confused, Inappropriate, Non-Agitated: Patient is able to respond to simple commands fairly consistently. However, with increased complexity of commands or lack of any external structure, responses are non-purposeful, random, or fragmented. Has gross attention to the environment, but is highly distractible and lacks ability to focus attention to a specific task; with structure, may be able to converse on a social-automatic level for short periods of time; verbalization is often inappropriate and confabulatory; memory is severely impaired, often shows inappropriate use of objects; may perform previously learned tasks with structure but is unable to learn new information;

VI. Confused-Appropriate: Patient shows goal-directed behavior, but is dependent on external input for direction; follows simple directions consistently and shows carryover for relearned tasks with little or no carryover for new tasks; responses may be incorrect due to memory problems but appropriate to the situation; past memories show more depth and detail than recent memory;

VII. Automatic-Appropriate: Patient appears appropriate and oriented within hospital and home settings, goes through daily routine automatically, but frequently robot-like, with minimal-to-absent confusion, but has shallow recall of activities; shows carryover for new learning, but at a decreased rate; with structure is able to initiate social or recreational activities; judgment remains impaired;

VIII. Purposeful and Appropriate: Patient is able to recall and integrate past and recent events and is aware of and responsive to environment, shows carryover for new learning and needs no supervision once activities are learned; may continue to show a decreased ability, relative to premorbid abilities, in abstract reasoning, tolerance for stress and judgment in emergencies or unusual circumstances.

The identification, categorization and scaling of general behavioral responses such as those in our scale, is not intended to elucidate specific categories of communication disorders. Instead the purpose of this type of evaluation is to establish the presence and pattern of change in such basic neuro-behavioral dichotomies as:

1. Response to external stimuli versus no response.

2. Gross undifferentiated response to stimuli versus differentiated response to stimuli.

3. Differentiated response to stimuli but no continued response after withdrawal of stimuli versus differentiated and sustained response after withdrawal of stimuli.

4. Sustained response to stimuli only if stimuli brought to patient versus sustained response on basis of patient's self-directed behavior.

5. Inappropriate versus appropriate responses to stimuli whether externally presented or self-initiated.

6. Inability to communicate because of cognitive/language dysfunction versus inability to communicate because of severe motor movement dysfunction.

The behavioral responses inherent in Items one through five above represent the manner in which the Levels of Consciousness Scale should be interpreted with respect to levels of information processing. In this regard, Item one represents reception of sensory stimuli versus no reception; Item two represents reception of stimuli but not in relation to specific sensory modalities; Item three represents response to specific sensory modalities and inability to retain it for purposes of processing; Item four represents ability to process information if information is continually presented versus ability to process information on a self-initiated basis; and Item five represents a qualitative evaluation of the patient's behavioral responses on Items two through four. Such a qualitative evaluation would be related to the accuracy, type, and form of a response in relation to a stimulus. The accuracy, type, and form of a response would form the basis upon which one describes the integrity of the patient's cognitive/communicative processes.

Item six is also very important. It represents the necessity of evaluating whether a patient's response or lack of response is related to an information processing breakdown or a motor output breakdown. For example, it is extremely important to distinguish between the patient who is an "akinetic mute" and the patient who is in some stage of coma. The former is, in fact, receiving and processing information but does not appear so because of the lack of motor response, while the latter may be receiving information at some level but not processing it.

We have found that, for patients at and between Levels II and VII, the rating scale is most useful when all disciplines interacting with the patient rate the patient on a daily basis at the time of treatment. It has been our experience that most patients at or above Level II will exhibit a range of behavior. There is usually a preponderance of behavior characteristic of one level and a scatter of behavioral responses both below and above that level. By determining the patient's range one is in a position to identify their most intact cognitive level, which behaviors signal regression in the face of stimuli and which indicate the ability to move to a higher level. It is on the basis of this information that one is able to construct the early phases of a treatment program. A program that presents stimuli in a manner that matches the patients most stable level of functioning as well as slightly challenging the next highest level simultaneously. In this way treatment functions to decrease the behavioral swings below the most intact level and increase the swings above. In time the next highest level becomes the patient's most functional level with a scatter of responses remaining from the previous level but now there is observed the beginning of abilities at the next highest level.

The use of a behavioral scaling technique such as this provides a means of systematically describing and categorizing the patient's level of cognitive/language functioning across time, be it a day, week or month. As such it provides, in the early phases of recovery, a more immediate and sensitive picture of the dynamics of the course of change. This type of assessment has several benefits. Systematic observation and assessment of the type, nature and quality of a patient's behavioral responses assists in estimating the level at which the patient is functioning in the hierarchy of cognitive processes. This information is critical to the determination of the most appropriate cognitive level toward which treatment should be directed. Behavioral scaling is also a means of beginning as early as possible to differentiate between those language impairment characteristics that are secondary to temporary interruption of cognitive/language processes, which reflect potential long term cognitive/language disorganization and those that may indicate the presence of a language disorder secondary to a focal lesion. Clear patterns of change emerge through daily to weekly charting. Through these patterns one is able to more objectively differentiate between the rapidly resolving, and therefore most probably temporary and reversible symptoms and the more slowly resolving and often decelerting language/cognitive symptoms that are characteristic of the diffuse and irreversible damage. Patients in this latter category are those who emerge from the previous global disruption of the phonological, semantic and syntactical bases of language to have language that is virtually intact linguistically yet still manifest expressive and receptive language dysfunction. Expressively such patients demonstrate a persistence of one or a combination of the following characteristics. Language expressions that are inappropriate in relation to a given situation, confabulatory, fragmented and/or incomplete, lacking in a logical sequential relationship to one another, circumlocutious and/or tangential, relevant to part of a stimulus but do not encompass the literal or implied whole concept, relevant only to the implied general concept but lacking in specificity relative to the parts of the concept. Auditory comprehension is observed to be impaired in a similar manner in this group. While they are able to grasp the meaning of specific words and sentence structures, they easily become auditorily confused and therefore experience periodic and random breakdown in their ability to comprehend the complete meaning of a message. The auditory confusion is triggered by such factors as auditory information that requires associative and/or inferential interpretation, auditory information that shifts rapidly from topic to topic and information that is presented rapidly or long in duration.

Behavioral scaling also provides an early means of identifying those patients who may also have a coexisting specific language disorder. The persistence of the more typical aphasic or apraxic characteristics at appreciably the same level of severity suggests the presence of a specific language disorder. In such cases not only will treatment need to be directed toward cognitive/language reorganization but also toward the specific language disorder as well. A third benefit of behavioral scaling is that the patients pattern of change will also generate information relative to the rate and direction of improvement. This provides information upon which one can determine when a patient's treatment program should be modified much closer to the time that such changes are appropriate and necessary.

In our experience a standardized aphasia test battery does not begin to yield useful information until the patient is functioning at Level V or above. Even at this level the still remaining high degree of confusion and disorientation considerably diminishes the validity of test results relative to the identification of specific language disorders. It is important, however, to present patients with stimuli relevant to the various communication skills in a categorical and systematic fashion. The failure of a patient to respond or a response that is completely without form and/or meaning is as significant as a response that fits into a more recognizable speech or language disturbance category. Tests administered to such severely involved patients will generate very important information regarding cerebral functioning under controlled, identifiable, and systematic conditions in contrast to the same patients functioning under free form and random conditions. The delineation of the difference between responses to structured versus unstructured stimulus conditions generates very important baseline data.

When a patient at this level of severity is administered a standardized test, the responses in the various behavior categories (auditory comprehension, auditory retention, visual comprehension, reading, language, speech, visuomotor abilities, and spelling) should be interpreted in relationship to the over-all severity of the patient's communication problem and/or cognitive status rather than in relation to specific stimuli within each category.

For example, the type and quality of responses of a confused and disoriented patient to the auditory disturbance subtests would be interpreted in relation to the ability to focus attention on a task and remember the instructions rather than to the auditory tasks themselves. In essence, the level of diagnosis for this type of patient would be to determine the stimulus conditions under which the patient becomes less confused and more oriented rather than to attempt to determine whether the problem is one of aphasia, apraxia, or an auditory disturbance.

As the patient moves from Level VI towards Level VIII it is not unusual to find that repeat testing indicates minimal to no deficits in all or the majority of categorical language abilities but at the same time observe that the patient is still having considerable difficulty using language to understand and convey the meaning of thoughts. This disparity between apparent linguistic competence on tests and performance in the natural communication environment is typically the result of two factors. First, the temporary disruption of neural activity that produced the global disturbances of language have, by now, remitted almost completely. Since most aphasia tests are oriented primarily toward the assessment of the categorical elements (i.e. phonology, semantic and syntactic) of language they now accurately portray the improvement in these areas of language dysfunction. This does not necessarily mean, however, that the patient has functional language abilities. Our tests do not assess in depth either the organizational structure of expressed discursive thought, the use of language as a verbal reasoning, associative, inferential or metaphorical communication tool or the auditory processing counterpart of these expressive language functions. Thus, it is entirely possible for a patient to do quite well on discrete identification, naming, sentence completion/understanding, and short answer tasks within the structured context of a test yet be unable to organize these very same language processes across time.

In many instances, then, the apparent presence of minimal to no impairment only reflects that the patient has reached the upper limits of that which a particular test was designed to assess. It is the quality of the language behavior, not its presence or absence, that now becomes of diagnostic and treatment significance. One must now evaluate to determine the presence of and differentiate between such language disorganization characteristics as: inappropriate, irrelevant, confabulatory, and fragmented language usage, language expressions that have no logical sequential relationship and/or are circumlocutious, tangential and concrete, as well as the intermittent and random occurrence of auditory confusion that is the receptive counterpart of these expressive characteristics. To accomplish this one must employ additional tests. Usually this becomes necessary when the patient is at Level VII and moving toward and beyond VIII. The following are a number of the tests that we use to assess the higher levels of language integrity: Wechsler Adult Intelligence Scale (WAIS) (1955) information, comprehension, similarities and vocabulary subtests; the Pictorial Absurdities, Verbal Absurdities, Pictorial and Verbal Opposites, Social Adjustment A and B, Free Association, Disarranged Pictures, Likenesses and Differences and Oral Directions Subtests of the Detroit Tests of Learning Aptitude (DTLA) (1959); Goldstein-Scheerer Object Sorting Test (1951); the Auditory and Visual Reception and Association, Auditory Closure and Sound Blending subtests of the Illinois Test of Psycholinguistic Abilities (ITPA) (1968); and Luria's (Christensen, 1975) tests of Understanding Logical Grammatical Structures and Understanding Thematic Pictures and Texts. As will be noted some of these tests were developed for and standardized on a children's population. Our intention in using them, however, is not to derive an age comparable score but rather to present controlled language tasks that provide us with the opportunity to assess the manner in which the patient deals with and responds to them. The assessment value lies in the clinical interpretation of the quality of the response and what that indicates regarding the type and nature of language disorganization.

Assessment of the patient's cognitive abilities should occur concurrently with our evaluation of language processes. The type and nature of the cognitive dysfunction will provide information as to why and how the patient is experiencing a breakdown in language organization. While a patient's level of cognitive functioning is evaluated by the behavioral scaling technique, it usually cannot be directly assessed until the patient reaches Level VII. The following are some of the tests that we use to assess the various cognitive abilities. Attentional, discrimination, temporal sequencing and retention span abilities: Visual Sequential Memory subtest of the ITPA (1968), WAIS (1955) Digit Span Subtest, Auditory Attention Span for Unrelated Words and Related Syllables, Visual Attention Span for Objects and Letters subtests of the DTLA (1959); Developmental Test of Visual Perception (Frostig, 1963); Southern California Figure-Ground Visual Perception Test (Ayres, 1966); Luria's (Christensen, 1975) Tests for Perception and Reproduction of Pitch Relationships and Perception and Reproduction of Rhythmic Structures, and the G-F-W Sound-Symbol Tests (Goldman, Fristoe and Woodcock, 1974) and G-F-W Test of Auditory Discrimination (Goldman, Fristoe and Woodcock, 1970). Immediate and recent memory abilities: Wechsler Memory Scale (Wechsler and Stone, 1945), Digit Symbol subtest of the WAIS (1955), Goldstein-Scheerer Stick Test (1945), Benton Visual Retention Test (1963), Luria's (Christensen, 1975) Mnestic tests, and the Goldman, Fristoe, Woodcock auditory memory tests (1974). Categorization, association, integration and synthesis abilities: Weigl-Goldstein-Scheerer Color Form Sorting Test (1945); Disarranged Pictures subtest of the DTLA (1959) and the Block Design, Object Assembly, Picture Arrangement subtests of the WAIS (1955) and the previously enumerated tests of higher level language organization.

The various cognitive abilities were arbitrarily placed in clusters because of the close interaction between them. However, from th standpoint of actual cognitive processing, there is not only a functional interaction within but between these clusters of cognitive abilities. Consequently one must remember that it is the interpretation of the pattern of deficits that leads to the determination of cognitive/language dysfunction not the score on specific tests. For example, one could not infer the presence of a problem with categorization, association and synthesis if a patient exhibits severe impairments of attentional and memory abilities even though the patient did very poorly on tests related to those higher level skills Here, one is undoubtedly observing a cause-effect relationship rather than areas of discrete impairment.

Finally, it has been our experience that the interpretation of the quality and pattern of both language and cognitive organization impairments is considerably aided by gathering information relative to factors that are not implicit in the tests themselves. Specifically, it is important to assess and identify the manner in which the patient approaches a given problem. We have found that each patient has an optimal and stable level of performance in relationship to the rate, amount, duration and complexity of stimulus input. Variations either above or below their optimal level of receiving and processing stimuli act to intensify their already impaired ability to remain organized. With respect to the patient's problem solving approach we have found it helpful to watch for the following characteristics: immediate recognition of solution, studies task before attempting solution, organized and systematic, impulsive or trial and error approach, develops alternate strategies when unsuccessful, overattendance to details, must be prompted to start as well as continue task, perseveration of approach across tasks, benefits from cues and correction, independently carries cues or corrections over to the next task. Information relative to the optimal manner of stimulus presentation as well as the patient's problem solving approach is critical diagnostic information. The behavioral rating scale and the tests yield information that tells us what the level of the problem is and what should and should not be treated. Knowledge about stimulus presentation and task approach tells how to treat the problem.

Our treatment approach is based upon the following postulates:

1. Treatment should be directed toward the reorganization of the cognitive processes rather than attempting to modify the abnormal language consequences of the cognitive disorganization.

2. As cognitive processes become reorganized there will be a commensurate reorganization of phonological, semantic, syntactic and verbal reasoning abilities.

3. The reorganization of cognitive abilities follows a predictable and systematic hierarchial sequence in which the reacquisition and stabilization of lower level processes is necessary to the emergence and stabilization of higher level activities.

4. Cognitive structure is maximized and behavioral responses become more organized when the treatment program progresses sequentially from the patient's highest level of cognitive abilities through all of the necessary steps subsequent to that level.

5. Treatment stimuli should be presented through the patient's

single most intact sensory modality and increased to other modalities only as increasing cognitive abilities support the ability to deal with multiple stimuli.

6. Regardless of the level of cognitive abilities toward which treatment is directed, the manner of stimulus input is critical to the elicitation of structured and appropriate behavioral responses. Consequently, one must manipulate the rate, amount, duration and complexity of stimulus input in a manner that is consistent with the patient's cognitive abilities at any given time.

The goal of treatment is to cause the patient to learn how to consciously process language stimuli in an orderly sequential manner. To this end the Speech-Language Pathologist uses treatment tasks that are specifically designed to cause the patient to: 1) Attend to the stimulus (attention); 2) Attend for a sufficient length of time to grasp its form and quality (attention span); 3) Suppress irrelevant stimuli (selective attention); 4) Recognize the differences between stimuli (discrimination); 5) Analyze groups of stimuli and determine the whole on the basis of the parts (temporal ordering, retention span, categorization); 6) Relate this information to past learned similar information (association/memory); 7) Associate and integrate this information with information from other areas of stimulus analysis (association/integration/memory); 8) Determine the most appropriate sequence of behavioral events by analyzing and synthesizing information derived from 6 and 7 above (analysis/synthesis/memory); 9) Transmit the sequence; 10) Attend to the output; 11) Compare the actual output with the intended output; 12) Determine if change is necessary; and 13) if necessary, produce modified response.

Depending upon their level of severity, some patients must begin at the level of first stabilizing attending abilities and sequentially working their way through each subsequent cognitive skill. Others may already possess a number of the lower level abilities. Consequently, their treatment begins at a higher level and progresses sequentially from that point. Still others may exhibit marginally functional abilities at all of these levels but they rapidly disintegrate under stress. Accordingly, for some this treatment process is carried out as a series of separate goals over a period of months. For others the progression through these thirteen steps occurs within a given treatment session while for others the goal may be to cause the patient to consciously apply the steps as a strategy for dealing with and solving a treatment task or possibly a discrete stimulus within a task. However, we have found that for those patients whose lower level cognitive skills (e.g. attentional, discrimination, temporal ordering, categorization) are functional, it is still necessary to present them with treatment tasks that cause them to consciously begin with attending abilities and progress to the level that is the focus of treatment. If treatment commences only at the level of deficit, the patient often experiences a weakening of the lower level skills because of the increased cognitive demands. Under such conditions the patient then rapidly has two cognitive tasks. They must try and deal with the original stimulus and simultaneously attempt to maintain the weakening subskills. Be beginning with the lower level skills the patient is provided with the external structure that will be necessary to deal with the tasks that are at the level of dysfunction. Even though treatment focuses on a particular cognitive function all functions are strengthened when the patient deals with the level of treatment focus. While the various cognitive abilities are displayed here in a manner suggestive of a hierarchical process this does not appear to be the way in which they function. On the contrary there seems to be a simultaneity of functioning of all processes. It is this simultaneity of functioning that provides the cognitive gestalt necessary to the processing of language data as a gestalt. Thus the purpose of focusing treatment on one area of cognitive function is not simply to strengthen that one function but also to assist the patient to be able to organize all of the other cognitive processes.

The therapeutic value of this approach does not lie in either the shear process of repetitively proceeding through these steps, though mass practice is extremely necessary, or in the stimuli that are used to elicit a response nor does it lie in the response itself. These three factors are simply the mediums through which the patient is taught cognitive strategies for processing language information. The general strategy is that they now must do something consciously that their brain previously did automatically. The secondary strategies arise from the concept that they must learn to evaluate their cognitive/language behavior in any given situation and consciously determine at what point in this hierarchy of thirteen steps they are experiencing a breakdown and then focus their attention on consciously manipulating the information through that particular stage. Within this context treatment tasks are oriented both towards strengthening weakened abilities and learning compensatory mechanisms. Treatment for any of these cognitive abilities must first be directed toward increasing the power of the ability and then, once power is established, and award increasing the quality of the skill. Power is improved by increasing the rate, amount and duration of stimulus input that a patient can handle while holding complexity constant. Quality of ability is enhanced by increasing complexity while holding rate, amount and duration constant. In that communication occurs to and from the patient in all treatment and non-treatment environments during rehabilitation, it is essential that this treatment strategy and approach be extended to all interactions that occur with the patient. For this reason the patient's communicative/cognitive rehabilitation program will be vastly strengthened if all rehabilitation team members approach the patient in a similar manner. While the tasks a patient is asked to perform will vary in accordance to the specific goals of each discipline it will be critical for all to be presenting the tasks and encouraging responses in a manner that appeals to the same level of cognitive abilities.

Several stimulus presentation parameters are critical to the success of treatment regardless of the level of cognitive/linguistic processing that is being treated. Using information from the previously described assessment approaches one should present stimuli at the rate, amount, duration and complexity that matches that which has been identified as a given patients optimal level of information processing. The task solutions should not require a higher level of problem solving that identified as the patient's most current problem solving approach. Treatment tasks should initially require non-verbal cognitive skills and move toward their linquistic counterparts when the patient demonstrates proficiency at the nonverbal level.

For example, the ability to attend and selectively attend to non-linguistic stimuli should exist or be fairly stable prior to presenting tasks such as identifying embedded target words presented auditorily or graphically; tasks that elicit the ability to categorize on the base of size, shape, weight, texture, etc. should be presented prior to the categorization of linguistic concepts, or tasks that require non-linguistic analysis and synthesis such as block designs should be presented prior to tasks that require the patient to synthesize part-whole language concepts such as occurs in story telling.

Treatment tasks should be presented in a manner that appeals to a sequence of analysis and response modalities rather than to all modalities simultaneously. We have found the following sequence quite helpful: tasks that are visual-visual (e.g. pointing to pictures that are like or similar to stimulus pictures), visual-motor (e.g. tracing, copying or supplying missing parts of visual stimulus), visual-auditory (e.g. identifying visual response to auditory stimulus), auditory-motor (e.g. producing a motor response to an auditory stimulus); and auditory-verbal (e.g. a verbal response to auditory stimulus).

As with the manner in which one progresses through the thirteen cognitive processes, a given patient's movement from non-linguistic to linguistic tasks and visual-visual to auditory-verbal analysis and response modalities will be dependent upon the severity of the dysfunction. For some these treatment parameters will represent the various sequential steps over a period of months while others will progress through them within a given treatment session or treatment task. The treatment value does not exist in the stimulus per se but rather in the clinician gradually increasing the patient's ability to handle higher and higher levels of rate, amount, duration and complexity of stimulus processing, more flexible problem solving approaches and therefore greater linguistic complexity. Treatment functions to challenge and channel spontaneous recovery, maximize residual function and compensate for lost abilities. It has been our experience that the critical therapeutic factor in all three of these language rehabilitation phases is the maintenance of the critical balance between the patient's most functional level of cognitive functioning and the type and manner of stimulus input. When the balance is maintained, the patient is able to process internal and/or external stimuli in the most organized manner and consequently utilize language processes at a more organized level. Clearly not all patients hold the prognosis that allows them to benefit from treatment. The severity of the brain damage, length of coma, age when injury occurred and pre-existing psychosocial problems all impact on the prognosis for the attainment of a high level of function. The greatest deterent to progress for those who hold a good prognosis is a treatment program that requires a higher level of cognitive functioning than the patient is capable of producing, appeals to all sense modalities simultaneously, is at a rate, frequency, amount, duration and complexity that is either too high or too low and attempts to elicit and modify language before the lower level cognitive abilities necessary to support it have been stablized. Treatment is a process of first stabilizing the most functional level and then gradually challenging abilities at the next highest level. At the outset the Speech-Language Pathologist creates the balance but ultimately this is what the patient learns.

## REFERENCES

Adams, R. and Sidmann, R.L. Introduction to neurophathology. New York: The Blakeston Division, McGraw-Hill Book Co., 1968.

Arseni, C., Constantinovici, A. and Iliesca, D. Considerations on post traumatic aphasia in peace time. Psychitria, Neurologia, Neurochirurgica, 1970, 73, 105-112.

Ayres, A.J. Southern California Figure-Ground Visual Perception Test, Los Angeles: Western Psychological Services, 1966.

Baker, H.J. and Leland, B. Detroit Test of Learning Aptitude, Indianapolis: Bobbs-Merrill, 1959.

Benton, A.L. The Revised Visual Retention Test, New York: The Psychological Corporation, 1963.

Brain, L. and Walton, J.N. Brain's diseases of the nervous system, 7th edition. New York: Oxford University Press, 1969.

Brock, S. Injuries of brain and spinal cord, 4th edition. New York: Springer Publishing Company, 1960.

Brooks, D.N. Memory and head injury. Journal of Nervous and Mental Disease, 1972, 155, 350-355.

Caveness, W.F. Introduction to head injuries. In Walker, E., Caveness, W., and Cutchley, M. (Eds.), The late effects of head injury. Springfield: Charles C. Thomas, 1969.

Christensen, A.L. Luria's neuropsychological investigation. New York: Spectrum, 1975.
Courville, C.B. Coup, contre-coup mechanisms of craniocerebral injuries: Some observations. Archives of Surgery, 1942, 45, 19-43.
Courville, C.B. and Amyes, E.W. Late residual lesions of the brain consequent to dural hemmorrhage. Bulletin Los Angeles Neurology Society, 1952, 17, 163.
Cronholm, B. Evaluation of mental disturbances after acute head injury. Scandinavian Journal of Rehabilitation Medicine. 1972, 4, 35-38.
Dye, O.A., Milby, J.B., and Saxon, S.A. Effects of early neurological problems following head trauma on subsequent neuropsychological performance. Acta Neurologic Scandinavia, 1979, 59, 10-14.
Fahy, T.J., Irving, M.H., and Millac, P. Severe head injuries. Lancet, 1967, 7514.
Field, J.R. Head injuries pathophysiology. Journal of the Arkansas Medical Association. 1970, 66, 340-347.
Frostig, M. Developmental Test of Visual Perception. Chicago: Follett, 1963.
Glasser, M.A. and Shafer, F.P. Skull and brain traumas: Their sequalae: Clinical review of 255 cases. Journal of American Medical Association, 1932, 98, 271-276.
Goldman, R., Fristoe, M. and Woodcock, R.W. G-F-W Sound Symbol Tests. Circle Pines: American Guidance Service, 1974.
Goldman, R., Fristoe, M. and Woodcock, R.W. G-F-W Auditory Memory Tests. Circle Pines: American Guidance Service, 1974.
Goldman, R., Fristoe, M. and Woodcock, R.W. G-F-W Test of Auditory Discrimination. Circle Pines: American Guidance Service, 1970.
Goldstein, K. and Scheerer, M. Goldstein-Scheerer Object Sorting Test. New York: The Psychological Corporation, 1951.
Goldstein, K. and Scheerer, M. Goldstein-Scheerer Stick Test. New York: The Psychological Corporation, 1945.
Greenfield, J.G. Some observations on cerebral injuries. Procedings Royal Society of Medicine, 1938-39, 32, 45.
Greenfield, J.G. and Russell, D.S. Traumatic lesions of the central and peripheral nervous systems. In Blackwood, W. (Ed.), Greenfield's neuropathology. Chicago: Year Book, 1963.
Groher, M. Language and memory disorders following closed head trauma. Journal of Speech and Hearing Research, 1977, 20, 212-223.
Hagen, C. and Malkmus, D. Intervention strategies for language disorders secondary to head trauma. American Speech-Language-Hearing Association Convention Short Course, Atlanta: 1979.
Halpern, H., Darley, F.L. and Brown, J.R. Differential language and neurologic characteristics in cerebral involvement. Journal Speech and Hearing Disorders, 1973, 38, 162-173.
Heilman, K.M., Safron, A. and Geschwind, N. Closed head trauma and aphasia. Journal of Neurology, Neurosurgery and Psychiatry, 1971, 34, 265-269.
Hooper, R. Patterns of acute head injury. Baltimore: Williams and Wilkins, 1969.

Horowitz, N. and Rizzoli, H.V. Complications following the surgical treatment of head injuries, Clinical Neurosurgery. Proceedings of the Congress of Neurological Surgeons, 1966, 277-287.

Jacobsen, S.A. The post traumatic syndrome following head injuries - Mechanisms and techniques. Springfield: Charles C. Thomas, 1963.

Kirk, S.A., McCarthy, and Kirk, W.D. Illinois Test Psycholinguistic Abilities. University of Illinois, 1968.

Levin, H.S., Grossman, R.G., Rose, J.E. and Teasdale, J. Long term neuropsychological outcome of closed head injury. Journal of Neurosurgery, 1979, 50, 412-422.

Lewin, W. The management of head injuries. Baltimore: Williams and Wilkins, 1966.

Mandleberg, I.A. and Brooks, D.N. Cognitive recovery after severe head injury. Journal of Neurology, Neurosurgery and Psychiatry, 1975, 38, 1121-1126.

Meyer, J.S., and Denny-Brown, D. Studies of cerebral circulation in brain injury. II. Cerebral concussion. Neurophysiology, 1955, 7, 529-544.

Miller, E. Simple and choice reaction time following severe head injury. Cortex, 1970, 6, 121-127.

Miller, H. and Stern, G. The long term prognosis of severe head injury. Lancet, 1965, 225-229.

Russell, R.W. Cerebral involvement in head injury. Brain, 1932, 55, 549-603.

Russell, W.R. and Smith, A. Post-traumatic amnesia in closed head injury. Archives of Neurology, 1961, 5, 4-17.

Schilder, P. Psychic disturbance after head injuries. American Journal of Psychiatry, 1934, 91, 155-188.

Smith, E. Influence of site of impact on cognitive impairment persisting long after severe closed head injury. Journal of Neurology, Neurosurgery and Psychiatry, 1974, 37, 719-726.

Strick, S.J. Diffuse degeneration of the cerebral white matter in severe dementia following head injury. Journal of Neurology and Psychiatry. 1956, 19, 163.

Thomsen, I.V. Evaluation and outcome of aphasia in patients with severe closed head trauma. Journal of Neurology, Neurosurgery and Psychiatry. 1975, 38, 713-718.

Tomlinson, B.E. Pathology. In Rawbothm, G.F. (Ed.), Acute injuries of the head, 4th Edition. Edinburgh, 1964.

Walker, A.E., Kabros, J.J. and Case, T.J. The physiological basis of concussion. Journal of Neurosurgery, 1944, 1, 103-116

Walker, E., Caveness, W. and Critchley, M. (Eds.) The late effects of head injury. Illinois: Charles C. Thomas, 1969.

Wechsler, D. Wechsler Adult Intelligence Scale. New York: The Psychological Corporation, 1955.

Wechsler, D. and Stone, C.P. Wechsler Memory Scale. New York: The Psychological Corporation, 1945.

Weigl, E., Goldstein, K. and Scheerer, M. Color Form Sorting Test. New York: The Psychological Corporation, 1945.

# COGNITIVE PERCEPTUAL MOTOR EVALUATION RESEARCH FINDINGS FOR ADULT HEAD INJURIES[1]

Diane L. Meeder, OTR, Clinical Supervisor

Occupational Therapy Neurology Services

Santa Clara Valley Medical Center

## INTRODUCTION

Historically, the early Greek view of the mind was simply that the mind is an organ that dealt with pure ideas. Plato in his time denied that it had anything to do with sensation, and Aristotle felt the mind was governed by the psychic powers, associated with motion and sensation, believing the physical seat of mental life to be in the heart and not the brain (Wilson, 1964). In the eighteenth century, the theory of the phrenologists became popular when Franz Joseph Gall, a Viennese physiologist assumed that the bumps on man's skull represented the parts of his brain that were well-developed (Wilson, 1964). He divided the brain into thirty-seven areas, identifying each as a personality trait such as "self-esteem or gaiety."

More recently, localization theory and right and left hemispheric dominance or specialization have been studied. The neural representation of behavioral functions cannot be ascribed to localized to discrete areas of the central nervous system (Luria, 1973). For example, the right and left hemispheric advantage theory, representing a refinement of hemispheric specialization, suggests that cerebral hemispheric functioning is systematically integrated, with one having an advantage over the other for certain functions (Moore, 1981). The left hemisphere can be considered to be more specifically localized and the right more holistic and integrative in function. Substantial research suggests that the role of the lower central

[1]This study was supported in part by Research Grant #RSA 13-p-5956-9-03 from the National Institute for Handicapped Research, Department of Education, Washington, D.C., 20202.

nervous system in perception and cognition cannot be underestimated. For example, the reticular activating system promotes general attention and alertness and performs functions that are central to adaptive or perceptive processes. Recent memory, linked to, in part, hippocampal functions can further be considered to play a critical role in those cognitive processes which relate to perceptual motor skills.

Most of the early work concerning perception and cognition was done in relation to the infant and child. As a result, many of the evaluations done initially to test the perceptual status of the adult cerebrovascular accident (CVA) patient were adapted from tests designed for use with children. In the past ten years there has been an attempt in the field of Occupational Therapy to eliminate the use of tests designed for children and to develop test batteries specifically for adult populations. Compounding this problem are the recent advances in the management of head injury, thus adding the need for the establishment of assessment and treatment tools specific to the adult head injury individual, separate from the stroke victim.

It is necessary to define the adult head injury individual on dimensions and evaluation strategies separate and unique from (although related to developmental acquisition) instruments already being used for the CVA patient. Occupational Therapy test batteries need to have established adult norms separate from those assessments used with stroke patients or children with learning disabilities. More importantly, normal recovery trends for head injury need to be studied and charted in order to get a clearer picture of what deficits are encountered and at what stages they might resolve. An attempt has been made in this study to establish what cognitive perceptual motor problems do in fact exist in adults with head trauma and to establish what the phases of recovery for these functions appear to be.

Cognitive perceptual motor skills involve the integration of sensory, motor, perceptual and cognitive modalities into a meaningful mode to create successful interactions with the environment. Perceptual motor skills should be considered as building blocks or significant components of cognition. It is important to consider the relationship between perceptual motor and cognitive functions. A perceptual motor skill can be generally described as "the ability to receive, integrate, and organize sensory stimuli in a manner which allows for the planning of purposeful movement" (Mosey, 1973). A cognitive skill as defined by this latter investigator is "the ability to perceive, represent, and organize objects, events, and their relationships in a manner which is considered appropriate by one's cultural group." As a result of a federal research grant given to Santa Clara Valley Medical Center (SCVMC) in San Jose, California by the National Institute for Handicapped Research, the Occupational Therapy Division has been studying the effects of head trauma for the past four years. The research herein described was conducted in a large rehabilitation center where there is a fifteen bed in-patient head injury unit. In addition, SCVMC has an acute neurosurgery service where acute head trauma patients are seen. After discharge the patients are re-assessed at regular intervals, as long as ten years post injury. Many of the cognitive perceptual motor (CPM) evaluation tools that the Occupational Therapy Department now uses were developed for the Head Injury Grant Project in order to systematize data collection and establish more objective baselines for measuring recovery trends. The findings in this paper are preliminary in nature as the final research analysis and project report are currently, at the time the present manuscript was composed, in preparation (Cope, 1981).

There have been many attempts to classify the consequences of head injury. The levels of consciousness evaluated in the standard neurological examination exemplifies one such attempt (Gilroy and Meyer, 1969). The Glasgow Coma Scale (Teasdale and Jennett, 1974) and the eight levels of awareness used by Rancho Los Amigos Hospital (Rancho Los Amigos Hospital Head Trauma Rehabilitation Seminar, 1977) are well known methods for attempting to evaluate and categorize behavioral sequelae of head injury. Given that head injury is a complex disability where not only the mechanism of trauma, but the resulting disability may vary considerably, an attempt was made by the Occupational Therapy division at SCVMC to define head injury in more general terms.

## Definition of Primary and Advanced Head Injury Patients

The term primary was used on the head injury unit at SCVMC to describe the patient who was functioning at a more basic or low level. This definition may be used when the patient evidenced any one or a combination of the following sequelae (Baum and Meeder, 1981):

(1) Severe motor impairment. The patient was generally dependent due to severe spasticity, abnormal reflexes, or loss of motor control.

(2) Severe Impairment of Perceptual Motor Skills. The patient may have had very poor gross visual skills or other perceptual motor skills which prevented him from being involved in self care or higher level functional activities.

(3) Decreased Functional Cognition and Behavior. The patient had cognitive/behavioral deficits and may have had extremely poor judgment, decreased safety awareness, problem solving and memory impairment resulting in dependency for functional tasks even though physically he may have been intact.

Generally, the primary patient is very dependent or requires maximum assistance, either physically, cognitively, perceptually, or for all three domains. A person may have severe motor involvement with cognitive perceptual abilities intact. This is very frustrating for the primary patient with severe motor deficits because he is "locked in" to his limited bodily functioning and cannot communicate nor control any aspect of his environment. On the other hand, the person who has severe cognitive perceptual deficits, but who has good motor skills (for example is able to ambulate) may still be considered a primary patient because he cannot perform self care activities nor function safely without verbal cues and constant supervision. Memory may be so impaired that the patient shows limited generalization from therapy. This patient is often referred to as the "walking wounded," having good motor function, but poor cognitive abilities.

The term <u>advanced</u> was applied to the head injury patient who may have had cognitive, perceptual, motor, and behavioral deficits, although they were not sufficiently significant so as to cause total dependence in activities of daily living. The occupational therapist must be able to relate the neurophysiological problems to the functional impairment at this stage. The advanced patient, unlike the primary patient, has the potential to make an adaptive response and achieve some generalization of learning in therapy toward achieving a functional, and not just a pre-functional goal. The advanced patient's overall level of awareness is higher and he has a better ability to control more aspects of himself and his environment. (Baum and Meeder, 1981).

The use of terms like advanced and primary are admittedly not descriptively precise, but rather provide a global index of impairment status. A given patient does not, obviously, spontaneously go from a primary to advanced status, but rather typically progresses gradually. It was the specific intent of the present research to describe that progression in terms of cognitive perceptual motor variables.

## METHODOLOGY

### <u>Subjects</u>

A total of 61 subjects were included for study. These 61 head injury subjects were evaluated with CPM evaluation measures two, four six and twelve months post-injury. The patient population was divided into three groups based on their scores derived from the Glasgow Coma Scale (Teasdale and Jennett, 1974). These three groups were then compared, at the four post-injury intervals, on measures of cognitive perceptual motor skills. The coma classification can be summarized as follows:

| Length of Coma | N | Range |
|---|---|---|
| ≤ 7 days | 15 | 1-7 Days |
| 8 - 31 | 27 | 9-30 |
| < 31 | 19 | 33-225 |

The following summative data describes these patient's demographic and diagnostic characteristics:

| Age | |
|---|---|
| 15-20 years | 35.5% |
| 21-25 years | 26.3% |
| 26-30 years | 5.3% |
| 31-35 years | 13.1% |
| 36-40 years | 7.9% |
| 41-45 years | 2.6% |
| 46-50 years | 2.6% |
| 51-55 years | 3.9% |
| 56-60 years | 2.8% |

| Sex |
|---|
| Female 29% |
| Male 71% |

| Cause of Injury | |
|---|---|
| Auto | 53.3% |
| Diving | 0 |
| Motorcycle | 14.3% |
| Sports | 4.9% |
| Work | 2.6% |
| Home | 1.4% |
| Pedestrian | 7.9% |
| GSW | 2.6% |
| Altercation | 6.5% |
| Other | 6.5% |

| CAT Scan Results | |
|---|---|
| Normal | 23% |
| Left hemisphere | 13% |
| Right hemisphere | 18% |
| Bilateral hemisphere | 34% |
| Not done | 12% |

| Glasgow Outcome Scale at Time of Admission | |
|---|---|
| PVS | 11% |
| Severe | 67% |
| Moderate | 16% |
| Mild | 0 |
| Unknown | 6% |

Premorbid Learning Disability 8%

| Education | | | |
|---|---|---|---|
| High School or less | 30% | Post Graduate | 4% |
| High School | 19% | Technical/Trade | 10% |
| Some College | 19% | Unknown | 15% |
| College Graduate | 7% | | |

Time From Date of Injury to Rehab Admission

| | |
|---|---|
| 0-21 days | 12% |
| 22-60 days | 34% |
| 61-120 days | 29% |
| 121-180 days | 15% |
| more than 181 | 10% |

## The Cognitive Perceptual Motor Evaluation

Many components of the cognitive perceptual motor (CPM) evaluation used by the Occupational Therapy Division at SCVMC evolved from the Hemiplegic Evaluation used at Massachusetts Rehabilitation Hospital in Boston (Wall, 1979). Recently, the Occupational Therapy Department at SCVMC did a major revision of their CPM evaluation protocol with plans for publication in progress.

Both the qualitative and the quantitative aspects of assessment must be comined in the evaluation of the neurologically impaired adult. The qualitative aspect uses observations of behavior in an analytical, descriptive and more subjective fashion. Traditionally, in the past, Occupational Therapists have used qualitative assessment, which states the given problems a patient might have, but is difficult to measure over time in a more formal manner. Quantitative assessment, which the CPM evaluation incorporates, is more numerical and statistical utilizing scores to measure behavior over time. It allows for a more objective comparison of the patient's progress, and through statistical analysis can allow for the comparison of the relationship between test variables. On the other hand, no matter how much the evaluator quantifies a test, qualitative observations are still essential. The CPM evaluation used by Occupational Therapy includes in the protocol: a) procedures for administering the test, b) verbal directions to be given to the patient, c) observation guidelines, and d) methods for scoring.

The cognitive perceptual motor evaluation utilized at SCVMC can be outlined as follows:

Gross Visual Skills

Visual Attentiveness
Ocular Pursuit
Homonymous hemianopsia
Visual-spatial neglect
Line Bisection

Praxis (Motor Planning)

Simple Praxis
Graphic Praxis
Two dimensional constructional praxis
Three dimensional constructional praxis

Body Scheme

Draw-A-Person Test
Body parts identification
Right-left discrimination
Body puzzle
Face puzzle

Depth Perception

Blocks
Wands
Skiing picture

Form Perception

Simple formboard
Parquetry design

Size Discrimination

Graded cylinders

Part-Whole Discrimination

Hooper Visual Organization Test

Spatial Perception

Ayres Position-in-Space Test

Visual Figure Ground Perception

Ayres Figure Ground Test
Frostig Figure Ground Test
Functional Figure Ground Test

The present study includes data derived from only measures of visual attentiveness, ocular pursuit, graphic praxis, figure ground perception, position-in-space perception and depth perception.

RESULTS

It should be noted that the group used at each time interval was not the same group of 15, 27, or 19 patients (as determined by length of time) coma, but rather a mean score for all patients at the four time epochs of two, four, six, and twelve months post-injury. For the most part, the patients constitute the same group. However, not all of the patients may have been testable at any given time period due to medical complications or transfer to another facility. The data presented in the present chapter are preliminary findings and do not reflect the final conclusions of the Head Injury Project.

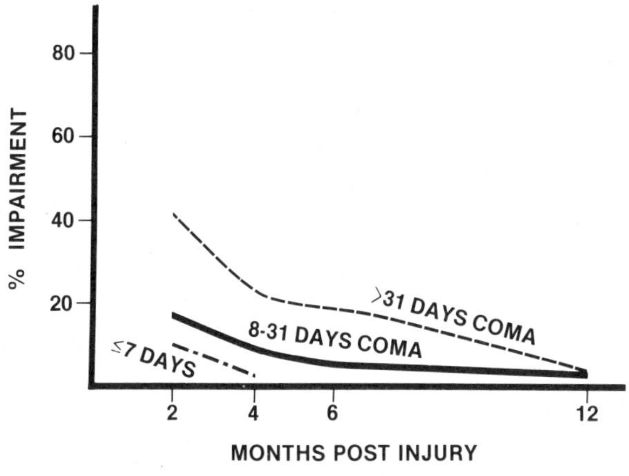


Figure 1. Visual Attentiveness

Table 1. Statistical Comparisons (t-tests) at 1 Year Post-Injury

| Variable | Short vs. Long | | Moderate vs. Long | |
|---|---|---|---|---|
| | t | p | t | p |
| Visual Attentiveness | 1.282 | n.s. | .373 | n.s. |
| Ocular Pursuits | 2.646 | .05 | 1.660 | n.s. |
| $\bar{X}$ Graphic Praxis | 2.000 | n.s. | 2.000 | .05 |
| Depth Perception | 1.520 | n.s. | 1.520 | n.s. |
| $\bar{X}$ Position-in-Space | 1.770 | n.s. | 2.251 | .05 |
| $\bar{X}$ Figure Ground | 2.730 | .05 | 2.510 | .05 |

## Visual Attentiveness

The first component of the evaluation concerned the evaluation of visual skills which included the five subtests previously listed. The first skill to be assessed was visual attentiveness which can be considered to represent one of the skills that lays the groundwork for the higher level CPM skills. Visual attentiveness was formally assessed using a 0-2 scale with 0 always representing an intact or no impairment status. The data presented in Figure 1 illustrates the recovery trends for visual attentiveness for the three groups, the composition of which was determined by the length of coma.

Table 2. Linear Regression Analysis Cognitive Perceptual Motor Variables

| | Months to Baseline in Rank Order | | | |
|---|---|---|---|---|
| Variable | $\bar{X}$ All Patients | ≤7 Days Coma | 8-31 Days Coma | >31 Days Coma |
| Visual Attentiveness | 11.3 mos. | 9.52 | 11.91 | 12.47 |
| Depth Perception | 13.14 | 9.50 | 11.59 | 18.34 |
| Form Perception | 13.29 | 10.35 | 11.03 | 18.50 |
| Body Scheme | 13.55 | 10.67 | 11.07 | 18.91 |
| $\bar{X}$ Praxis | 13.84 | 9.50 | 11.36 | 20.66 |
| Graphic Praxis | 14.0 | 9.95 | 11.44 | 20.61 |
| 2-D Praxis | 14.34 | 10.82 | 12.99 | 19.21 |
| Ocular Pursuits | 14.52 | 10.94 | 14.77 | 17.87 |
| 3-D Praxis | 14.65 | 10.88 | 14.78 | 18.29 |
| Size Discrimination | 15.42 | 10.58 | 11.13 | 24.56 |
| 3-D Spatial | 13.26 | 9.68 | 11.32 | 18.79 |
| Frostig Position-in-Space | 15.92 | 11.23 | 12.99 | 23.54 |
| Ayres Position-in-Space | 16.38 | 11.46 | 13.75 | 23.94 |
| $\bar{X}$ Position-in-Space | $\bar{X}$ 15.18 | | | |
| Frostig Figure-Ground | 12.49 | 10.27 | 10.69 | 16.51 |
| Functional | 13.65 | 10.11 | 11.15 | 19.71 |
| Ayres Figure-Ground | 26.75 | 9.89 | 13.25 | 57.12 |
| $\bar{X}$ Figure-Ground | $\bar{X}$ 17.63 | | | |

Table 3. Pearson r Correlation Comparison of CPM Variables at 2 months post injury.

| 2 Mo. Data r & p's Pearson r Correlation | | Visual Attentiveness | Ocular Pursuits | Graphic Praxis | Depth Perception | Ayres F.G. | Frostig F.G. | Func'l F.G. | Ayres PIS | Frostig PIS | 3-D |
|---|---|---|---|---|---|---|---|---|---|---|---|
| Visual Attentive-ness | r | | | | | | | | | | |
| | p | | | | | | | | | | |
| Ocular Pursuits | r | .6008 | | | | | | | | | |
| | p | .01 | | | | | | | | | |
| Graphic Praxis | r | .5408 | .2186 | | | | | | | | |
| | p | .01 | N.S. | | | | | | | | |
| Depth | r | .6480 | .4002 | .9741 | | | | | | | |
| | p | .01 | N.S. | .01 | | | | | | | |
| Ayres Fig-Grd | r | .4945 | .4532 | .7636 | .7409 | | | | | | |
| | p | .01 | .05 | .01 | .01 | | | | | | |
| Frostig Fig-Grd | r | .6322 | .3834 | .8144 | .8068 | .8672 | | | | | |
| | p | .01 | N.S. | .01 | .01 | .01 | | | | | |
| Func'l Fig-Grd | r | .6027 | .4451 | .9516 | .9660 | .7519 | .8066 | | | | |
| | p | .01 | .05 | .01 | .01 | .01 | .01 | | | | |
| Ayres PIS | r | .4519 | .3335 | .6974 | .8685 | .7283 | .7301 | .7872 | | | |
| | p | .01 | N.S. | .01 | .01 | .01 | .01 | .01 | | | |
| Frostig PIS | r | .5977 | .3773 | .7434 | .9157 | .7343 | .8513 | .8243 | .9358 | | |
| | p | .01 | .05 | .01 | .01 | .01 | .01 | .01 | .01 | | |
| 3-D | r | .5776 | .4545 | .9575 | .9512 | .8828 | .8181 | .9702 | .8920 | .8207 | |
| | p | .01 | .05 | .01 | .01 | .01 | .01 | .01 | .01 | .01 | |

As one can see from Figure 1, the group which had the shortest length of coma appears to intercept baseline or zero impairment at around four months post injury, the 8-31 day group at approximately six months post-injury, and the greater than 31 day coma group at around twelve months post-injury. Statistical comparisons of the differences in mean scores for visual attentiveness at one year in the short versus long coma, and the moderate versus long coma, were not significant (see Table 1). A regression analysis was done (see Table 2), and it was found that visual attentiveness was one of the earliest skills to "return" in adults with head injury, crossing baseline at 11.9 months in the 8-31 moderate coma group. The absence of a statistically significant difference between coma groups at one year for visual attentiveness may be secondary to the early "recovery" of this function. Correlational analyses (see Table 3) suggested that visual attentiveness correlated with all other CPM skills at the $p < .01$ level of significance. These results may indicate that the scores on these tests parallel one another and are highly correlated over time. These data also suggest that as one perceptual motor skill improves, visual attentiveness may also improve.

Ocular Pursuit

The next gross visual skill analyzed was ocular pursuits, which concerns the ability to track in multiple directions, that is horizontal, vertical, diagonal, right/left, left/right, clockwise, and counterclockwise. A 0-2 scale was used for rating ocular pursuits. Again, the qualitative aspect of assessment was used in addition to the quantitative measurement. For example, the observation guidelines listed ask the therapist to look for short visual attention span, jerky eye movements, excessive head movement, losing track of the object, nystagmus, overshooting, smoothness and speed of ocular pursuits.

The data suggest (see Figure 2) that coma length makes more of a difference for recovery of ocular pursuits than was seen for visual attentiveness, with the less than 7 day coma group crossing baseline before twelve months post, and the 8-31 and greater than 31 day groups lagging behind. Statistical comparison of means (see Table 1) demonstrated that the difference between the moderate and long coma groups for ocular pursuit at one year was not significantly different. However, comparison of the short versus long coma groups for ocular pursuit was significant at the $p < .05$ level. Therefore, ocular pursuit may represent a more complex skill than visual attentiveness involving more complex shifts of attention and sustained attention. It appears to not reach baseline as quickly as visual attentiveness. Regression analyses (see Table 2) show that ocular pursuit crossed baseline in the 8-31 days group at 14.8 months post-injury and 17.8 months in the greater than 31 day severe coma group. From the Pearson r correlation (see Table 3), the only CPM skills that ocular pursuit were highly correlated with at a

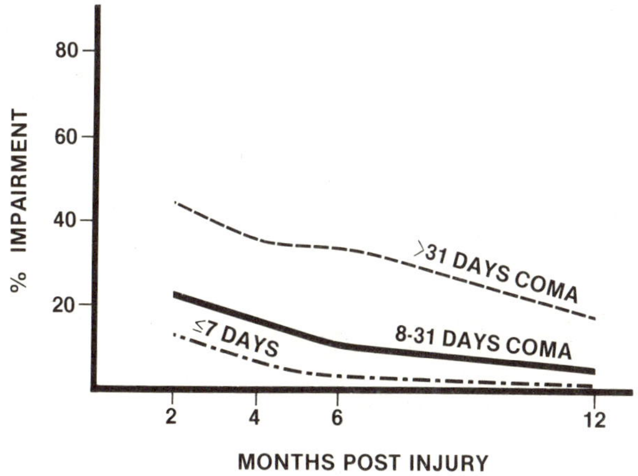


Figure 2. Ocular Pursuits

significant level included body scheme, figure ground perception, and position-in-space at two months post-injury. However, it should be added that further statistical analyses than herein described revealed that at 4 and 6 months post-injury measures of ocular pursuit were highly correlated ($p<.01$) with all other CPM skills. This may suggest that scanning related to more complex perceptual motor tasks involving other systems such as the tactile, kinesthetic, and vestibular sensory processing which help to develop visual skills.

## Praxis

The evaluation of praxis at SCVMC includes four separate measures, as outlined previously. Praxis was defined as the ability to carry out a complex or skilled movement regardless of paralysis, sensory changes, or decreased understanding. Graphic praxis was the one test out of this battery selected for the present data analysis. Graphic praxis was evaluated using simple and complex designs, where the patient was asked to draw a cube, house, and clock designs. First, the patient was asked to perform the task from memory after seeing a cue card for ten seconds, and then he was asked to copy the drawings. If the patient was unable to perform the copy, he was then asked to do the drawing by imitation after a demonstration by the evaluator. Graphic praxis was scored using a 0-3 scale.

Coma length correlated more significantly with recovery trends over time for graphic praxis than for visual attentiveness or ocular pursuit (see Table 3). These results might be interpreted to suggest that praxis is a higher level perceptual motor skill and thereby took longer to cross baseline (see Figure 3). Statistical comparisons done at one year post-injury (see Table 1), comaring the moderate and severe coma groups, showed that the difference between the two groups

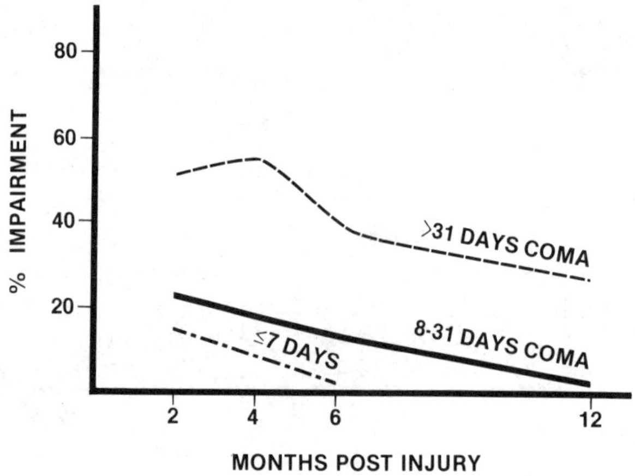


Figure 3. Graphic Praxis

were significant at the $p<.05$ level. The results suggest that the longer the coma, the longer it will take for improvement on graphic praxis skills. The results of the regression analyses (see Table 2) suggest that the greater than 31 day coma group in fact intercepts baseline or "zero" impairment at 20.6 months post-injury. Graphic praxis was also, quite interestingly found to significantly correlate (see Table 3) with all other CPM skills at the $p<.01$ level of significance at all time epochs. So perhaps, motor planning, which involves visual, as well as motor ability, is important for the development of other perceptual skills.

Depth Perception

This task was, again, rated on a 0-3 scale, where the patient was asked to point to the closest or furthest block, among several blocks placed on a table. The results of the regression analysis (see Table 2) suggest that dept perception was the second earliest skill to intercept baseline. The 8-31, moderate coma group crossed baseline at 11.6 months post-injury, and the greater than 31 day group at 18.3 months post-injury (see Figure 4). Statistical comparisons of group means revealed no significant differences between coma length groups. On correlation analysis (see Table 3), depth perception correlated highly ($p<.01$) to all other CPM skills for those measures of CPM skills herein studied.

Figure Ground Perception

One of the figure ground tests used was the Southern California Sensory Integration Tests (Ayres, 1976), which includes selecting three pictures out of increasingly complex backgrounds. This test was not standardized for adults, so the norms compiled by Siev and

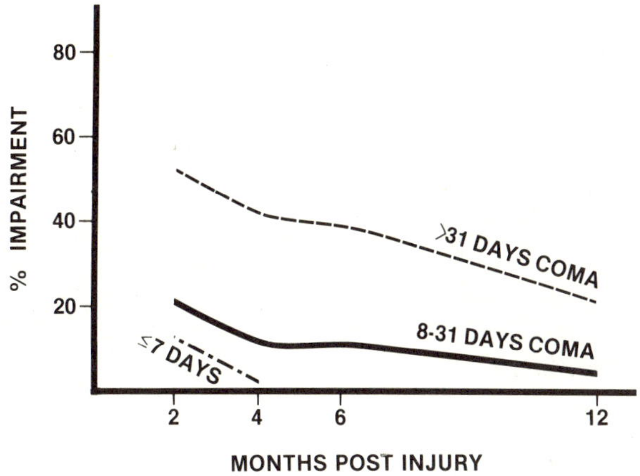


Figure 4. Depth Perception

Frieshtat (1976) were used within the context of a 0-3 scale. Figure ground perception is defined as "the ability to distinguish a foreground from a background" (Siev and Frieshtat, 1976). The second measure of figure ground perception used was the Frostig figure ground test which includes the ability to perceive and trace geometric shapes that are overlapping or placed on complex backgrounds. The Frostig was scored by the number of items correct out of a total of twenty items. Functional figure ground perception was tested lastly, which requires the patient to select and identify six objects from a full box of objects. Again, the patient's score was based on the number of correct items.

A comparison of the three figure ground tests reveals that the Ayres shows the highest percentage of impairment on all three coma groups (see Figure 5). Consequently, if the therapist evaluated a high level patient who passed the Ayres, the patient would not need to be assessed on the Frostig or Functional figure ground tests. The results of the regression analysis (see Table 2) suggest that the greater than 31 day coma group intercepts baseline on the Ayres figure ground test at 57.1 months post-injury, and on the Frostig test at 16.5 months post-injury. The Ayres, it would appear then, is a more sensitive test to more complex deficits, lending itself to measuring recovery over a longer period of time. Another important consideration in deciding which tests to administer is that the Ayres does not require motor efficiency whereas the Frostig requires motor ability of the upper extremities to perform. On the Pearson r correlation (see Table 3), at all time periods, it was found that all three tests are highly correlated to one another at the $p < .01$ level of significance. A t test done on a mean of the figure ground tests at one year post-injury for the moderate vs. long coma was significant at the $p < .05$ level.

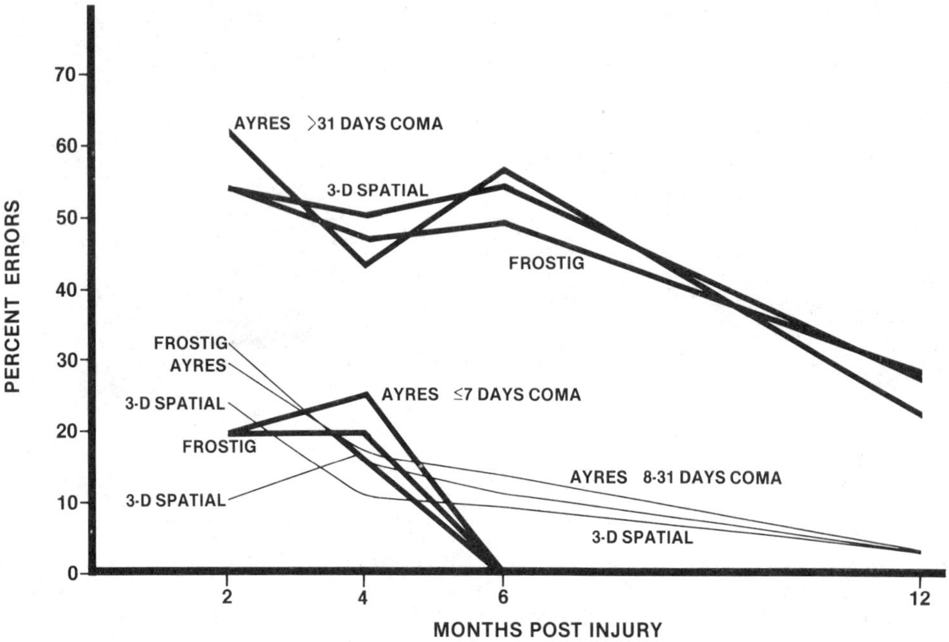


Figure 5. Position-In-Space Tests

Position-in-Space

The evaluation of position in space included three measures, the Ayres position-in-space test (Ayres, 1976) was used and measures the ability to perceive the position-in-space of objects from a selection of designs on cards. The Frostig position-in-space test (Frostig, 1963) assesses the patient's ability to distinguish from a series of pictures which is the "same as or different from" the rest. Neither test is standardized for adults and both are scored on a 0-3 scale on the basis of number of items correct. The last test used was the Three Dimensional Spatial Orientation task which tests the ability to place objects in relation to oneself or other objects, such as behind, in front of, or on top of the box. This test relies more on language ability, so it must be used selectively when testing individuals with aphasia. Again, a 0-3 scale was used based on the number of items performed correctly.

All three tests, as seen in Figure 6, were found to parallel each other highly in slope, and in fact on the Pearson r correlation, (see Table 3), correlated to one another at all time periods at the $p < .01$ level of significance. The regression analysis (see Table 2) illustrates that the Ayres and Frostig tests intercept baseline at close to the same time in the slight, moderate, and severe coma

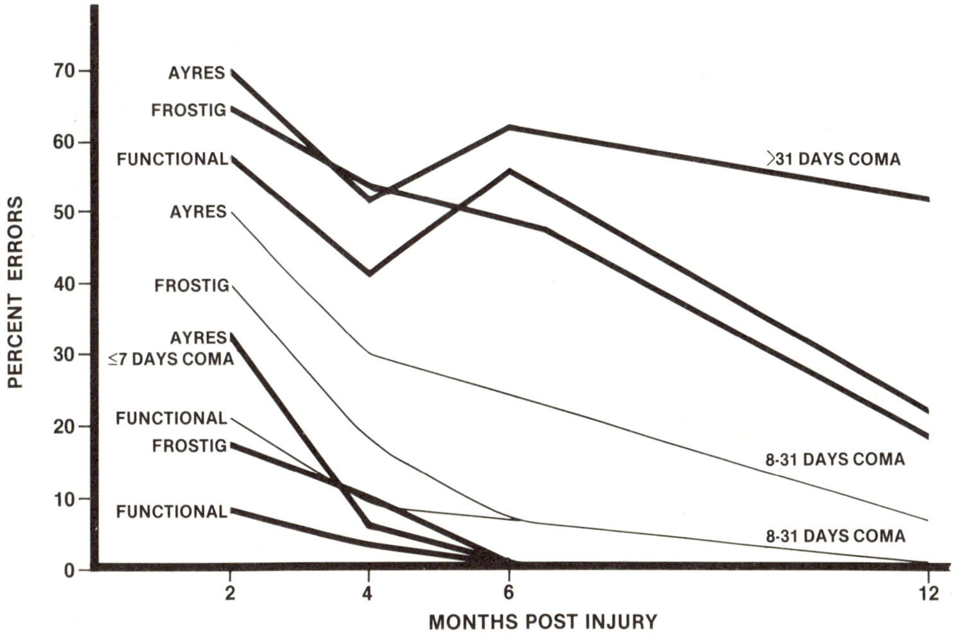


Figure 6. Figure Ground Perception Tests

groups: at eleven to twelve months in the less than or = 7 day group, thirteen to fourteen months in the 8-31 day group, and twenty-four months, or two years post in the greater than 31 day group. This indicates that either the Frostig or the Ayres tests may be used to measure spatial ability. These data suggest that only one of these two tests is necessary, and either one appears more sensitive and can be used over a longer period of time than the three dimensional spatial orientation task.

## DISCUSSION

As has been illustrated in the present results, the longer the coma, the slower the rate of recovery on all CPM variables. The short coma group consistently intercepts baseline on the regression analysis much sooner than the moderate or long coma groups. These data suggest that as a function of length of coma the clinician can project some general guidelines for when a specific CPM function approaches baseline or "zero impairment."

For example, visual attentiveness reaches baseline by one year post injury (see Table 2) in all three coma groups, and is the earliest CPM skill to "return" in adults with head trauma. It appears that most of the CPM variables on the regression analysis intercepted baseline by 12-14 months post-injury for the short and moderate coma groups. However, the majority of the CPM variables for the long coma group took the projected 18-24 months to reach baseline. The Ayres figure ground perception variable stood out from the rest in taking 57.12 months to intercept baseline in the long coma group.

For the most part, CPM skills are highly correlated with one another over time at all time epochs. As one CPM skill improves, another skill also improves as seen on the Pearson r correlational analyses (see Table 3). These results may suggest that treatment of one deficit area will in fact impact another. For example, decreasing a patient's double vision, thereby increasing his depth perception may also improve his figure ground perception. Another example was that of graphic praxis where on the correlational analyses a high correlation to all CPM skills at all time periods was found, suggesting that perhaps motor planning forms an integral part in the development of other skills as it involves visual, motor, and spatial ability.

In comparing Ayres and Frostig tests, both of which were originally designed for children, it can be seen that the Ayres figure ground perception test takes much longer to cross baseline (see Table 2) than do the Functional or Frostig tests. These results might be interpreted to suggest that for application to assessment of the adult, the Ayres appears to be a more sensitive test to more subtle and complex deficits which can be used over a longer period of time to measure figure ground impairment, as it will not intercept "zero impairment" as quickly. In terms of position-in-space, it appears that either the Ayres or the Frostig may be used to test spatial skills as both correlate highly to one another at the $p<.01$ level and appear to intercept baseline at the same time for the three coma groups. Whether the Ayres or the Frostig tests are the best tests to use for adults remains to be seen. A comparison of these tests to adult norms and to the many standardized neuropsychological test batteries that have already been developed and validated would be useful.

The results of the linear regression analysis of the specific cognitive perceptual motor variables suggests that recovery of CPM functions follows a progression or a hierarchial sequence. This is <u>not</u> to say that it follows the developmental stages the infant goes through, for this would be a gross oversimplification. However, using Gesell's levels of infant development of perceptual motor skills (Gesell and Amatruda, 1964) as <u>one</u> comparison out of many, some parallels can be drawn from the infant to the adult (see Table 4). For example, a mean of visual attentiveness is the first skill to intercept baseline at 11.3 months and on Gesell's scale, the first skill the infant develops is infant gaze at hand. This is not to suggest that the infant brain can be equated to the adult brain, nor that recovery in adult head injury will always follow a developmental sequence. It must be noted that each individual patient presents with different behavior, and that Gesell's is just one developmental theory out of many. It does suggest that perhaps the restructuring of the functional brain systems following trauma does follow a hierarchy. The finds of the present research, in combination with the experience gleened through our four years of clinical effort have resulted in the formulation of some tentative assumptions regarding the treatment of head injury.

## General Principles of Treatment of Cognitive Perceptual Motor Skills

There is no cookbook approach which is applicable for the amelioration of CPM deficits. However, there are some general principles

Table 4. Rank Order of CPM Skills Based on Regression Analysis ($\bar{X}$ of 3 Coma Groups)

| ADULT HEAD INJURY PATIENTS | $\bar{X}$ OF MONTHS | NORMAL DEVELOPMENT (GESELL) |
|---|---|---|
| VISUAL ATTENTIVENESS | 11.3 MOS. | INFANT: INFANT GAZE AT HANDS |
| DEPTH PERCEPTION | 13.14 | INFANT SEES NEARNESS OF OBJECTS |
| FORM PERCEPTION | 13.29 | 4-5 MONTHS: COORDINATES VISION WITH MANIPULATION |
| BODY SCHEME | 13.55 | 1 YR.: DEVELOPS VISUAL SPACE, MOUTH AND TACTILE SPACE |
| GRAPHIC PRAXIS | 14.0 | 2 YRS.: MARKS HORIZONTAL AND VERTICAL LINES |
| 2-D PRAXIS | 14.34 | 2-1/2 YRS.: START OF SPATIAL RELATIONS |
| OCULAR PURSUITS | 14.52 | 3 YRS.: FAR SPACE IN RELATION TO SELF |
| 3-D PRAXIS | 14.65 | 4 YRS.: SENSE HEIGHT, WIDTH, DEPTH SIMULTANEOUSLY, DRAWS CROSS AND SQUARE |
| SIZE DISCRIMINATION | 15.42 | 5 YRS.: FORM PERCEPTION, OBLIQUES, COLORS WITHIN LINES |
| POSITION-IN-SPACE | 15.18 | 6-8 YRS.: HIGH LEVEL VISUAL MOTOR ACTIVITY |
| FIGURE GROUND PERCEPTION | 17.63 | |

of treatment which may be of assistance. It must be remembered that each person with a head injury is unique and must be approached individually. Some general guidelines for treatment include:

1. Follow sequential steps or a progression. This does not mean take the adult through all the developmental steps the infant went through, but rather to sequence treatment in a hierarchy, ensuring that the patient gain some basic skills before moving on to more complex tasks.

2. The human organism works as a whole and skills cannot always be developed element by element or the individual will acquire splinter skills, isolated to the clinical situation with little functional and real transfer of training.

3. Visual perception of the external world and successful interaction is partially dependent on perception of one's internal self, for example, one's own body and body scheme.

4. Complex motor tasks are dependent on mastery of basic motor planning and mastery of more gross motor patterns. For example, dressing the lower extremities requires balance, spatial relations, body scheme, and good reciprocal motions.

5. Equilibrium reactions are important for visual-motor maturation. The extraocular muscles are skeletal muscles that are facilitated via connections of the vestibular nuclei with the cranial nerve nuclei.

6. The tactile system is primal in activating the reticular system upon which attention, perception, and learning are dependent (Moore, 1981).

7. Motor skills and perception are intimately interdependent. It is also very difficult to separate language and cognitive abilities.

8. Sensory integrative processes involving visual, auditory, tactile, kinesthetic, and vestibular input are critical to the later developmental of the cognitive processes.

9. One must provide controlled, structured, and normalized multi-sensory input, followed by demanding an adaptive response. The therapist may need to work on a more automatic level initially.

10. The approach in general must have goals prioritized, be consistent, repetitive, and well-structured by all team members. Many aspects of therapy provide external supports or cues that must be faded gradually with the ultimate

goal of patient internalization of his own scheme for eliciting the behavior and integrating it on an automatic level.

## SUMMARY

The evaluation of cognitive perceptual motor skills in the adult head injured individual is a complex and lengthy process for the Occupational Therapist. Such an evaluation not only needs to be quantitative and measureable, but should include qualitative features such that assessment can readily be applied to treatment. Preliminary research findings suggest that the "return" of CPM skills in adult head injury patients follows a hierarchial sequence. It has also been found that coma length does make a difference for recovery of some CPM functions and that recovery of these skills continues well beyond one year post-injury. Some skills, such as visual attentiveness are noted to "return" early and some, such as figure ground perception, late. This implies that there may be critical periods for treatment of CPM deficits. For example, the clinician may want to focus on the early returning skills initially in establishing the treatment regime, and then as the foundation is laid, concentrate on more complex or later returning skills.

The head injury population, unlike other disability groups, cannot easily be categorized. However, grossly defining the patient's functional level in conjunction with the herein described general principles of treatment are provided so as to attempt to give some order and structure to the clinician working with this complex disability group. The evaluation and treatment of adults who have sustained a head injury is a very challenging field where unexpected outcomes are not uncommon. Hopefully, future predictions, previously an empirically unfounded task, can now potentially be made with some data reference. These findings impact potentially not only communication with family members, but they are relevant to issues of third party payment and length of stay in the hospital or rehabilitation setting. It is hoped that the present study has contributed to the objective measurement of recovery from adult head injury.

## REFERENCES

Ayres, J. Southern California sensory integration tests. Los Angeles: Western Psychological Services Corporation, 1977.

Baum, B.A. and Meeder, D.L. Head injury in adults. In: L. Pedretti (Ed.), Occupational Therapy: Practice skills for physical dysfunction. San Francisco: C.V. Mosby, 1981.

Cope, D.N. Head injury project final report. National Institute for Handicapped Research, Department of Education, 1981.

Frostig, M. Developmental test of visual perception. Chicago: Follett Publishing Corporation, 1963.
Gilroy, J. and Meyer, J.S. Medical neurology. New York: McMillan, 1969.
Luria, A.R. The working brain. New York: Basic Books, 1973.
Moore, J. Hemispheric specialization. The Bay Area Sensory Symposium, Stanford Children's Hospital, 1981.
Mosey, A. Three frames of reference. Thorofare, New Jersey: Charles B. Slack, 1970.
Rancho Los Amigos Hospital Head Trauma Rehabilitation Seminar. A monograph published by the Professional Staff Association of Rancho Los Amigos Hospital, Downey, California, 1977.
Siev, E. and Frieshtat, B. Perceptual dysfunction in the adult stroke patient. Thorofare, New Jersey: Charles B. Slack, 1976.
Teasdale, G. and Jennett, B. Assessment of coma and impaired consciousness. Lancet, 1974, 2, 81-83.
Wall, N. Hemiplegic evaluation. A manual published by the Occupational Therapy Department of Massachusetts Rehabilitation Hospital, Boston, 1979.
Wilson, J.R. The mind. New York: Life Science Library, Time Inc., 1964.

# COGNITIVE AND NEUROPSYCHOLOGICAL ASPECTS OF AFFECTIVE CHANGE FOLLOWING TRAUMATIC BRAIN INJURY

Lance E. Trexler, Ph.D.

Coordinator, Neuropsychology Service
Medical Psychology Department
Community Hospital of Indianapolis

## INTRODUCTION

The functional information processing capability of the central nervous system (CNS) may be systematically related to the type and severity of disturbance of affective behavior following traumatic head injury. This hypothesis rests upon the assumption that affective behavior consists of an "appropriate cognitive state plus a certain degree of arousal" (Valenstein and Heilman, 1979, p. 415). Further, one might hypothesize that inappropriate affective behavior, following head injury, is therefore related to alterations of an "appropriate" cognitive state and/or a disturbance of arousal mechanisms. Cognition, however, can be considered to represent a number of interrelated processes including attention, memory and ability to learn, among others. The formation of cognitive states involves the perception and processing of current environmental information as well as the processing and accessing of internally, neurally represented information. Further, the neural representation of information is most likely related to (1) the extent to which a behavioral (affective) repertoire has been learned and (2) the functional integrity and accessability of that information.

Cognition and arousal cannot be considered, however, to function as independent processes. The extent to which a particular stimulus is arousing depends upon one's previous experience with that stimulus (and the consequences of that experience) and, concomitantly, the corresponding cognitive interpretation of the significance of that stimulus. The degree of significance, or the contextual saliency, of the stimulus is similarly related to the level of arousal which was previously associated with this particular stimulus. Consequently, degree of arousal and cognition can be viewed as dynamically interacting processes, which interact as a function of (1) previous experience and (2) the specific stimulus characteristics. Further, a review of the neural systems which largely mediate cognitive processes, arousal and emotional responses reveals a corresponding dynamic interaction, suggesting that (1) affective behavior is not mediated by any one particular brain structure and (2) affective changes following traumatic brain injury can follow from the dysfunction of a number of CNS processes.

The present chapter is concerned with reviewing the neural systems which mediate arousal and emotional responses, as well as the role of cortical influence in modulating these responses. Further, the role of cognitive processes in affective behavior will be discussed so as to lay a foundation for identifying clinical syndromes of affective disturbance in head injury and concomitantly, treatment strategies.

## NEURAL SYSTEMS MEDIATING EMOTIONAL BEHAVIOR

All levels, phylogenetically, of the central nervous system are involved in the mediation of affective behavior. Further, these levels of mediational representation cannot be considered unidirectional, but rather as dynamically interactive. This section of the present chapter is concerned with a brief review of what appear to be the three most relevant neural systems, namely the "reticular" activating system, the limbic system, the cortical modulatory influences, and their functional interrelatedness.

### Arousal and Activating Systems

Brodal (1981) points out that the "activating system is a functional concept, the reticular formation a morphological one, and it has been obvious for many years that these do not correspond" (p. 396). While the initial investigation (Moruzzi and Magon, 1949) of this "reticular activating system" cautiously referred to the anatomical specificity of this system as originating in the reticular formation of the brain stem, this functional system principally involves a network of cells in the pons, medulla and mesencephalon, with connections to and from diencephalic and telencephalic structures (see Figure 1). Anatomically, the reticular formation represents a relatively cytoarchitectually unique group of cells in the central areas of the brain stem and motor fiber bundles. In conjunction with limbic and thalamic structures, the activating system plays a role in the sleeping-wakefulness cycle (Green and Arduini, 1954) where reciprocal activation-suppression areas within the reticular formation and between the reticular formation and higher structures subserve a more subtle modulation of central arousal. Thatcher and John (1977) elucidate three main functional characteristics of the activating system where (1) diverse reticulocortical

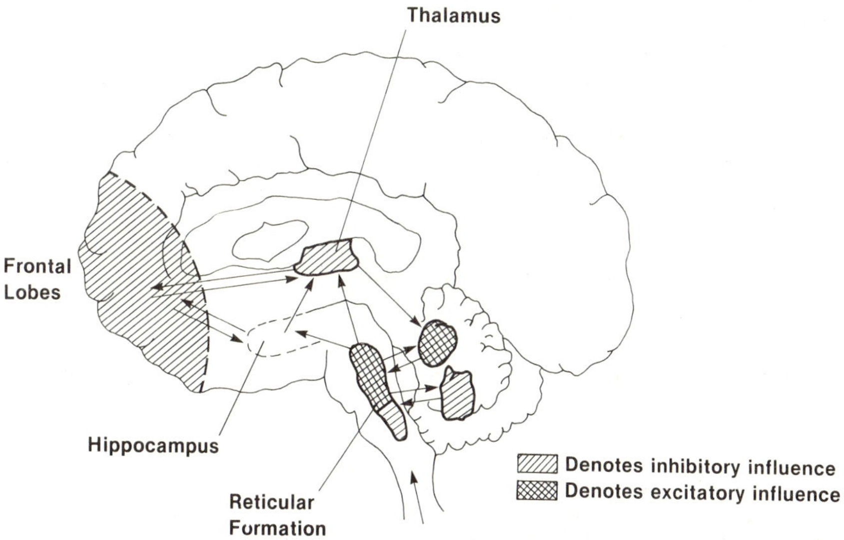


Figure 1. Reticular Activating System

projections regulate the level of excitation of the cerebral cortex, (2) feedback information from principally thalamic sensory relay nuclei, limbic structures (especially the hippocampus) and cerebral cortex modulate brainstem reticular formation activity and (3) reciprocally excitatory-inhibitory ascending and descending inter-relations subserve the processes of habituation and orienting responses. This bi-directional hierarchical balancing of arousal and central activation permits the organism to adjust attentional mechanisms according to its biological and environmental demands. The balancing of habituation/orienting responses is a requisite for learning, where differential levels of central arousal are elicited by relevant and irrelevant stimuli, as subserved by phylogenetically multi-level excitation-inhibition interactions. The activating system's relationship with the thalamus permits for the attenuation of one sensory modality and the inhibition or suppression of another as a function of the information value of the stimuli. Therefore, information which is of little significance or highly redundant is ignored, whereas highly salient and/or novel data is attended to. This information impinges upon the central nervous system via sensory data as a function of the relationship between the thalamus and the brainstem reticular formation. It is this relationship which led Thatcher and John (1977) to define attention as "the focusing of perceptual mechanisms upon inputs in particular sensory modalities or upon the specific configuration of stimuli which correspond to a unique event in the environment" (p. 91). It is also important to note that these processes occur without conscious effort to the extent that when performing a given task, attentional vigilance and selectivity occurs relatively automatically.

The balancing of attentional shifting mechanisms also involves a specific and a general or non-specific activating system where specific activating systems tend to be modality specific and where general activating systems influence overall central excitation. With the onset of a novel stimulus generalized activation is likely to occur which is initiated by the midbrain reticular formation (Lindsley, Bowden and Majoun, 1949). Following repeated stimulation and habituation, the lower brainstem may eventuate an inhibitory response through the non-specific activating system, which facilitates the effects of specific activating systems (Gastaut, 1958). The non-specific thalamic reticular nucleus also "feedbacks" information to other specific and non-specific thalamic nuclei as an integrative function of thalamocortical and corticothalamic activity (Scheibel and Scheibel, 1967). Further, with repeated stimulation, specific activating systems, which ultimately influence primary sensory cortex via sensory-specific thalamic nuclei, mediate central activation (Jasper, Naquet and King, 1955), while the influence of the non-specific activating systems decrease. These processes serve as the neural substrate for orienting and habituation responses and it is the dynamic interaction of the non-specific and specific activating systems which may partially subserve attention shifting or selective attention.

The involvement of the limbic system also contributes to attentional processing, and at this level an introduction of cerebral structures which are also intimately involved in emotional behavior occurs. Whether or not an orienting response occurs in response to a stimulus to some extent depends upon the organism's previous experience with that stimulus. The neural representation of previous learning is an extraordinary topic in and of itself, but let it suffice to say that the hippocampus has an important role in the comparing and contrasting of a given stimulus relative to learned, encoded information and hippocampal lesions result in an inability to store new information (Penfield and Milner, 1958). The extent to which a given stimulus "matches" previously learned stimuli determines the magnitude of an orienting response and it is the hippocampus, in conjunction with other limbic structures, which modulates the dynamic, spatially and temporally, balance of the orienting response and habituation (Thatcher and John, 1977).

The reticular-hippocampal relatedness is relevant for affective and non-affective stimuli. However, the neural mediation of affect involves several other structures and systems, principally including the hypothalamus and portions of the limbic system. The hypothalamus functions in numerous capacities and has multiple nuclei. For the purpose of the present discussion, its functions will be briefly reviewed. The hypothalamus is organized anatomically and neurophysiologically to maintain a homeostatic balance of opposite motivational-emotional processes. Fear and flight responses, pain and pleasure, eating and cessation of eating (Epstein, 1960), placidity and rage responses (Kessler, 1941) are a few of the affective behaviors partially subserved by the hypothalamus and the control of affective reactions based on any sensory modality of stimulation may be a function of particularly the ventromedial hypothalamic nuclei (Wheatley, 1944). As the highest center for control of the autonomic nervous system, hypothalamic functions are important for the regulation of gastrointestinal, cardiovascular and neuroendocrine systems. (Rickles, 1972). The hypothalamus receives afferent impulses through the medial forebrain bundle originating from the septum and the amygdala, which are important centers of the limbic system. Further, the hypothalamus receives input from the thalamus which may originate in the orbitofrontal cortex.

## The Limbic System

The limbic system is similarly complex and its relevant structures (hippocampal formation, amygdala, septum, and portions of the cingulate cortex) form a feedback loop involving the fornix, anterior portions of the thalamus and the medial forebrain bundle. Figure 2 represents a, albeit greatly simplified, schematic of the interrelatedness of these structures. The activity of the hypothalamus, amygdala, septum, hippocampus and cingulate cortex collectively subserve affective experience and when those experiences are synchronized or integrated with events in the external environment and involve some goal-directed component, the tertiary frontal cortex plays an

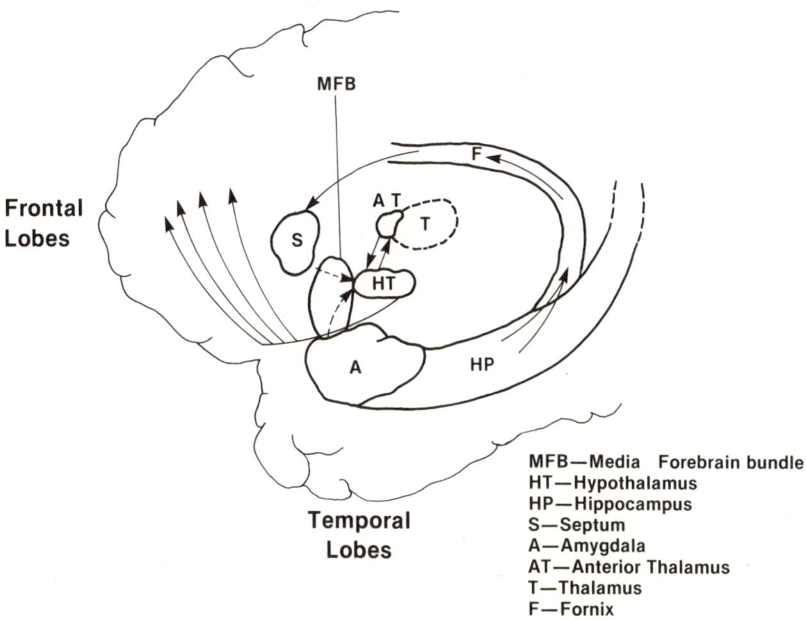


Figure 2. Schematic Summary of Limbic System.

important (possibly involving inhibitory and sequential planning influences) role. The contribution of the more phylogenetically advanced structures appears to add a modulatory influence to particularly affective expression, in context of the information received from more primitive limbic system structures. One principal feature of the limbic system involves the balancing of opposite emotional states which may occur within and between structures. The activity of especially the septum and the amygdala illustrate this reciprocal balancing. Rage, (Brady, 1960), flight reactions (Gloor, 1960) and confusion have been noted to occur with amygdaloid stimulation and lesions of the amygdala result in docility. In contrast, Brady and Nauta (1953) and Woods (1956) found that abalation of the septum resulted in essentially a disinhibition of amygdala activity, or rage and aggressive behavior. Consequently, amygdaloid and septal functions appear to represent bipolar influences, which impinge on the hypothalamus. In summary, the amygdala appears to exert a facilitory or excitatory influence and the septum an inhibitory influence on the hypothalamus, via the medial forebrain bundle. Afferent activities of particularly the orbitofrontal and basal cortex of the frontal lobes from the hypothalamus initiates the environmental (internal-external) synchronization of these affective processes which is then "feedback" into the limbic system primarily through the anterior nuclei of the thalamus.

The ascending and descending activating systems, in conjunction with limbic processes, coordinate levels of arousal associated with affective experience and expression. The extent to which these processes influence attention then depends upon the intensity of affective processing and the degree of interference on attention shifting mechanisms.

<u>Relevant Cortical Influences</u>

There appear to be primarily two mechanisms through which the functions of the cerebral cortex influences cognitive-affective behavior. The first mechanism concerns relatively specific areas of cortex which play a role in the modulation of arousal and attentional processes. Secondly, the role of the cerebral cortex in information processing, and the concomitant laterlized asymmetries, influences predominantly the expression and perception of affect.

Cortical functions can act to either facilitate or inhibit limbic and activating systems. However, especially the frontal cortex appears to be more directly involved in the modulation of the limbic system, particularly the medial and orbital surfaces of the prefrontal cortex (Pribram, 1973). Luria (1980) concludes that lesions of the lateral surfaces of the frontal lobes result in a "deautomation of motor, speech, and intellectual acts while states of consciousness and memory functions remain relatively intact" (p. 265). Contrastingly, lesions of the mediobasal surfaces of the frontal regions "are characterized by disturbances mainly of the emotions and personality, disturbances of consciousness, of memory processes, and the selectivity of psychological functions...(p. 266). The disturbances described as associated with lesions of the mediobasal frontal cortex may be suggestive of the role of these cortical areas in the modulation of arousal and attention, through corticofugal feedback, which appears to be largely inhibitory in nature. Valenstein and Heilman (1979) have suggested that the affective disturbances associated with frontal lesions may be resultant from essentially a disinhibition of septal area and amygdala functions. Further, these latter authors propose that patients with lesions of the dorsolateral surfaces of the frontal cortex have disturbances of "phasic arousal" where they fail to respond with degree of arousal which would be expected to a stimulus in context of appropriate cognition.

Differential characteristics of the left and right cerebral hemisphere information processing capability may be related to the perception of affect. The right cerebral hemisphere appears to subserve the perception of the affective tonal characteristics of spoken language (Haggard and Parkinson, 1971; Tucker, Watson and Heilman, 1977). Some research also suggests that there is an asymmetrical hemispheric mediation of arousal, which may be related to perceptual processes. Holloway and Parsons (1969) postulated that injury of the cerebral cortex would increase autonomic arousal secondary to a disinhibition of cortical influences. However, Morrow, Vrtunski, Kim and Boller (1981) and Heilman, Schwartz and Watson (1978) have found that right cerebral hemisphere injured patients evidence lowered levels of autonomic arousal (as measured by galvanic skin response) relative to left hemisphere patients. Morrow et. al. (1981) found that left hemisphere patients also however had lower levels of arousal than controls, in contrast to Heilman et. al. (1978) and Trexler and Schmidt (1981).

The foregoing briefly reviewed research suggests that not only subcortical, but cortical, functions are involved in the central mediation of cognitive-affective behavior. The parameters on which this complex multi-dimensional (bi-polar opposite representation for different affective states), multi-level (phylogenetically) interaction operate can be viewed as cognitive processes.

## THE ROLE OF COGNITION

Affective behavior differs from other forms of behavior to the extent that it is associated with arousal. Affective behavior is also intertwined with the processes of motivation, although this interrelatedness is not the specific focus of the present chapter. It should be noted, however, that many of the previously reviewed neural systems subserving attention, arousal and emotionality are intrinsic to motivational processes. More, or at least equally complex, however, is the relatedness of affective behavior and cognition. If affective behavior is comprised of a cognitive state and arousal, as Valenstein and Heilman (1979) have suggested, an analysis of both components is warranted.

Arousal is a relative concept however. The degree of arousal associated with great pleasure can be comparable to the arousal experienced with great discomfort. The difference may be considered to be cognitive in nature. The interpretation of arousal responses determines whether or not we label the experience as "pleasureable" or "painful." This interpretation, like the interpretation of any other stimulus, is based upon (1) the specific stimulus characteristics, (2) the context in which the stimulus occurs, and (3) previous learning. Previous learning becomes relevant to the experience of emotion to the extent that it has influenced the formation and development of cognitive processes and to the extent that it is recalled. Memory, therefore, becomes an important cognitive process which is relevant to affective behavior. (The reader is urged to review Wyer and Carlston, 1979, for a very illuminating examination of social learning phenomena and cognition.) This line of reasoning requires that we examine the nature of cognitive processes to understand the relatedness of the neurophysiology of arousal and attention to affective-cognitive behavior.

Cognition can be considered to be present at all levels of processing mediated by the CNS, except perhaps with exception of spinal reflexes and physiologic homeostatic mechanisms. Cognition can further be considered to represent a number of processes, as opposed to functions. A function has a specific and circumscribed goal, in terms of both spatial and temporal characteristics. Consider for a moment visual functions. A visual stimulus will elicit the response of retinal cells which in turn initiate an afferent neural response through the optic pathways, the lateral geniculate nuclei and eventually to the visual cortex. Once the neural representation of the visual stimulus has reached the level of the cerebral cortex, it can then be interpreted in terms of (1) the salient features of the stimulus, (2) the context in which it occurs and (3) the organism's previous experience with this particular stimulus. Visual functions are essentially the "contents" of the stimulus and the "contents" are stored in memory. The processes which organize and modulate the visual functions are cognitive. The cognitive process of attention, for example, determines the degree of cortical arousal elicited by this visual stimulus as a function of stimulus saliency, novelty and the significance of the stimulus relative to its internal representation (memory). Consequently, visual functions are concerned with making perceptual "sense" of the stimulus and transforming the corresponding neural representation into organized neural activity. It is through these functions, therefore, that the stimulus is recognized Cognitive processes can be considered to influence these recognition functions in that they modulate the "attention" devoted to this particular visual stimulus and relate the neural representation of this stimulus to the overall purpose and goals of the organism at that time.

This conceptualization suggests that cognition and function dynamically interrelate to produce the qualitative and quantitative aspects of the experience of a given stimulus. This conceptualization differs from those suggesting that cognition is concerned with only "higher level" mental operations. Further, cognition cannot be localized in the CNS, but rather can be viewed as a general capacity of the CNS, whereas functions are relatively localized and lateralized. Further, cognitive processes cannot be considered "hierarchical" either in the psychological or neuropsychological sense in that levels of processing occur simultaneously involving cortical and subcortical activity, in contrast to sensory-perceptual functions which are clearly hierarchical.

Since the present chapter is concerned with emotion and cognition, no attempt will be made to exhaustively review all aspects of cognitive processing. So as to illustrate the relevance of cognition in emotional behavior however, attentional processing will be discussed as an important component of the processes which can be associated with arousal and therefore affective in nature.

## Attentional Cognitive Processing

Attentional processes exemplify cognitive processes in general in that the evidence supports the contention that there are a number of levels of attention and that attention is modulated as a function of (1) specific stimulus characteristics, (2) the environmental context, and (3) learning history. Before addressing these more complex aspects of attentional processing, several relevant parameters of attention will be addressed.

Moscovitch (1979) describes effort and selectivity as relevant parameters of attentional control processes, where effort is conceptually related to a quantitative dimension of attention. This quantitative dimension of attention is related to the complexity, familiarity or novelty and significance of the stimulus. Selectivity refers to the extent to which a given stimulus or one stimulus, in context of others, is selected for primary processing. This latter qualitative dimension implies that the CNS has a limited information processing capacity and that certain stimuli take precedence (in context of the organism's overall need to adapt) over others. This competitive selectivity process exemplifies the interaction between central processes and functions.

Levels of processing can be illustrated within the cerebral cortex itself, which are hierarchically organized in spatial and temporal dimensions. Hubel and Wiesel (1962, 1963) have shown that neurons in the primary visual cortex responded to more basic components of visual stimuli whereas the secondary visual cortex functioned in a more integrative manner; the activity of the secondary cortex was less stimulus bound in terms of the correspondence between the psychophysical properties of the stimulus relative to the neurophysiological activity. Consequently, using the example of vision, there appears to be a process-function interaction where certain irrelevant features of the total stimulus configuration are filtered out through attention processes in context of visual functions. Further, this function-process interaction occurs within and between levels of processing, whether it be sub-cortical or cortical, and between sensory modalities.

Selectivity can be considered to operate directly as a function of (1) interference and (2) expectancy effects. Interference refers to the infringement of processing demands necessitated by one stimulus on the processing of another, more central and salient stimulus. This infringement is dependent upon the automaticity with which the competitive stimulus is processed. Hicks (1975) and Lomas and Kimura (1976) have shown that complex motor responses, as executed with the right hand, interfered with the concurrent verbal activity whereas verbal activity actually facilitated the performance of very simple and non-directed motor behavior (Kimura, 1973; Kinsbourne, 1972). In this context Walley and Weiden (1973) advanced a theory to the effect that recurrent lateral inhibition, the suppression of neighboring cortical regions following activation of a particular zone, accounted for the observed decriment in processing of a stimulus which was highly similar in terms of stimulus characteristics relative to the processing of a proceeding stimulus. These latter authors also suggest that arousal facilitates recurrent lateral inhibition. The expectancy effects of selectivity of attention refer to the processing of a stimulus based on (1) information which immediately proceeded the onset of the stimulus and, concomitantly, (2) a probabilistic expectancy of what the nature of the forthcoming stimulus would be, based on previous learning. Klein, Moscovitch and Vigna (1976) have proposed that attentional factors determine which hemisphere of the cerebral cortex processes a given stimulus as a function of expectancy effects, the properties of the stimulus itself, and functional asymmetries of the right and left cerebral hemispheres.

Selectivity of attentional processing was considered in terms of interference and expectancy effects. The other parameter of attentional processing briefly treated concerned that of effort, which was essentially related to the quantity of attention centered on or devoted to a particular stimulus. It should be noted that both selectivity and effort concern the capacity of the CNS to process information and probably represent mechanisms which serve to maximize the processing efficiency of the CNS. Further, these mechanisms facilitate the organism's internal organization and representation of its external environment, the generation of responses and a meaningful adaptation to the evolving and changing bombardment of stimulus information. As stated earlier in this section, these parameters of attentional processing are operational as a function of (1) specific stimulus characteristics, (2) the environmental context, and (3) the organism's previous experience with similar stimuli, and serve as modulatory controls of cerebral activity. The extent to which attentional processes modulate cerebral activity can now be directly addressed.

Stimulus Characteristics and Contextual Information. Stimulus characteristics which are relevant to the corresponding attentional processing vary along many continuums and do not fall into isolated categories. Further, only with specialized conditions are any two stimuli exactly the same; our natural environment varies along too many parameters for a given stimulus to occur under the same conditions, twice. It can also be argued that even with the occurence of two identical stimuli, under identical circumstances, the interpretation of that stimulus is different by virtue of the observer's previous experience with the stimulus itself. Nonetheless, an examination of some of the relevant stimulus characteristics may be meaningful.

Stimuli can, obviously, vary in terms of function; visual, auditory, tactile, olfactory, gustatory and kinesthetic stimuli are all characteristically different psychophysically and the intact CNS reliably differentiates them. At this very basic level an interaction between attentional processing and CNS function exists, as modulated by more complex cognitive processes. Stimulus characteristics become quite important when considering the attentional processing of individuals with lesions of the CNS. Brain damage or dysfunction, contingent upon the location, may differentially affect the attentional processing of a given stimulus; e.g., auditory neglect following temporal lesions, visual inattention and neglect following occipital lesions, or possibly a general or global neglect following right hemisphere lesions (Heilman, Schwartz and Watson, 1978). Finally, the intensity and duration of any given stimulus will affect attentional processes. Stimuli of high intensity may elicit more CNS arousal than stimuli of low intensity. Depending upon the nature of the stimulus and rate of habituation, the onset of a stimulus as compared with repetitive presentation, may elicit the greatest quantitiy of attentional effort.

Contextual factors most likely play the largest role in determining the influence of attentional processes on our interpretation and overall regard of a given stimulus. A stimulus contains identical characteristics in terms of its quantitative features only in a rare or contrived circumstance, and even less often under the same circumstances. Variations in the context in which a stimulus occurs gives rise to the qualitative features of a stimulus, which include the saliency, relevance and contextual dependence or contextual independence of the stimulus. The saliency of a given stimulus refers to several quantitative features such as intensity or duration relative to what is congruent with or compatible with other stimuli in the perceptual field. The extent to which stimulus one ($S_1$) is viewed as salient depends upon whether or not it is similar or dissimilar to stimulus two ($S_2$), or novel relative to what might be expected. The expectancy factor occurs as a function of previous learning, which can be thought of as an internally represented context. The relevance of a stimulus can be addressed on several levels: $S_1$ as relevant to $S_2$ either temporally, spatially or functionally, $S_1$ as relevant to an internal context, and $S_1$ as relevant to the ongoing commitment of CNS activity, organization and purpose or direction when $S_1$ occurs. Contextual dependence and independence relates to the extent to which $S_1$ must be associated with $S_2$, $S_3$, $S_4$, etc. to be recognized and elicit effort. Those stimuli which can be considered contextually independent elicit attention in and of themselves regardless of the circumstances, whereas contextually dependent stimuli do not evoke sufficient attentional processes to be recognized as independent from the overall percept. The concept of contextual independence and dependence can be related to an internal context, the neural representation of previously learned information. Battig (1979) and Jacoby and Craik (1979) refer to similar characteristics in memory processes.

## Internal (Neural) Representation and Learning History

One's previous experience, as encoded and stored in the central nervous system, serves as a referent from which to attend to and interpret any new stimulus. While extraordinarily relevant, memory processes significantly interface with attentional processes and differentiating the two is most likely more academic than functionall accurate, a review of memory processes goes beyond the scope of the present chapter. (The interested reader is encouraged to see Cermak and Craik, 1979, for a thorough exploration of this topic.) Nonetheless, there are several aspects of learning history and the corresponding neural organization of information which are important, especially as they relate to cognitive-affective behavior.

The extent to which a given behavior has been repeated obviously influences the level of encoding of that behavior. The more repetitious the behavior the less volitional attention (Luria, 1973) requir to execute the processing and response formulation of that behavior. Responses to environmental stimuli can be "overlearned", meaning that (1) there exists a high probability of their reoccurence and (2) the response may become stimulus bound. A stimulus bound response refers to the evocation of an organized sequence of behavior which occurs relatively automatically with little contribution of higher-order processing. The lowest level of a stimulus bound behavior is a spina reflex. It may be the case that more complex forms of organized behavior are similarly processed, including social-affective behavioral routines, as a function of the extent to which they have been "overlearned." The automaticity of stimulus bound behavior enables the organism to process other information and speeds response generation. However, this efficiency of processing potentially comprises the perception of subtle differences between situations. In other words, inattending to certain idiosyncratic differences in stimulus configurations is adaptive so as to expedite processing, although at the expense of some "fine tuning" in stimulus-response synchronization. The extent to which we inattend to certain details of a stimulus is dependent upon our previous experience with that stimulus and the consequences that followed. Behavior appears to be "inappropriate" when the response does not meaningfully synchronize with the stimulus configuration and significant or relevant variants (relevant to previous learning) have been ignored.

Affective behavior (expression) represents an interaction between learned response patterns, the cognitive-affective state and the configuration of the stimulus. It is obvious that learned affective response patterns are unique to the individual and represent the consequences of an environment-individual interaction. Furthermore, it may be the case that "overlearned" cognitive-affective repertoires determine affective behavior patterns seen following traumatic brain injury. Affective behavior patterns are also obviously influenced by the integrity of perceptual mechanisms to the extent that the individual is capable of accurately "perceiving" the relevant stimulus characteristics (previously discussed as cortical influences). Finally relevant cognitive functions, as briefly herein discussed, play a

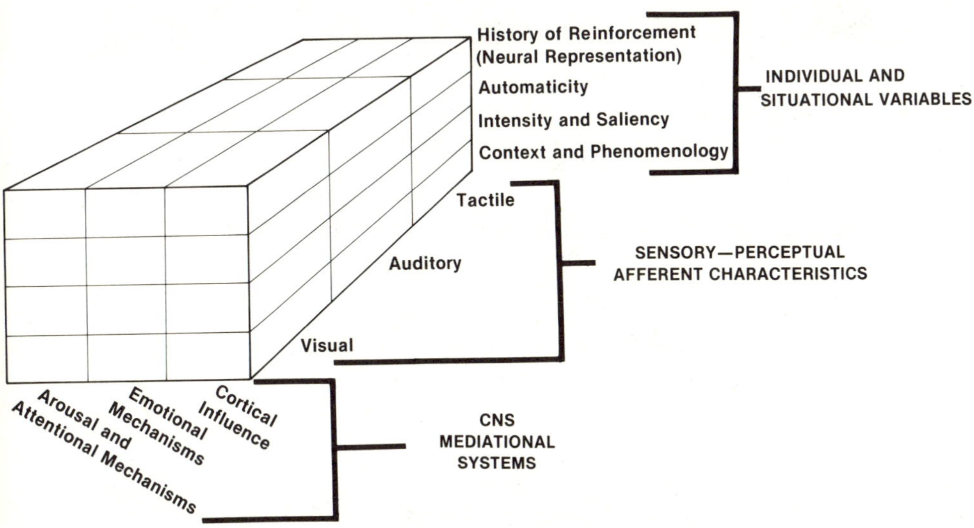


Figure 3. A conceptual model exemplifying the relevant variables and processes subserving affective behavior.

critical role in understanding cognitive-affective behavior following trauma to the central nervous system. Figure 3 represents a schematic of the relatedness of these processes.

## CLINICAL SYNDROMES OF COGNITIVE-AFFECTIVE BEHAVIOR FOLLOWING TRAUMATIC BRAIN INJURY

It is in fact the explicit intent of this chapter to attempt to make sense of what sometimes appears to be the totally unpredictable, unexplicable and inconsistent behavior characterizing traumatic head injury. Through a review of relevant neurophysiological systems which are likely to become dysfunctional in head injury and a thorough examination of cognitive processes, some clarity may emerge such that perhaps a meaningful taxonomy of cognitive-affective behavior following traumatic head injury could be devised. Such a taxonomy may provide (1) a common perspective from which to view these characteristics and (2) some suggestion as to appropriate interventive strategies. The present section of this chapter is such an attempt.

The following taxonomy illustrates relevant cognitive-affective dysfunction on two bi-directional dimensions. It is not presumed that these two dimensions are comprehensive in scope, but rather provide a conceptualization from which derivations can be developed. It is also not presumed that these dimensions are independent from each other, but rather probably systematically interact as a function of location, severity and chronicity of injury. Finally, while the taxonomy may elucidate cognitive-affective disturbance following traumatic head injury, the herein described interventive recommendations (which are probably applicable to post-acute patients) are totally untested and represent intuitive hypotheses rooted solely in clinical experience, certainly riddled with theoretical and methodological assumptions. As a consequence, these recommendations are tentative in their entirety and at best perhaps represent hypotheses to be systematically investigated.

The treatment of cognitive-affective disorders may need to include teaching the traumatic head injury patient (1) an awareness or recognition of the disorder, (2) self-monitoring strategies or an ability to profit from environmental feedback and (3) skills, abilities or compensatory strategies which can functionally replace previous, less appropriate, responses. It is not presumed however, that treatment should necessarily follow the order in which the above aspects of treatment are listed. Finally, many of the suggested interventive strategies are utilizable with relatively intact, post-acute patients. However, simplifying and structuring the herein described strategies, utilizing the same principles, may facilitate the utilization of those treatment strategies for more acute or more severely injured patients.

Inhibition-Disinhibition Dimension

This dimension is descriptive of the traumatically injured patient's propensity to either under- or over-react to particularly emotional stimuli. Further, this dimension concerns the characteristic impulsivity and/or hypoarousal of traumatic brain injury. The continuum from inhibition to disinhibition can manifest within and between patients. Inhibition of responses may be associated with hypoarousal and an inability to spontaneously initiate a behavior. Further, at this end of the continuum, the traumatically injured patient's behavior can be characterized by a lack of response to very salient stimuli in the environment, and yet perhaps be accompanied by a high probability of what would be considered to be an over-reaction to insignificant stimuli. This difficulty in modulating arousal results in symptoms of disinhibition as well. The impulsivity characteristic of disinhibition appears to be spontaneous and without warning, perhaps resulting in agitation or combativeness. As opposed to an impairment in an ability to initiate appropriate behavior, symptomatology of disinhibition includes the initiation of inappropriate behavior, where the behavior is typically considered to be inappropriate because of the degree (excess) of affective arousal associated with the circumstances.

Both inhibition and disinhibition can be seen as adaptive cognitive-affective behaviors for the traumatically head injured patient. It may be the case that inhibition responses occur when the patient is experiencing an overwhelming bombardment of stimuli and inhibition (hypoarousal) represents one process to limit the influx of information, thereby preventing disinhibition. Conversely, disinhibition may represent a process which facilitates arousal in response to a need for the organism to situationally adapt. We have observed a number of patients who performed poorly on a given task until they become overtly somewhat agitated and "inappropriately" aroused (disinhibited). As a consequence, disinhibition may represent a cognitive-affective response to task demands which exceed the patient's capability to process information. The facilitation of arousal states may, hypothetically, improve information processing leading to a more adaptive response generation.

If inhibition and disinhibition are viewed as adaptive responses, from the perspective of the patient's cognitive-affective processing capabilities, intervention should not attempt to eliminate these coping responses without providing more "appropriate" alternative strategies. The use of major tranquillizers for the treatment of agitation may represent, consequently, an attempt to eliminate one of the few mechanisms of adaptation available to the patient. In other words, agitation may represent the final stage of unmodulated arousal, initiated (that is, increased arousal states) so as to facilitate capacity for information processing. The use of a major tranquillizer may therefore effectively prohibit an adaptive (albeit socially undesireable and inappropriate) response. Further, the use of such medications certainly does not provide the patient skills or strategies with which to increase capacity for information processing.

The treatment of inhibition-disinhibition disorders should address the three components of interventive strategies previously described, including (1) a recognition of the impairment, (2) self-monitoring and (3) specific strategies for altering behavior. Teaching brain injured patients to be aware of or recognize impairments of inhibition disinhibition modulation typically requires a multi-faceted approach. One strategy which we have found helpful involves educating the patient about the consequences of brain injury with regard to information processing capacity and subsequent adaptive arousal states. We have typically been able to find real life examples for each patient where they were not able to process all of the information impinging upon them and then elucidate their response, either inhibition (withdrawal) or disinhibition (hyperarousal). After providing some basic information to one particular head injury patient about the limiting effects on information processing of head injury, she inquired as to whether or not this might be related to why she could not talk to her husband while he was washing the dishes. This served as a perfect example, as her husband could not understand why, when they were talking in the kitchen, his wife always seemed to become angry. It seems probable that the verbal stimulation of conversation in addition to the visual-auditory stimulation of his washing the dishes was, collectively, more than the patient could adequately process. Her anger response may have, therefore, reflected a disinhibition of arousal mechanisms. It was frequently the case however that her arousal was excessive resulting in a heated argument and more stimulation, again, than she could adequately process. Finally, she would often then inhibit, resulting in non-communicative withdrawal, confusion and self-derogatory beliefs, when she was no longer able to even approximate a meaningful assimilation of the information. For patients unable to associate the educational information regarding the consequences of brain injury (explained, of course, in very simple and basic terms), the use of in vivo situations may be helpful. We have at times purposely over-stimulated patients with complex information so as to tax their information processing capability, and to point out at the time the effect on arousal states. The use of video-taping the in vivo experiment as well as providing systematic feedback regarding level of arousal through biofeedback instrumentation may also be quite educational. Once the patient has become aware that they have difficulty in processing information and modulating and attaining optimum levels of arousal, the intervention then needs to concern itself with a maintenance of this awareness and development of self-monitoring strategies.

Teaching head injury patients to self-regulate on an inhibition-disinhibition dimension may represent one of the most significant concerns of rehabilitation, expecially with respect to long term social adaptation. However, it may be the case that for many of the acute or post-acute severely injured patients, these strategies of intervention will not be possible. In this case, it will be necessary for the external environment to monitor the patient and provide very direct, simple feedback to the patient as to appropriate responses. Specifically, when a patient becomes excessively inhibited or disinhibited it would be appropriate for a responsible person to direct the patient to "relax for a moment, close your eyes if you want and calm down" when he or she becomes or better yet, is becoming disinhibited. A short and soft, but direct, statement is typically best with the suggestion to limit (closing one's eyes) informational stimuli. In the case of prolonged inhibition responses, the environment should provide an increase in the intensity and amount of information and attempt to facilitate arousal, perhaps by talking about something which is known to be relatively affectively-laden for the patient. These patients who cannot internally modulate, however, their level of arousal may benefit from the use of central stimulant drugs (Trexler, in preparation).

Teaching families the basic information processing-arousal mechanisms associated with traumatic head injury, as well as suggestions for intervention, may prevent or minimize the degree of secondary familial emotional disturbance typically encountered post-hospitilization. Initially, traumatic head injury patients require external cueing to elicit a self-monitoring response. Further, those patients with severe memory dysfunction may require prompting as to what exactly it is that they are to self-monitor. To address this latter problem, it would be appropriate to have the patient write (if possible) on either a sheet of paper, or better, on a frequently visible poster that he is to (1) stop what he is doing, (2) ask himself if he understands what is transpiring in his environment, and, if possible, (3) evaluate his level of arousal. Patients sometimes find useful the Subjective Units of Distress Scale (Wolpe, 1973), where they are to rate on a scale from zero to 100, zero being no distress at all, their general level of distress. Providing the patient with a folder, with basic information as to exactly what they are to self-monitor, Subjective Units of Distress Scale rating forms, and paper for diary notes as to what was going on in their environment resulting in inhibition or disinhibition can be very helpful.

The stimulus cueing of self-monitoring behavior can be achieved through a number of means, depending upon the patient's environmental circumstances. Initially, it will be necessary for nursing staff or family members to remind the patient to self-monitor. Further, pairing self-monitoring behavior with behaviors which are frequent and routine such as eating, taking medication or going to therapy may be helpful to strengthen the probability of self-monitoring behavior. We have sometimes used brightly colored self-adhesive file dots affixed on the patient's watch to serve as reminders to self-monitor information processing capacity and level of arousal. For those patients with severe memory deficits, it will be necessary for them to overlearn what these stimulus cues are reminding them to do. In general, however, those considerations of self-monitoring as outlined by Mahoney and Arnkoff (1978) and Hollon (1981) should be addressed. The use of self-instructional training (Meichenbaum, 1977; Wilson, 1978) and inoculation training paradigms (Meichenbaum and Novaco, 1978) are also highly recommended as strategies to teach patients the maintenance of self-control behaviors, for those patients who are capable of processing relatively complex information.

Those patients who can learn to self-monitor can benefit from several specific interventive strategies, with the goal of training skills and abilities to replace marked inhibition-disinhibition responses. Inoculation paradigms have already been mentioned (Meichenbaum and Novaco, 1978) and incorporates (1) the anticipation of environmental conditions which have historically elicited particularly disinhibition and (2) self-control responses like self-induced relaxation. The use of relaxation training, perhaps biofeedback-assisted, is therefore appropriate as an interventive strategy for disinhibition disorders. The critical concern however involves teaching the patient to identify the occasions when the skills derived through relaxation or biofeedback training are applicable. The identification of those situations should be learned during the self-monitoring phase of intervention. Systematic desensitization procedures (as reviewed by Murray and Jacobson, 1978) are applicable for expecially patients with over-learned disinhibition responses to specific arousal-inducing stimulus conditions. Direct and in vivo modeling techniques (Barrios, Cox and Trexler, 1982) may also be of considerable import in providing the traumatically brain injured patient with a more adaptive skill repertoire. Procedures to facilitate arousal and directly address inhibition of information processing and arousal have not historically been of clinical concern and there is therefore little literature concerning this topic. Patient's with hypoarousal can sometimes be prompted to increase arousal by using more direct, intense stimuli. Interventive strategies concerned with facilitating arousal in the traumatically head injured population with deficits in modulating arousal need to be developed and researched.

### Stimulus Bound - Distractible Dimension

This dimension of cognitive-affective behavior refers to more subtle behavioral disturbances than in the case of the inhibition-disinhibition dimension and concerns, primarily, dysfunction of especially selective attention or attention shifting mechanisms. Stimulus bound behavior represents one end of a continuum of behaviors which can be characterized by an inability to shift attention from either one particular stimuli or from one feature of a complex stimuli. Stimulus bound behavior can further be described as an impairment of what might be referred to as contextual attention, a dynamic interchange between attentional focusing on relevant and ignoring of irrelevant stimuli as a function of the saliency of the stimuli (in context of its spatial and temporal environment) and the organism's general state. Stimulus bound behaviors are typcially evoked automatically, that is, without conscious premeditation or planning. As a consequence, many observed stimulus bound behaviors characteristic of traumatic head injury represent overlearned, frequently repeated behavioral patterns and tend to occur only in the presence of the conditioned stimulus. Further, these stimuli can be either external or internal (e.g., thoughts, feelings). Perseveration therefore represents one class of stimulus bound behavior, typically elicited by internal cues. These behaviors seem impervious to habituation.

Distractible behavior conversely relates to an inability to focus attention on any one stimulus and appears to reflect undiffern-tiated and unselective orienting responses. At this end of the continuum, distractible behavior can be characterized by an indiscriminant attentional effort (as conceptualized by Moscovitch, 1979) where irrelevant stimuli may elicit the same attentional effort, quantitatively, as does relevant stimuli. As suggested earlier, impairments of selectivity of attentional effort may occur as a function of interference (which can most likely be temporal in nature) and expectancy effects. The importance of expectancy effects are obviated by the traumatically head injured patients' propensity to act before they have received all of the instructions or relevant information (impulsivity) and to perseverate, behaviorally, when external situations do not recapitulate what they expect. In contrast to stimulus bound behavior, distractible behavior is characterized by premature habituation, if it occurs at all.

Stimulus bound and distractible cognitive-affective behaviors both impair learning, and as a consequence patients with impairment on this dimension have difficulty in generating alternate response sets and benefiting from environmentally provided feedback. Affective behavior is often impaired as resultant from stimulus bound and/or distractible behaviors. Patients with difficulties in shifting attention processes or in contextual attention typically, as a compensatory strategy, develop what appear to be very rigid and obsessive-compulsive behavioral patterns. Any alteration in physical setting, sequence or situational variable often elicits anger or irritability for patients with either stimulus bound or distractible behavior. This response may result from an increase in arousal, as described in the inhibition-disinhibition dimension, so as to facilitate information processing and attentional shifting. Continued distractibility seems to also be associated with chronic anxiety.

Many patients appear to become quite stimulus bound with regard to negative physical consequences of their injuries. In addition to frequently perseverating about scars, motor impairment or minor difficulties with language (these deficits are prototypically of much less significance that the patient's degree of cognitive impairment), the perseverative thoughts are often quite self-depreciatory, lending to chronic anxiety states, depression and a serious compromise of self-concept. The extent to which these latter emotional states arise from cognitive-affective changes or from post-injury social learning is difficult to differentiate and a matter for future clinical investigation. It is certainly the case, nonetheless, that patients who continue to perseverate on either topics which are associated with relatively high levels of arousal and on overlearned behavioral repertoires do not elicit consistent positive reinforcement from their environment. A particular patient on our inpatient rehabilitation unit would ask the nursing staff every five minutes whether or not he could call his mother, which happened to be a toll call. This desire to call home appeared to be motivated by a feeling of anxiety in being separated by a considerable distance, from his family. It was frequently the case that when the nursing staff would discourage his request he would become irritable, fail to appreciate the reasoning as to why he could not call every five minutes, and on one occasion became disinhibited-aggressive, threatening and confused. The rigidity in response set (calling home) to alleviate anxiety was impervious to habituation. In this case it appeared that the stimuli which elicited a stimulus bound response were internal in nature (anxiety and fear), overlearned (historically typical for this patient) and not amenable to feedback. As might be expected, nurses did not treasure the opportunity to care for or be around him. Perhaps it was the case that this relatively covert social rejection increased his need to call home and precipitated depression (manifested by spontaneous frequent crying). It should also be noted that this particular patient oscillated between stimulus bound and distractible behaviors, the former typically emotional in content.

Patients who exhibit persisting stimulus bound behavior do not at least in the present author's experience, typically have great difficulty in recognizing their propensity to perseverate, but are typically not aware that they are stimulus bound. As a consequence, some of the same interventive strategies described in the inhibition-disinhibition dimension for increasing awareness and recognition of deficits can be used. Further, it is very difficult to teach patients to self-monitor stimulus bound behavior. As a consequence we have tended to utilize direct interventive strategies.

Regardless or whether or not the behavior under question is highly affective or not, exercises oriented at developing patient skills in alternative response generation may be helpful. This exercise typically involves asking the patient to write down or verbalize as many alternative responses (responses other than those on which they have been perseverating), with or without prompting, to a given situation as possible. Based upon this list, then, the patient is to choose the response he thinks would be most adaptive and why.

This type of intervention may work most optimally in a group setting. This approach optimally modifies some of the historically reinforced cognitive expectancy effects. Teaching stimulus bound patients to generate alternative responses when the content is highly affective most likely requires some relaxation training as well. Cognitive rehabilitative training (especially as discussed by Gross in Chapter 6 of the present volume) oriented at facilitating attention shifting is critical. Providing succinct feedback which is not overly complex and in a manner which is compatible with the patient's information processing capability may similarly be important. Further, the way in which patients process feedback should be validated through questioning, as many patients with stimulus bound-distractible cognitive-affective disturbances misperceive feedback and miss the most critical and salient components of feedback. All of this to say that we should be quite explicit in giving feedback and confirm with the patient his interpretation of that feedback.

Interventive strategies for disorders at the distractible end of this continuum should, again, address the three components previously described including (1) developing an awareness or recognition of the disorder, (2) self-monitoring strategies and (3) direct training to develope skills, abilities or compensatory behaviors. Supportive confrontation is typically sufficient for relatively distractible patients to become aware of their inability to focus attention on any one task or stimulus although this, in most cases, requires repetition. Further, overtly illustrating performance decrements on tasks on which they attended poorly relative to tasks on which they attended well is sometimes helpful. Self-monitoring of distractibility can be achieved through several strategies, although they require an informed and cooperative staff. As highly distractible patients are quite vulnerable to the effects of interference, staff conversation with the patient should be short and succinct, followed by an inquiry of the patient as to the reason, meaning or purpose for the communication or conversation. Only after each portion or significant component of the conversation has been fully processed should the conversation continue. In this context, it is of course appropriate to eliminate as many of the distracing stimuli as possible. Through tracking each portion of verbal discourse, patients often recognize that they have difficulty with attending and discoursing. Engaging in structured conversation and clarifying each salient component of the conversation serves as an externally facilitated monitoring strategy. Systematically and repetitively conversing in this manner may decrease distractibility. Another strategy which has been clinically useful involves teaching the patient to ask a question (the content, although not the appropriateness, is irrelevant) whenever he enounters a staff person. If the patient does not spontaneously ask a question, he is reminded to do so. The extent to which the staff person's response was processed by the patient can then be validated using the above described form of structured conversation. Finally, as most highly distractible patients have difficulty in finding words, it is often helpful to use verbal prompting and then have them repeat the sentence, including the word(s) which were prompted. This latter strategy may help the patient more clearly identify his thought in its totality and not lose his sequence of thoughts due to a word finding deficit.

Interventive strategies concerned with alleviating distractibility should probably begin with techniques oriented at lengthening span of attention for configurally simple stimuli; which modality of senory stimuli depends upon the patient. As span of attention increases, it may then be appropriate to increase the complexity of the presented stimuli and to include a component of attention focusing in context of distracting stimuli. Again, some of the procedures outlined by Gross in Chapter 6 of the present volume have been found to be clinically useful. In our laboratory we have also found the use of a custom programmed micro-computer to be useful in treating attentional deficits. Finally, preliminary evidence suggests that central stimulants reduce distractibility in highly distractible patients (Trexler, in preparation).

As can be seen from the above described interventive strategies, they do not appear to be highly "affective" in content. However, these suggested approaches to the treatment of stimulus bound-distractible dimension disorders are applicable to situations which are quite emotional in nature as well. In fact, it is probable that patients with marked dysfunction on this dimension evidence their difficulties the most when the content of their verbal behavior is affective in content. It may therefore be clinically appropriate to utilize some of the strategies outlined in the inhibition-disinhibition dimension (e.g., relaxation training). It is assumed however, that much of the affective components of these cognitive-affective deficits are secondary to an impairment of cognitive (attentional) processes.

In summary, the inhibition-disinhibition and stimulus bound-distractible dimensions may provide a crude taxonomy of cognitive-affective disorders in closed head injury. They are based on a review of the neurophysiological mechanisms mediating arousal, attention and emotions and clinical observations of patients with traumatic head injury. The described strategies of intervention are obviously tentative. It was the intent of the present chapter to provide a conceptualization of cognitive-affective disorders from which the reader can design and implement treatment approaches which are ideosyncratically meaningful, as compared to a "cookbook" of techniques which would likely not fit the dynamic and interrelated processes characteristically impaired by traumatic head injury.

REFERENCES

Barrios, F.X., Cox, M.D. and Trexler, L.E. Behavior therapies. In: H.S. Moffic and G.L. Adams (Eds.), A clinician's manual on mental health care: A multidisciplinary approach. Menlo Park: Addison-Wesley, 1982.

Battig, W.F. The flexibility of human memory. In: L.S. Cermak and F.I. Craik (Eds.), Levels of processing in human memory. Hillsdale, New Jersey: Lawrence Erlbaum, 1979.

Brady, J.V. and Nauta, W.J. Subcortical mechanisms in emotional behavior: Affective changes following septal forebrain lesions in the albino rat. Journal of Comparative Physiology and Psychology, 1953, 46, 339-346.

Brodal, A. Neurological anatomy: In relation to clinical medicine, Third edition. Oxford: Oxford University Press, 1981.

Epstein, A.N. Reciprocal changes in feeding behavior produced by intrahypothalamic chemical injections. American Journal of Physiology, 1960, 199, 969-974.

Gastaut, H. The role of the reticular formation in establishing conditioned reactions. In: H.H. Jasper, L.C. Proctor, R.S. Knighton, W.C. Noshay and R.T. Costello (Eds.), The reticular formation of the brain. Boston: Little, Brown, 1958.

Green, J.D. and Arduini, A. Hippocampal electrical activity in arousal. Journal of Neurophysiology, 1954, 17, 533-557.

Haggard, M.P. and Parkinson, A.M. Stimulus and task factors as determinants of ear advantages. Quarterly Journal of Experimental Psychology, 1971, 23, 168-177.

Heilman, K.M., Schwartz, H.D. and Watson, R.T. Hypoarousal in patients with the neglect syndrome and emotional indifference. Neurology, 1978, 28, 229-232.

Hicks, R.E. Introhemispheric response competition between vocal and unimanual performance in normal adult human males. Journal of Comparative and Physiological Psychology, 1975, 14, 23-33.

Hollon, S.D. Cognitive-behavioral treatment of drug-induced pansituational anxiety states. In: G. Emery, S. Hollon, and R. Bedrosian (Eds.), New directions in cognitive therapy: A casebook. New York: Guilford Press, 1981.

Holloway, F.A. and Parsons, D.A. Unilateral brain damage and bilateral skin conductance levels in humans. Psychophysiology, 1969, 6, 138-148.

Hubel, D.H. and Wiesel, T.N. Receptive fields, binocular interaction and functional architecture in the cat's visual cortex. Journal of Physiology, 1962, 160, 106-154.

Hubel, D.H. and Wiesel, T.N. Receptive fields of cells in striate cortex of very young, visually inexperienced kittens. Journal of Neurophysiology, 1963, 26, 994-1002.

Jacoby, L.L. and Craik, F.I. Effects of elaboration of processing at encoding and retrieval: Trace distinctiveness and recovery of initial context. In: L.S. Cermak and F.I. Craik (Eds.), Levels of processing in human memory. Hillsdale, New Jersey: Lawrence Erlbaum, 1979.

Jasper, H.H., Naquet, R. and King, E.E. Thalamocortical recruiting responses in sensory receiving areas in the cat. Electroencephalography and Clinical Neurophysiology, 1955, 7, 99-114.

Kessler, M.M. Spontaneous and reflex emotional responses differentiated by lesions in the diencephalon. Proceedings of the Society for Experimental Biology and Medicine, 1941, 47, 225-227.

Kimura, D. Manual activity during speaking. I. Right-handers. Neuropsychologia, 1973, 11, 45-50.

Kinsbourne, M. Eye and head turning indicates cerebral lateralization. Science, 1972, 176, 539-541.

Klein, D. Moscovitch, M. and Vigna, C. Attentional mechanisms and perceptual asymmetries in tachistoscopic recognition of words and faces. Neuropsychologia, 1976, 14, 55-66.

Lindsley, D.B., Bowden, J.W. and Magoun, H.W. Effect upon the EEG of acute injury to the brainstem activating system. Electroencephalography and Clinical Neurophysiology, 1949, 1, 475-486.

Lomas, J. and Kimura, D. Intra-hemispheric interaction between speaking and sequential manual activity. Neuropsychologia, 1976, 14, 23-33.

Luria, A.R. The working brain. Middlesex, England: Penguin Press, 1973.

Luria, A.R. Higher cortical functions in man, Second edition. New York: Basic Books, 1980.

Mahoney, M.J. and Arnkoff, D. Cognitive and self-control therapies. In: S.L. Garfield and A.E. Bergin (Eds.), Handbook of psychotherapy and behavior change: An empirical analysis, Second edition, New York: John Wiley, 1978.

Meichenbaum, D. The nature of internal dialogue - foundations of a theory of behavior change. In: Cognitive behavior modification: An integrative approach. New York: Plenum Press, 1977.

Meichenbaum, D. and Novaco, R. Stress inoculation: A preventative approach. In: Spielberger and Sarason (Eds.), Stress and anxiety, Volume 5. Washington: Hemisphere Publishing Corp., 1978.

Morrow, L., Vrturski, B., Kim, Y. and Boller, F. Arousal response to emotional stimuli and laterality of lesion. Neuropsychologia, 1981, 19, 65-71.

Moscovitch, M. Information processing and the cerebral hemispheres. In: M.S. Gazzaniga (Ed.), Handbook of behavioral neurobiology: Volume 2 on neuropsychology. New York: Plenum Press, 1979.

Murray, E.J. and Jacobson, L.I. Cognition and learning in traditional and behavioral therapy. In: S.L. Garfield and A.E. Bergin (Eds.), Handbook of psychotherapy and behavior change: An empirical analysis, Second edition. New York: John Wiley, 1978.

Penfield, W. and Milner, B. Memory deficit produced by bilateral lesions in the hippocampal zone. Archives of Neurology and Psychiatry, 1958, 79, 475-497.

Pribram, K.H. The primate frontal cortex - executive of the brain. In: K.H. Pribram and A.R. Luria (Eds.), Psychophysiology of the frontal lobes. New York: Academic Press, 1973.

Rickles, W.H. Central nervous system substrates of some psychophysiological variables. In: N.S. Greenfield and R.A. Sternback (Eds.), Handbook of psycholophysiology. New York: Holt, Rhinehart and Winston, 1972.

Scheibel, M.E. and Scheibel, A.B. Structural organization of nonspecific thalamic nuclei and their projection toward the cortex. Brain Research, 1967, 6, 60-94.

Thatcher, R.W. and John, E.R. Foundations of cognitive processes. Hillsdale, New Jersey: Lawrence Erlbaum, 1977.

Trexler, L.E. The effects of central stimulants on behavioral, psychophysiological and psychometric parameters of arousal and attention in traumatic head injury: Three case studies. Manuscript in preparation.

Trexler, L.E. and Schmidt, N.S. The treatment of the emotional consequences of brain injury: Arousal responses and perception of complex affective stimuli. Paper presented at the European Meetings of the International Neuropsychological Society, Bergen, 1981.

Tucker, D., Watson, R.T. and Heilman, K.M. Affective discrimination and evocation in patients with right parietal disease. Neurology, 1977, 27, 947-950.

Valenstein, E. and Heilman, K.M. Emotional disorders resulting from lesions of the central nervous system. In: K.M. Heilman and E. Valenstein (Eds.), Clinical neuropsychology. New York: Oxford University Press, 1979.

Walley, R.E. and Weiden, T.D. Lateral inhibition and cognitive masking: A neuropsychological theory of attention. Psychological Review, 1973, 80, 284-302.

Wheatley, M.D. The hypothalamus and affective behavior in cats. Archives of Neurology and Psychiatry, 1944, 52, 296-316.

Wilson, G.T. Cognitive behavior therapy: Paradigm shift or passing phase? In: J.P. Foreyt and D.P. Rathjen (Eds.), Cognitive behavior therapy: Research and application. New York: Plenum Press, 1978.

Wolpe, J. The practice of behavior therapy. Oxford: Pergamon Press, 1973.

Woods, J.W. Taming of the wild Norway rat by rhinocephalic lesions. Nature, 1956, 170, 869.

## CONCLUDING REMARKS

Lance E. Trexler, Ph.D.

Coordinator, Neuropsychology Service
Medical Psychology Department
Community Hospital of Indianapolis

In the foregoing section a diversity of conceptualizations regarding the structural and organizational nature of brain behavior correlates, the associated effects of cerebral insult and the relevant implications for treatment are presented. The commonalities and differences reflect the complexity of the topic at hand as well as our relatively primitive state of the art. This section obviates an exploratory epoch in the pursuit of knowledge concerning the nature of cognition, the cerebral and environmental determinants, and the effect of damage to the central nervous system (CNS). A thorough reading of the foregoing section leaves one wondering if (1) the authors were addressing the same organism and the same functional repertoire of the CNS, (2) the topic at hand entails such complexity that varying perspectives are possible, or (3) both. These disparate analyses should not serve to predicate pessimism, however. Rather, the content of this section may be seen as a conceptual foundation for many lifetime's of investigation and collectively may represent a whole meritorious of thought provocation. If there were only one opinion on the nature of cognition, and its dysfunction, we run the risk of not knowing what we don't know. Further, it is assumed that each of the authors believe that their conceptualization and ensuing treatment efforts have resulted in some desireable effect on patients with cerebral dynsfunction which is, in and of itself, of import.

There are several issues which I perceive to be critical in the analysis of conceptualizing cognitive rehabilitation on which the foregoing chapters can be compared. The first issue concerns the model of cognition, its normal and abnormal derivations, and, again, its relevance for the treatment of cognitive impairment following brain insult. Secondly is the issue of the scope of cognition. Essentially, this issue concerns a definition of cognition and to what extent cognition relates to cerebral functioning, in toto. Thirdly, the model, within a certain circumscribed scope, of cognitive functioning is a critical issue, where cognitive functions may be viewed as (1) hierarchial in nature with certain more basic cognitive functions requisite to "higher-order" cognition and to some extent localizable in the CNS or as (2) essentially non-localizable and comprised of non-reducible processes which dynamically interrelate.

The extent to which models of normal cognitive functioning resemble models of abnormal cognition may be questionable. On one hand we can utilize a subtractive approach to understanding the consequences of brain injury, where the organization of brain behavior relationships is preserved less some circumscribed neuropsychological function. This appears to be the position of Craine, although he talks in Principle Six about "a process through which a brain-damaged patient learns how to learn." How, in Craine's conceptual formulation, neurotraining addresses these impaired cognitive processes is not obvious, however. Further, the approach offered by Craine seems to argue against dynamic formulations of cognition in considering his emphasis on deficit-specific training and habituation through repetition. Rather, the conceptualization advanced by Craine can be viewed as an atheoretical behavioral approach to modifying deficits in cognitive functioning in context of intact or normal cerebral functions. The conceptualization offered by Piasetsky and his colleagues is different from that of Craine in that (1) it is not atheoretical and (2) it articulates a developmental, reductionistic formulation of brain behavior operations. Nonetheless, the conceptualization provided by Piasetsky et al., is decidedly compartmentalizing, although the scope of his models must be taken into account. It is not explicit, however, in the case of Craine or Piasetsky et al., what is "cognitive" and what is not. In marked contrast are the formulations of Gross. His conceptualizations address the integrative and synthetic aspects of cerebral processes, while acknowledging specific deficits. Nonetheless, the chapter presented by Gross eloquently captures the behavior prototypical of patients with cerebral injuries and provides some framework for understanding their cognitive dysfunctional processes. While the concepts of the organic syndrome and the concretic personality are somewhat tentative and globally descriptive, Grosse's analysis is unique in that it provides an understanding of abnormal cognition as opposed to normal cognition. As suggested by Lurian formulations, insult to the central nervous system may force a re-organization of all brain behavior processes in context of an impairment of specific and circumscribed functional repertoires, not merely a loss of behavioral routines localizable to those areas damaged. Hagan also points to a general disorganizaton of cognitive processing which subsumes language. It appears that on one hand we have Craine and to some extent Piasetsky concerned with essentially reductionistic aspects of central processes and Gross and Hagan providing a conceptualization much more dynamic and integrative in nature. Obviously, empirical research validating either view is absent.

These diverging views may in fact be related to the scope of brain behavior correlates subsumed by cognition. Hagan clearly states, at least in the case of traumatic brain injury, that impairment of language is typically secondary to a dysfunction of cognitive processes, although may be accompanied by specific dysphasic symptomatology. This suggests therefore that he is viewing cognition as a more general set of cerebral processes related to language functioning. Similarly, Meeder relates perceptual motor functions to cognition. Her inclusion of empirically acquired data represents a decided asset to the present volume, although the interrelatedness of cognitive processes and perceptual motor functions was not explicitly addressed. Hagan acknowledges a co-existence of language-cognitive disorganization and the interrelatedness for cognitive-perceptual motor functions may, through a reading of Meeder, be assumed. Finally, Trexler has attempted to relate cognition to affect. Collectively, the foregoing chapters suggest that cognitive processes are, in scope, related to language, perceptual motor and emotional components of brain behavior mechanisms. This is obviously affected by one's definition of cognition. Nonetheless, these chapters are suggestive of, at a minimum, an interrelatedness between cerebral processes, which may argue against compartmentalizing any one set of cerebral functions, both conceptually and therapeutically. In this context, cognition is typically thought to represent processes which are "higher-order" relative to other more basic, presumably less conscious, cerebral functions. However, the content of the foregoing chapters argue against this notion, where in contrast, cognitive processing appears to be integral to all "levels" as well as to a wide scope, in terms of content, of CNS activity. It can be concluded, however, that when embarking upon cognitive rehabilitation, what one rehabilitates is a matter of conceptual definition and scope.

The third issue which permeates these chapters concerns, as previously mentioned, the organization of cognitive processes, and the concomitant implications for intervention. With the exception of Gross, there is the explicit assumption that there is a hierarchy of cognitive functions which may or may not be related to their developmental acquisition. This assumption is also related to the simplicity and complexity of brain behavior functions, where "higher-order", more complex functions at the apex of a hierarchy. These hierarchial models appear to be static however, as if cognitive processes did not occur over time, nor do they articulate how compartments (assumably localizable functions) interrelate throughout the course of cognitive processing. On the other hand, the very dynamic model of Gross does not explicitly address the content of processing, the incorporation of specific and circumscribed neuropsychological deficits. In this context, it was obvious throughout the chapter by Trexler that, at least with respect to arousal and attentional mechanisms, phylogenetically "higher" centers of the CNS modulated the activity of "lower" centers, but that "lower" centers provided the information to "higher" centers for modulation.

Consequently, a reciprocal interaction between levels of processing, in space and time, was suggested. It would seem appropriate that further conceptual efforts attempt to integrate the hierarchial-static and the process-dynamic models.

In considering how we conceptualize what we are treating, I think that it is critical that we ask ourselves whether or not we are thinking of normal cognition or abnormal cognition. Further, if we are thinking of abnormal cognition, the research by Thomas and Trexler as presented in Chapter 3 should be considered, where it was suggested that models of abnormal cognition may be different for different diagnostic groups. In other words, the impaired functions and processes typical of, for example, closed head injury may not resemble those characteristic of cerebrovascular accident. These considerations I believe represent a significant empirical challenge.

# PART III: INTERVENTIVE STRATEGIES

# THE SYSTEMATIC REMEDIATION OF SPECIFIC DISORDERS: SELECTED APPLICATION OF METHODS DERIVED IN A CLINICAL RESEARCH SETTING[1]

Eugene B. Piasetsky, Ph.D., Yehuda Ben-Yishay, Ph.D., Joseph Weinberg, M.A., and, Leonard Diller, Ph.D.

The Institute of Rehabilitation Medicine
N.Y.U. Medical Center, N.Y.

The ultimate goal of rehabilitation is to maximize the patient's ability to function within a normal environment. Cognitive rehabilitation is a major component of this effort. Among the many disabilities which may befall an individual, disturbances in thinking, perceiving and acting are among the most confining. Research in cognitive rehabilitation may be seen as addressing these problems at two levels: 1) seeking methods by which to remediate primary cognitive domains so as to promote the broadest basis for independent functioning; and, 2) seeking methods by which to remediate the functional foundations of important activities of everyday life so as to enhance the individual's sense of personal satisfaction and allow him to experience a productive lifestyle. As scientists, we are inexorably drawn to seek out, understand and influence the primary processes which govern human behavior. As clinicians, we are governed by the mandate to apply our knowledge in order to best serve our patient's needs. These seemingly obliquely related directives, when blended together, form the logic underlying a unified research effort. The two training programs I will be describing illustrate this point. They represent diverse orientations to the problem of cognitive rehabilitation, owing, in large part, to the unique characteristics of impairment associated with the patient populations addressed. Ultimately, both converge in terms of principle objective. The

[1] The preparation of this paper and the research cited therein were supported in part by grant 10236-08-N1NCDS and the designation of the Institute of Rehabilitation Medicine, New York University Medical Center, as a rehabilitation research and training center by the National Institute of Handicapped Research (RT-1/RD92, 93).

first program was initiated in response to a need manifested in distubances in specific behaviors among right brain-damaged patients in a rehabilitation setting. The second program was initiated in response to an observed deficiency among traumatic head-injured patients in the basic mediation of an interchange with the environment. The first, then, began with specific behavioral objectives in view, while the second sought to provide patients with the basic means through which behavioral objectives might ultimately be addressed.

Despite the differences in initial orientation of the two programs, the design of each reflects the application of a standard and systematic developmental logic (Diller, 1976). Once the problem has been defined it is operationalized into a set of representative tasks. A set of training principles is developed by defining those stimulus and response properties which influence patients' performance. Finally, the training principles are expressed in terms of systematic and graded "cuing" procedures, through which training will be effected. The specific manner in which training is to be applied is, finally, determined in consideration of the special clinical needs of the patient population addressed. Evaluating the efficacy of treatment is planned so as to be consistent with the broad-based objectives of the rehabilitation process.

## TREATING PERCEPTUAL DISORDERS IN RIGHT BRAIN-DAMAGED (RBD) STROKE PATIENTS

The treatment program was developed in a series of clinical research studies conducted over a period of 10 years at the Institute of Rehabilitation Medicine. It addresses a range of perceptual problems commonly associated with damage to the right cerebral hemisphere and attributable, in large part, to an underlying disorder in spatial attention and visual scanning (Diller, Ben-Yishay, Gerstman, Goodkin, Gordon and Weinberg, 1974). The primary syndrome associated with perceptual problems in RBD patients has alternatively been labelled unilateral neglect of space or hemi-inattention. It is principally characterized by a marked propensity to ignore information arising from the left side of space. In studying the problem, Diller et al. (1974) found that neglect *per se* was only one of the anomalies of visual behavior which characterized perceptually impaired patients. Employing a pair of letter cancellation tasks, they identified three characteristics of impaired performance which a remediation program needed to address: 1) *Visual neglect*, as evidenced in a tendency to begin cancelling targets on each line of print at some point other than the left-most margin; 2) *Erractic and errored scanning*, as evidenced in a tendency to skip over segments along each line, cancelling targets which were spaced relatively far apart while missing those in-between; 3) *An excessively fast rate of performance*, evidenced within the context

in order to help the patient recognize a common basis for what he may well be experiencing as a multitude of separate functional losses. In addition, some simple procedures have been devised to provide patients with objective evidence of their problem while simultaneously demonstrating the potential remedial value of the training (Weinberg and Diller, 1977). One procedure is to lay out an assortment of coins and bills in a semi-circle in front of the patient. The patient is instructed to pick up the money and hand it to the trainer. Invariably, the patient will fail to pick up the money which was situated to his or her left. The trainer then instructs the patient to turn his head to the left. In doing so, the patient discovers the money he neglected and is introduced to a manner of searching the environment which yields success. The use of "discovery" as a tool for fostering awareness is repeatedly employed throughout the training. In doing so, the patient develops and maintains the necessary motivational impetus for active participation in the training. Without this, little in the way of meaningful learning will take place.

The first goal is to cause the patient to look towards the neglected side and establish this behavior as a pre-requisite to scanning the environment. An apparatus (the "scanning machine") was devised to facilitate the accomplishment of this goal. The apparatus consists of a black elongated oval board (78 inches long and 8 inches wide) studded with two rows of ten colored lights and affixed with a target which traverses its periphery. Activation of lights and movement of the target is controlled on a separate panel monitored by the trainer. The target may be moved through a continuous range of speeds and the lights may be activated singly or in pairs, and in any desired sequence. In training, the scanning machine is employed in several ways:

1) Compensating for visual neglect: Establishing a left-field anchor. The patient is positioned directly in front of (at a distance of from 35 to 55 inches) and centered on the apparatus. The target is initially centered and the patient acknowledges seeing the target by pointing to it. The patient is instructed to follow the target as it traverses slowly into the neglected field. Head movements are encouraged in the early stages to maximize teaching but are to be phased out as the training progresses. This procedure is repeated over a 10-15 minute period each day, steadily increasing the depth of penetration of the neglected field. Individual light targets may be illuminated for the patient to "discover", providing him with feedback as to his progress and serving as external anchors for directing his gaze. Once the patient is able to consistently follow the moving target to the left-most edge of the apparatus, it is stabilized in that position and becomes an anchor point for the second application of the "scanning machine";

2) Searching (Gross Scanning). The trainer activates the

colored lights and instructs the patient to scan the apparatus and identify how many and/or which lights have been illuminated. The patient's behavior is monitored in two ways: a) all scanning trials must be initiated by locating the stabilized target anchor; and, b) the scanning sequence (i.e., reporting of targets) must be performed in a left-to-right direction. If the patient hesitates at the beginning of a training trial, he is provided with a "sharp" "alerting" cue of "look left".

3) Tracking. This exercise involves the use of the moving target. The patient practices following the target across the top of the machine, in both a left-to-right and a righ-to-left direction. The trainer monitors where the patient is looking during the exercise so as to offer immediate cues at the first sign of "jerky" movements or "wandering".

As the patient comes to master the principles of anchoring to the left side and scanning from left-to-right, the patient is trained to transfer these principles to paper and pencil tasks. This next phase of training serves to further improve the patient's scanning abilities and prepare the patient to apply these abilities to reading (Weinberg, Diller, Gordon, Gertsman, Lieberman, Lakin, Hodges and Ezrachi, 1977). In conjunction with continued practice on the "scanning machine", the patient is trained to systematically scan and cancel targets on a numerical analog of the visual cancellation task. Initially, the patient is provided with a maximum of external cues by which to guide his scanning. A bold red vertical line is drawn on the left margin of the cancellation form and is established by the trainer as a scanning anchor. If needed, red numbers are placed to the left and right of each line of targets to serve as additional anchors. In practicing the principles of scanning on this task, patients' tendency work too rapidly is highlighted in so far as it manifestly interferes with their ability to meet the more discrete scanning demands of the task. Training in cancellation focuses on two issues: 1) That the patient begin each scan by finding the left-most border and proceed from left-to-right; and, 2) that he scan each target individually at an even and appropriate pace. Simply telling the patient that they are moving too fast has no effect. Instead, a steady pacing rate is established by having the patient call out each number as it appears in sequence on the line of print. As soon as the patient skips a number, he is brought back to it. Calling out numbers may also be combined with placing a small dot beneath each number, intensifying the patient's active participation in the training exercise. As the patient becomes more proficient in his scanning on this task, both the anchoring and the pacing cues are systematically removed (faded). Finally, the patient practices scanning without the benefit of cues. The final step in this training sequence is to apply the skills learned in performing the cancellation exercises to reading. Using paragraphs of varying length, selected from large print and regular print N.Y. Times and Reader's Digest, the patient is practiced at systematically scanning each line of print. Anchoring cues are provided and, with the patient reading aloud, pacing may be monitored. As was the case in the cancellation exercises, maximum cuing (red line and numerical anchors) is provided initially and is then systematically removed.

Training in sensory awareness and spatial organization (VIP II). Training patients to compensate for visual neglect and to scan their visual environment amelilorated some of their visual-perceptual problems. However, while their performance on a number of visual tasks improved (most notably those related to academic performance), performance on others was unaffected (Weinberg et al., 1977). Included among those tasks on which patients failed to improve, was the bisection of lines. It was also observed that, while patients no longer evidenced a gross disturbance in visual exploration and scanning, they continued to exhibit a lateral distortion in where they located their body midline. In recognition of the presumed importance of body reference in making spatial judgments, a training package was designed to address this issue (Weinberg, Diller, Gordon, Gerstman, Lieberman, Lakin, Hodges and Ezrachi, 1979).

Training in sensory awareness is directed at re-aligning the patient's somatosensory reference (body space) and re-coordinating the referential relationship between body space and extra-personal visual space. This establishes the foundation for remediating problems in spatial organization. Training in spatial organization is directed at teaching the patient to effectively use his visual-somatosensory reference in making spatial judgments (size estimations).

Training in sensory awareness seeks to achieve two inter-related goals: 1) train patients to attend to and to locate sensory stimulation in relation to their body midline; and, 2) train patients to relate the location of sensory stimulation to a corresponding location in extra-personal visual space. To facilitate training, an apparatus (The "Maniken") was designed to replicate the upper portion of the human back. It measures 35 centimeters wide at the shoulders and rests on a table at wheelchair level. The apparatus is studded with twelve lights, which are divided equally between the left and right halves and arranged symetrically relative to the midline of the apparatus. Directly beneath each light is a pressure sensitive circular switch. The lights and switches are arranged so that they form three horizontal patterns (rows), each comprised of four lights. Individual rows are separated by five centimeters. The upper-most row, corresponding to a level just above the shoulder blades, contains one light on either side of the maniken's midline (five centimeters apart) and one light approximately in line with each shoulder blade (ten centimeters away from the "midline" lights). The second row contains lights at each of the two lateral positions (i.e., in line with the shoulder blades) and a light next to each of these (five centimeters away towards the midline). The third row duplicates the pattern of the first. The apparatus is connected to a console containing 12 switches, corresponding to the lights on the maniken. Depressing a switch on the console "activates" the corresponding pressure switch on the maniken. When the apparatus is turned "on" all lights are illuminated. "Activating" a switch will cause the respective light to temporarily extinguish when its switch is touched. This is used to provide the patient with immediate feedback as to his success in localizing a position on the apparatus.

Prior to training, the patient's ability to perceive stimulation at each of the 12 positions on his back is probed. Training is attempted so long as the patient is able to sense single stimulation in at least two positions on their impaired side. Training consists of drawing the patient's attention to a location on his back and referring that location to others and his midline. Verbal cues are provided in training to help the patient learn and retain somatosensory anchors. In addition, patients are trained to locate on the maniken, comparable positions to that touched on their back by the trainer. The patient indicates his choice by touching a switch on the maniken's back. If correct, the corresponding light will temporarily extinguish. If incorrect, the light remains on. Training is provided for individual locations, beginning with those on the unimpaired side, and progresses to simultaneous locations on each side and across the midline.

Training in spatial organization involves the use of five plexiglass rods of differing lengths (10, 15, 20, 25, and 30 centimeters) and two small plexiglass cylinders. In training, one rod is placed at a distance of 45 centimeters from the patient and he is instructed to estimate the length of the rod by placing the two cylinders at a similar distance apart. The patient is instructed to scan the length of the rod and use his body as a reference for estimating its length. The patient then scans the distance between the rods as he has placed them and compares that distance to the length of the rod. Once final "adjustments" have been made, the patient is given the stimulus rod in order to assess his performance. The trainer assists the patient in evaluating the feedback obtained by comparing his estimate with the rod. The trainer specifically notes tendencies to over or underestimate the length. With the trainer's assistance, the patient considers what compensatory measures need be taken and the task is tried again. Training progresses through increasingly longer rods and in three different locations: directly in front of the patient (centered on the body); to the right (unimpaired side); and, to the left (impaired side).

<u>Training in pattern organization and sequential analysis (VIP III)</u>. This training was designed for the mild-to-moderately impaired patient who do not exhibit gross impairments in visual

exploration, scanning or somatosensory reference. Such patients will typically perform well on simple visual tasks (such as visual cancellation, W.R.A.T. Reading, line bisection) but be unable to sustain this level of performance on more complex visual tasks (such as Raven's Colored Progressive Matrices). Moreover, these patients will tend to evidence an attentional bias (i.e. position preference) on a specially constructed picture-matching test (Piasetsky, 1981). Training is directed at two objectives: 1) Provide the patient with a strategy for appraising the overall nature of a visual stimulus; and, 2) cause the patient to adopt a systematic method of appraising elements of detail within a visual stimulus (Weinberg, Piasetsky, Diller and Gordon, under review).

Training in pattern organization involves two related training procedures. Both are designed to teach the patient to appraise the overall nature of visual stimuli by anchoring their attention around elements located in the left visual field (that contralateral their side of lesion):

1) Locus of Words. Using paragraphs of varying lengths (5 - 20 lines), patients are trained to impose a gross system of spatial coordinates on the passage. Cuing, in the form of transparent overlays which divide the passage into upper/lower and left/right halves, is provided during the course of training. Patients are trained to incorporate the system of coordinates in order to systematically recall the name and location of anywhere from 2 - 8 pre-determined words. The maximum number of words which a patient is asked to recall never exceeds the limit of their verbal free recall, assessed at baseline. In this training procedure, the critical training dimension is the patient's recall of location. Training focuses on the patient's ability to organize the location of words into pattern-cues within the paragraph. Training follows a sequence in which the number of words to be recalled is increased within each successive paragraph length.

Dot configurations. This procedure was designed as a companion to the locus of words exercise. It consists of dot patterns which are presented within a frame which corresponds to either the 5-line paragraph or the 20-line paragraph. Patients are trained to localize individual dots and also to form meaningful gestalts. Forming gestalts is trained for each half-field separately (left vs. right; upper vs. lower) and the entire field. Patients demonstrate their use of organization strategies by reproducing patterns in empty frames.

Training in sequential analysis was designed to teach the patient to systematically and carefully examine visual material. Patients are trained to examine sets of similar visual stimuli and compare them with a target stimulus. In most instances, one of the stimuli being compared will be identical to the target stimulus.

Training is directed at establishing the manner in which the analysis is performed and only secondarily at whether a correct match is found. Patients are trained to perform a clockwise appraisal of each stimulu choice, comparing them with the target on a detail-by-detail basis. All details are considered. A variety of stimuli are used, including meaningful (i.e., clock face) and non-meaningful ones (irregular silhouette shapes). The principal considerations during training are: 1) that the patient carry out a systematic and thorough examination of each of the stimulus choices; and 2) that the patient inhibit any tendencies to be impulsive and rush through the analysis. Even when it has been determined that a particular choice is different from the target, the patient is trained to continue the search, noting each remaining similarity and difference in detail.

## REHABILITATION OF ATTENTIONAL DISORDERS IN TRAUMATIC BRAIN-INJURED ADULTS

The Orientation Remedial Module (ORM) was developed by Ben-Yisha and his associates (Ben-Yishay et al., 1978; 1979; 1980) to address problems in alertness and attention found in persons who have sustained a severe head trauma. It is provided as part of a comprehensive remedial-rehabilitation program for head trauma patients who, despite conventional rehabilitation efforts, remain unable to resume functional social and occupational lives. Participants in the progra receive 20 weeks of intensive remedial training, beginning with the ORM and progressing through increasingly more demanding domains of cognitive functioning. In addition, participants take part in supervised and highly structured peer group "discussions" in which a range of personal and social-interpersonal issues are addressed. Participants in the program must be one year post-injury, have participated in a standard rehabilitation program, and be sufficiently free of gross problems in language and speech so as to be able to participate in the group discussions. All participants receive a comprehensive evaluation at approximately one month prior to entering the program and again at the time of entry. In addition to the comprehensive evaluation, participants are tested on tasks which directly relate to the training he will receive.

The term attentional disorder is used here to represent a class of problems involving patients' ability to mediate an effective interchange with the environment. Ben-Yishay refers to these as overlay phenomena, which he considers to be clinical manifestations in the basic levels of consciousness. Included among these clinical manifestations are: insufficient alertness; distractibility; problems in selective attending; disturbances in concentration or the ability to sustain a mental effort; and, delayed or poorly modulated responsiveness. To the extent to which these disturbances prohibit access to the patient's critical faculties, they represent a major obstacle to the effective diagnosis and treatment of the more substantive aspects of the patient's functioning. It is for this reason that the amelioration of attentional disorders constitutes the logical and imperative first step in the overall remedial-rehabilitation program.

The Orientation Remedial Module consists of five component exercises which were designed to form an overlapping hierarchy in demand complexity. Each exercise was constructed to address a critical dimension of the generic domain of attention/arousal. Each employs an instrument and set of procedures which were devised to be naturally engaging, so as to evoke in the patient a desire to perform. Additionally, the instruments and procedures were constructed to inhere with sufficient versatility so as to allow for selective and graded cuing. The goal of providing this module is two-fold: that the five exercises, delivered in sequence, will produce a cumulative enhancement in the patient's levels of alertness, attention and concentration; and, that, upon completion of the module, the patient will be a sufficiently good "consumer of his environment" to permit training in more substantive areas.

Training the patient to attend and react to environmental "signals"

As the first exercise in the sequence, this training seeks to stimulate the patient's general level of arousal and enhance attention, concentration and responsiveness. The reaction-time paradigm serves as an effective milieu within which to accomplish these objectives. It embodies, at a most basic level, the unified process implicit in an active engagement of the environment (i.e., seeking and interpreting the signal (s) -- for which to -- select and apply appropriate action (s) ). In this first exercise, the demands placed upon the patient are simplified along two dimensions:
1) Both the signal and the appropriate action are simple, well-defined and unvarying; and, 2) The signal is external to the patient.

The instrument employed in this training exercise is a visual reaction time apparatus which has been specially modified for use as a training tool (The "Attention Reaction Conditioner"). It consists of a vertical display board containing eight colored lights arranged in a wide semicircle. Centered at the base of the board is a small white signal light which the patient responds to by depressing a disc positioned in front of the display board. Activation of the colored lights is contingent upon how fast the patient responds to the signal light. They provide the patient with simple and direct feedback as to his performance and are used by the trainer so as to provide the patient with an incentive to respond more quickly. In addition to two pre-programmed conditions, the instrument has a provision which allows the trainer to control how many colored lights the patient obtains for his response. This allows the trainer to work with patients whose level of arousal and attention is relatively low. In each of the two pre-programmed conditions, the number of colored lights activated by the patient's response is electronically controlled. Under the "slow" condition, a response latency of between 450-550 milliseconds illuminates all eight lights. One less light is illuminated for each additional 100 millisecond increment above 550 milliseconds. So, for example, under the "slow" pre-programmed condition, a response latency of between 550-650 milliseconds illuminates seven lights, while a response latency of between 650-750 milliseconds illuminates six lights, and so on. Response latencies in excess of 1350 milliseconds will not illuminate any lights. A similar principle governs the activation of lights under the "fast" pre-programmed condition. Response latencies of up to 200 milliseconds light up all eight lights. One less light is illuminated for each additional 50 millisecond increment above 200 milliseconds. Under the "fast" condition, a patient must respond within 600 milliseconds in order to obtain any lights.

The patient is introduced to the exercise with the explanation that the task he will be performing helps people to "concentrate" better. Reference is also made to helping him improve other important skills such as avoiding "distractions" and responding with "maximum speed" and "efficiency". Each training session begins by having the patient perform ten trials of the task under the "fast" pre-programmed condition. After each trial, both the patient and the trainer count the number of colored lights the patient has illuminated. This procedure is repeated after each training trial as well, in order to insure that the patient is attending to the feedback. The trainer records the results of the daily testings in order to chart the patient's progress. Training begins under the feedback condition (manual, "slow" pre-programmed, "fast" pre-programmed) judged most appropriate on the basis of the patient's performance at baseline testing. As the patient increases the number of lights he attains under a feedback condition, indicating a reduction in reaction-time, he is advanced to a more demanding condition of feedback. The trainer may assist the patient by offering "readiness and response" cues while providing a source of social reinforcement, praising his performance and encouraging him to try to light up more lights than before. Training is discontinued when the patient reaches ceiling (i.e., eight lights under the "fast" condition) or plateaus.

## Training the patient to time his response in relation to changing environmental cues

This exercise focuses on training the patient to more effectively "screen out" distractions and use available environmental cues to determine the most appropriate time to respond. During the course of performing the training task, the patient is faced with a set of stimulus cues (markings on the face of a "clock-like" device) and must select and remain focused on the appropriate one. In the early phase of training, the patient's cue to respond is a direct one.

As training progresses, the patient's cue to respond is a referred one and the patient must adjust his choice of referred cue so that his response will continue to achieve the desired result.

The instrument employed in training (The "Zeroing Accuracy Conditioner") is an oversized "clock-like" device with a single sweep hand. The face of the device contains 60 hash marks evenly spaced about its circumference. The number "0" appears at both the "12 o'clock" and "6 o'clock" positions, and the number "15" appears at both the "3 o'clock" and "9 o'clock" positions. The device is connected to a flat metal box on which is mounted a button. When the button is depressed, and for as long as pressure on it is maintained, the sweep hand will be in motion. The direction in which the sweep hand moves (clockwise or counter-clockwise) and the speed of its movement (ranging from 1 - 28 revolutions-per-minute) can be controlled by the trainer. Because of the size of the sweep hand relative to that of the electric motor which powers it, lifting one's finger off the button will not instantly stop the hand's motion. It will, rather, tend to "coast" to a stop. How much the hand will tend to "coast" is directly related to how fast it is moving. At a low speed, the hand will stop at virtually the moment that the patient lifts his finger off the button. This enables the patient to stop the hand at a particular marking by lifting his finger off the button as the hand reaches that marking. At higher speeds, however, the tendency for the hand to "coast" to a stop must be taken into account. To stop the hand at a particular marking, the patient must engage in a process of experimentation: observe how far the hand coasts; determine the right moment at which to lift his finger so as to compensate for the coast; watch the device and determine whether he has been successful and adjust accordingly. On subsequent trials, at the same speed, the patient will have to remember when to lift his finger or make the necessary correction.

The patient is introduced to the exercise with the explanation that the task he will be performing is another one which helps people "concentrate" better, avoid "distraction" and "respond quickly". He is also told that the task will provide him with "practice in decision making" and "timing his responses". In introducing the patient to the task, the trainer demonstrates the coasting effect and informs the patient that he must allow the hand to go around at least once but not more than three times before lifting his finger off the button. Prior to each training session, the patient performs twelve trials of task. The training is individualized according to the patients performance in testing. At slower speeds, training focuses on basic timing and avoiding distractions. At faster speeds, training focuses on anticipating the best moment, before the hand reaches the designated marking, at which to act. The patient is provided with feedback as to his performance by counting the number of markings between the designated target and where the hand actually came to rest. The trainer may assist the patient in determining the optimum "release point" at faster speeds and, as always, provides praise and encouragement. Training is discontinued when the patient plateaus.

Training the patient to be actively vigilant

The third exercise in the sequence seeks to train the patient to actively scan his environment, seek out the presence of signals and identify them. In the two previous exercises, while the patient was required to actively engage his environment, the environment was essentially "brought to" the patient. In this exercise, the patient must contend with two stimulus sources, which cannot be simultaneously monitored, and a variety of specific stimuli.

The instrument employed in this exercise (The "Visual Discrimination Conditioner") consists of a long horizontal display panel containing two moveable (4 x 4 inch) cubes. The cube on the left side of the panel contains a one-inch digital display and the cube on the right contains five colored lights. When maximally separated, the distance between the two cubes is 30 inches. Under normal conditions, a person seated two feet from the center of the panel can detect the onset of stimuli on both sides, while looking at the center of the display panel. However, if no preparatory warning is given, accurate discrimination of the specific stimulus presented (color, number, or both) requires that the individual laterally scan and look at the stimulus source(s). The cubes can be activated separately or together. The time interval between successive stimulus presentations is controlled by the trainer. The length of time each stimulus presentation lasts (stimulus "on" duration) can be manually controlled or electronically set to one-second duration.

The nature of the instrument is explained to the patient. He is told that it provides "two kinds of information", numbers on the left side and colors on the right. An example of each is demonstrated for the patient and he is told that it will be his responsibility to report what he sees at both sides of the instrument. The patient is cautioned to remain "constantly vigilant" since the instrument may light up a number, color, or both. Each training session begins by testing the patient's performance on the task at maximum separation and at one-second stimulus duration. A total of thirty-six test trials are obtained: 12 unilateral left; 12 unilateral right; 12 bilateral/simultaneous. Unilateral presentations are randomized by side while the bilateral presentations occur in sequence. A record is kept of the patient's overall performance and is provided as feedback upon completion of testing.

Training is tailored to the patient's needs according to his performance on initial testing. Training involves several elements:

1) Systematically increasing the distance between the two cubes until a maximum separation is achieved. Under the simplest condition, the cubes would be situated side-by-side at the center of the display panel; 2) varying the quality and helpfulness of the preparatory cues provided to the patient. A most-helpful cue might pre-warn the patient which side(s) will be activated and provide a "count-down" to the stimulus onset; 3) feedback is provided after each training trial as to whether the patient noticed the presence of a stimulus and whether he identified it correctly; and, 4) praise and encouragement to be more vigilant. Training is discontinued when the patient's performance at testing is errorless or when the patient plateaus.

Training the patient to estimate time

This exercise is particularly significant in that it seeks to train the patient to respond to internalized cues. The instrumentation employed is relatively simple, consisting of a ten-second stopwatch which is capable of measuring time to the nearest 1/100th of a second. The stopwatch is mounted on a small stand with an activating lever which enables the patient to start or stop the watch whether it is facing him or turned away.

The patient is introduced to the task with the explanation that the exercise is designed to improve "mental control" and "concentration". Prior to each training session, employing a standard stopwatch, the patient's ability to estimate time periods ranging from two to 12 seconds is tested. Training is conducted in stages and, with the exception of minor modifications to meet individual needs, is uniform. The logic of the exercise is to train the patient to internalize the rhythm of the watch through the use of timed body movements. The steps followed are: 1) synchronizing back and forth swaying movements of the upper body with the observed movements of the stopwatch hand; 2) synchronizing swaying movements with the imagined movement of the stopwatch hand; 3) synchronizing head movements with the imagined movements of the stopwatch hand; and, 4) "keeping time" with the imagined movements of the stopwatch hand while the body remains still. Less physically impaired patients would begin the task using finger tapping in place of swaying movements of the upper body. On training trials in which the watch is facing away from the patient, synchrony of movement is applied to estimating the passage of a specific time period. The patient is provided with feedback as to the accuracy of his performance and, as always, is praised and encouraged to do better. Training is discontinued when the patient plateaus in testing.

Training the patient to synchronize with complex rhythms

This is the final exercise in the sequence and, accordingly, involves the patient's integration of previously trained skills.

The stimuli for this exercise are series of morse code-like tones systematically distributed over time. For the patient to achieve success on this exercise, he must: attend to the rhythm formed by the sequence of tones; internalize it; and, anticipate each "beat" so that his responses are in phase with the stimulus.

The instrumentation for this exercise include: a casette tape recorder; cassettes; a telegraph key; a dc two-channel event recorder; and, an electronic display panel containing two lights and a provision to generate morse code-like pulses. The display panel is the primary training instrument (The "Rhythm-Synchrony Conditioner"). It is designed to be capable of simultaneously presenting a pulsed rhythm through two different outputs. One output is channelled through the tape recorder, producing an auditory representation of the rhythm; the other output is channelled to one of the lights on the front of the display panel. This permits the trainer to present a rhythm to the patient, simultaneously in the auditory and visual modes. A second feature of the training instrument is that the rhythm which the patient taps out on the telegraph key can be visually displayed by the second light on the panel.

As is the case with each of the training exercises, the patient's first exposure to the task is in a testing situation. Because of the imposing nature of the task's complexity, care is taken to "fortify" the patient in preparation for testing. The patient is instructed as to what he is to do. He is told that he will hear three different rhythm patterns, that there will be a period of silence in between each pattern, and, that patterns go from easy to complex. He is told that his job is to "duplicate the sound pattern on the telegraph key" and is cautioned to pay attention to two things: "tap the key in sychrony with the beeps" he hears, "start at the same time"; and, "maintain the duration of each tap for exactly the length of time" he hears it. The task is demonstrated for the patient and he is encouraged to "meet the challenge" while being re-assured that "no matter what the results of the test" his performance on this "complex task" can be improved by "systematic training". In testing, the patient listens to and attempts to synchronize with three taped rhythm series. Each series consists of 60 tones. The output from the tape recorder and the patient's performance (via the telegraph key) are fed into the event recorder which provides a graphic display of the two sources simultaneously. This display is analyzed by the trainer to determine if: 1) the patient responded to each tone; 2) the patient began his response within 100 milliseconds of the onset of the tone; 3) the patient held down the telegraph key for the same duration as that of the tone. Each tone of each series is graded in this fashion. This is translated into a score by assigning 1-point for each of the three analysis variables. The patient, then, may receive a maximum of 3-points for each tone. The scores for the tones are summed, yielding a value from 0 to 540. This value is recorded and used to monitor the patient's progress.

Training is carried out in stages. Special modifications may be introduced into the training procedures to accommodate the needs of individual patients. For example, patients who exhibit particular difficulties in manipulating the telegraph key are provided with special remedial training in producing long versus short-duration presses, separately and in sequence. Standard training involves the use of visual feedback in directing the patient's responses. The patient is provided with a visual representation of a tonal sequence (on the display panel) and monitors his own performance in relation to it. The patient is correct when "his" light is illuminated in unison with "instrument's" light. Training is discontinued when the patient plateaus.

We have herein reviewed training methods developed at the Institute of Rehabilitation Medicine, New York University Medical Center, derived for utilization as remedial procedures to ameliorate circumscribed aspects of the consequences of stroke and traumatic brain injury. Evaluation and investigation of the benefit of these remedial procedures can be found in the series of Monographs published by the Institute of Rehabilitation Medicine and in articles published in professional journals as listed in the references of the present chapter. Nonetheless, these herein described remedial procedures represent a portion of the focus of an ongoing clinical research effort concerned with the treatment of cognitive consequences of insult to the central nervous system.

## REFERENCES

Ben-Yishay, Y. et al. Working approaches to cognitive deficits in brain damaged. Rehabilitation Monograph 59, New York: Institute of Rehabilitation Medicine, New York University Medical Center, 1978.

Ben-Yishay, Y. et al. Working approaches to cognitive deficits in brain damaged. Rehabilitation Monograph 60, New York: Institute of Rehabilitation Medicine, New York University Medical Center, 1979.

Ben-Yishay, Y. et al. Working approaches to cognitive deficits in brain damaged. Rehabilitation Monograph 61, New York: Institute of Rehabilitation Medicine, New York University Medical Center, 1980.

Diller, L. A model for cognitive retraining in rehabilitation. Clinical Psychologist, 1976, 29, 13-15.

Diller, L., Ben-Yishay, Y., Gerstman, L., Goodkin, R., Gordon, W. and Weinberg, J. Studies in cognition and rehabilitation. Rehabilitation Monograph 50, New York: Institute of Rehabilitation Medicine, New York University Medical Center, 1974.

Diller, L., and Weinberg, J. Evidence for accident-prone behavior in hemiplegic patients. Archives of Physical Medicine and Rehabilitation, 1970, 51, 358-363.

Piasetsky, E. B. A study of pathological asymetries in visual-spatial attention in unilaterally brain-damaged stroke patients. Doctoral Dissertation. City University of New York, 1981.

Weinberg, J., and Diller, L. Hemi-inattention in rehabilitation: The evolution of a rational remediation program. In E. A. Weinstein and K. P. Friedland (Eds.), Advances in Neurology, Volume 18. New York: Raven Press, 1977.

Weinberg, J., Diller, L., Gordon, W., Gerstman, L., Lieberman, A., Lakin, P., Hodges, G. and Ezrachi, O. Visual scanning training effect on reading-related tasks in acquired right brain damage. Archives of Physical Medicine and Rehabilitation, 1977, 58, 479-486.

Weinberg, J., Diller, L., Gordon, W., Gerstman, L., Lieberman, A., Lakin, P., Hodges, G. and Ezrachi, O. Training sensory awareness and spatial organization in people with right brain damage (RBD). Archives of Physical Medicine and Rehabilitation, 1979, 60, 491-496.

Weinberg, J., Piasetsky, E. B., Diller, L., and Gordon, W. Treating perceptual & organization deficits in non-neglecting right brain damaged stroke patients. Journal of Clinical Neuropsychology, in press.

# TECHNIQUES AND APPLICATION OF SIMULTANEOUS INFORMATION PROCESSING

Yigal Gross, Ph.D.
Psychology Department
Bar Ilan University and the Unit for Neuropsychological Treatment and Rehabilitation
Ramat Gan, Givatayim, Israel

Zila Ben-Nahum, M.A.
Unit of Neuropsychological Treatment and Rehabilitation
Givatayim, Israel

Gabriel Munk, M.A.
Rehabilitation Center
Shiba Hospital
Tel-Hashomer, Israel

## INTRODUCTION

The previous chapter outlined a theoretical approach to interventive neuropsychology, which does not focus on individual symptoms of brain-damaged patients, but rather on the concretic quality of their personality. We concluded with a statement which defines the goal of the treatment as training the patient to divide his attention between figure and ground in his experiential field, so that not only the figure is processed and coded, but, to a lesser extent, also the ground. The focus of the present chapter is to initially focus on some general and practical considerations and assumptions, from which the herein described treatment or interventive strategies were developed.

At the outset, it should be stated that the intervention principle which we outlined allows us to develop any number of different techniques. The strategies herein reviewed were selected in order to demonstrate a representative sample of techniques, each aimed at different stages in the treatment, and different levels of patients. Another purpose of this selection is to stimulate the reader's creative thinking so that unique and individualized treatment methods could be devised which fit the individual patient, as well as the therapist.

Initially, some general clinical principles of intervention will be addressed.

1. The utmost purpose of the treatment is to introduce hope and self-esteem to the patient, who might otherwise be in a state of helplessness and self-despise.

2. The hope and self-esteem which we want to help the patient develop should be based on accurate reality testing. This is particularly difficult in traumatic brain injury in which a sudden change has occurred involving the very system which is supposed to perceive, evaluate and act upon its evaluation of that change.

3. We, as therapists, have the difficult task of delineating for the patient his loss of abilities, the different ways in which his world has changed, and also his potential are the aspects of his world which provide for him a firm basis from which he can operate. The difficulty of this latter task is twofold. On the one hand, we are dealing with very sad life events, and we have to deal with, at least, our intense emotions. On the other hand, we have to conceive of ways in which we can clarify to the damaged brain patient the various ways in which he has changed. We will deal only occasionally with the emotional aspects, but will devote some attention to the patient's recognition of his cognitive disabilities and the effects they have on his life.

4. In order to help the patient recognize his disability, three different conditions have to exist: (A) the aspects of the disability which should be dealt with first should be those which are relatively not emotionally loaded; (B) the process should include a well-blended mixture of frustrations and successes, punishments and rewards; (C) the disability should be demonstrated through concrete experiences rather than through abstract discussion.

5. While performing training on any given task, the patient should be made aware of any similar difficulties he might exhibit in everyday life. Consequently, errors of impulsivity, for example, exhibited during training might be discussed in context of other situations in which he may be impulsive. The intent of this consideration is to promote the generalization of any strategy which the patient might learn in training to his environment.

One possible way to enable the patient to recognize his

disabilities is through training him to overcome them. But in order for him to be motivated to participate in training, he has to admit, in the first place, that he is having problems. How do we get around this vicious circle? The patients seem to have solved the problem by the very fact that they indeed come to us with a complaint, at least in some cases. Usually, they are willing to admit to problems in memory. We have found that this is so even in those cases when the patient does not have really serious memory problems. Apparently, it is easier for the patient to view his memory as a faculty which is external to his personality, while he cannot do so with "thinking" or emotional abilities. We suggest to start with training tasks which seem to be related to memory training, while their actual purpose is to train contextual processing. We further suggest to begin with such tasks which are not at all similar to real-life situations, in which the patient has been experiencing painful and repeated failures and frustrations. Finally, we suggest that we ensure that the patient can be convinced his performance on the task is improving through his effort.

## INTERVENTIVE TECHNIQUES

As a first example a method which seems to be very simple and directly related to memory will be described.

### Interference Resistance Training

This method presents many opportunities for the patient to define for himself, with the help of the therapist, the functional problems he has, and realize that he is actually able to improve on his initial performance. All we need is a piece of paper on which are presented rows of random digits, random geometric figures, or random anything.

Using the example of numbers, this task is performed by the therapist successively covering two or more of the numbers, depending upon the capability of the patient, such that as the next number in the sequence is covered the most remote or last number is exposed. It is the task of the patient to indicate which number will be revealed with each successive step. The performance of this task requires that the patient attend to the digit which is being covered at each step, remember the number(s) which was previously covered and name the next digit to emerge. These three components of this

3 7 2 5 3 3 7 6 5 2 0 1 3 5 8 6
2 0 4 8 0 5 6 4 8 9 4 7 4 2 9 1

Figure 1. Stimulus configuration used for Interference Resistance Training.

△□□X◊△□○△○□X○□
○△□□X□○X□◊△△○□

Figure 2. Stimulus configuration used for Interference Resistance Training.

task may correspond to the memory processes of encoding, storage and retrieval. The task requires attentional processes to encode and store stimuli to which we do not immediately respond, and respond to and consequently immediately forget stimuli which are not currently in our immediate external environment. The patient's difficulties in storing that which is not overtly and immediately responded to, is attested to by the fact that the patient might say aloud <u>not</u> the digit which is about to appear from under cover, but either the one which had to be entered into memory storage, or another one of the covered digits. In a sense, the patient has difficulty in ignoring temporarily some parts of the stimulus situation in order to come back to them at a later stage. He also has a problem in recording not only the digit, but also its ever-changing position.

Two remarks have to be made here before we go on to describe another kind of technique. Primarily as in many other training tasks, we begin to work with the task in a manner which demands little so as to not promote another failure experience. We begin the treatment with a comment about the fact that the patient ought not be discouraged by the apparent simplicity of the exercise. We then may proceed with the simplest task: covering a digit for some time, and asking the patient to recall it. We would move on very quickly to the next step, which is concealing two digits, and then introduce non-relevant interference; for example, ask the patient to pay attention to the two digits we are about to conceal, conceal them, and then ask for his address, name, phone number, etc., and, of course, the two concealed digits. If and when the patient is performing this task well, we begin to introduce relevant interference. Now we may ask the patient to memorize two digits while he is reading aloud several others. Only at this stage will the patient be ready for the actual training. Again, we begin gradually. We begin by concealing one digit, moving the covering object, and requesting the patient to guess consistently the concealed single digit. Then we will proceed to conceal two digits, requesting the patient to guess the digit which is to be uncovered when the covering object is being moved.

## Conditional Responses

This interventive technique utilizes an instrument which is a 60 X 60 centimeter panel on which are two sets of twenty lights each. The two sets are arranged in two diamonds, one within the other. The internal set is made of randomly arranged colored lights and the external diamond configuration is made with all white signal lights. The signal lights are lit automatically, one after the other, in a clockwise fashion, at an adjustable rate (usually a one per second cycle is appropriate). A set of twenty micro-switches arranged in a diamond shape on separate 20 X 30 centimeter panel are connected to the colored lights in a corresponding arrangement. The patient is seated in such a way that he sees the panel with the lights in front of him, while his hand can comfortably operate the micro-switches. Pressing one of the micro-switches on the small panel illuminates the corresponding colored light.

During the practice sessions the patient would be required to put on the light which corresponds to the lit signal light, so that when the top signal light is on, he will put on the top colored light, and then when the signal moves to the second signal position, he will put on the second colored light. This task requires some training until the patient performs reliably. Now we can introduce some conditions which will require the patient to make a decision as to whether or not he should put on the colored light at each position. Having a conditional response requires, almost by definition, a contextual operation, since the patient has to attend to a response set or a preprogrammed strategy while he is attending to external relevant stimuli. This might serve as an introduction to the patient's use of himself as a criterion for making decisions as to whether, if, and how he should respond. The conditional arrangements we usually work with are the following:

1. Skip every other light;

2. Skip a particular color, which should change from time to time so the patient can experience overcoming his tendency to perseverate;

3. Skipping two colors;

4. Follow the signal at one-step delay, e.g., when the signal light is in the third position, the second color light should be illuminated. This task proves to be rather difficult for patients, probably because they have to attend to one position and operate another.

Using all of these conditions, we may produce another variable which we feel is extremely important. We ask the patient to perform the task at hand while engaging in discussion, being asked simple questions, such as what is your name, or (in later stages of training), to perform an arithmetic problem. It is made clear to the patient that the most important part of the task is the operation of the instrument, and he should answer questions only if and when he realizes that he could do so without distracting his attention from this task.

There are several important aspects of these tasks. First, there is an obvious requirement for a division of attention and effort. Second, the level of attention and the processing mode which are allocated to each part of the total situation is constantly changed by the patient in order to achieve optimal performance level. Finally, and probably most importantly, the patient learns to introspect, and to use information he obtained through the introspective process to guide his behavior. For example, he should learn to adjust the speed in which he is bombarded with information to the rate at which he can absorb it.

At this point I would like to review a very preliminary study we have done in order to test the effects of the two training techniques which I have just reviewed. The interested reader is referred to Ben-Nachum (1978) and copies can be obtained from the first author of the present study for details of this study.[1] We took four patients and testing them in three conditions: (1) before training began, (2) after 10 hours of experimental training using the techniques described above, and (3) after ten hours of control training. The control training included two tasks. The first being the memorization of a gradually increasing number of colored bulbs operated by the trainer. The second task was memorizing sentences consisting of an increasing number of words. In both control tasks the instrument was used as a timer so that the patient had to delay his response until the signal light reached a given position. The familiar figure matching test (FFMT), the digit symbol sub-test of the Wechsler Adult Intelligence Scale and digit span (forward and backwards), paired associates, and passages of the Wechsler Memory Scale were administered pre- and post-training to all subjects. The order of the experimental and control training was alternated between patients.

The data presented on Table 1 and Figure 3 reveal that while both training conditions resulted in an improvement relative to baseline performance, the experimental training procedures appear

Table 1. Psychological Test Performance at Baseline and Following Two Training Conditions.

| | TIME FFMT | ERRORS FFMT | DIGIT SYMBOL | ASSOCIATE LEARNING | MEMORY OF PASSAGES | DIGITS BACKWARD | DIGITS FORWARD |
|---|---|---|---|---|---|---|---|
| BASE LINE | 601" | 9, 7 | 19 | 11 | 11 | 3, 2 | 5, 2 |
| AFTER CONTROL TRAINING | 406" | 8, 2 | 30, 5 | 14, 2 | 14 | 4, 3 | 5, 7 |
| AFTER EXPERIMENTAL TRAINING | 487" | 3, 7 | 30, 5 | 13 | 15, 5 | 5, 3 | 6, 8 |

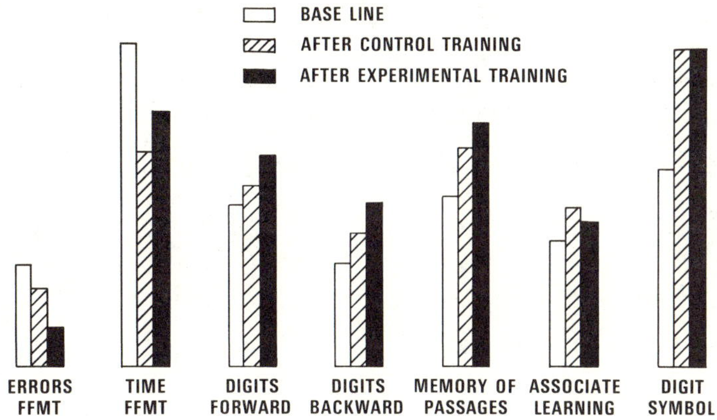


Figure 3. The performance of four patients on criterion tests before training, after control training and after experimental training.

to have affected the greatest improvement on cognitive functions as assessed by these measures. Table 2 illustrates the percent change, relative to baseline, following the two training conditions. While certainly tentative, these preliminary data are supportive of utility of the experimental training procedures herein described.

The Empathic Dialogue

The principle of simultaneous information processing is applicable to more than tasks principally oriented at cognition, but to social-affective situations as well. The present exercise facilitates the integration of many cognitive processes while engaging in conversation. Let us analyze the conversation situation from the point of view of simultaneous processing. A person says something to another

Table 2. Percent Change in Psychological Test Performance following Two Training Condition.

| | TIME FFMT | ERRORS FFMT | DIGIT SYMBOL | ASSOCIATE LEARNING | MEMORY OF PASSAGES | DIGITS BACKWARD | DIGITS FORWARD |
|---|---|---|---|---|---|---|---|
| BASE LINE | 601" | 9.7 | 19 | 11 | 11 | 3.2 | 5.2 |
| AFTER CONTROL TRAINING | -33% | -15% | +60% | +35% | +27% | +35% | +10% |
| AFTER EXPERIMENTAL TRAINING | -17% | -63% | +60% | +18% | +40% | +70% | +30% |

person. He might then turn his attention to a second person, and review in his own mind the impact of the communication had on that person. For example, when I see my daughter coming back from school wearing a long face, I may decide to ask her, "Is anything wrong?" Knowing her, and the fact that she is in a terrible mood, I may expect her to feel that I am attacking her in my question. In that case I may expect her to burst into tears, blaming me for not being compassionate. She might also do something else. She might resort to a passive-aggressive attitude, and bitterly say, "Nothing." In a real interaction situation, I have to evaluate if indeed I want my daughter to feel as if she was attacked by me, to which I would respond by feeling guilty. If the answer is negative, I may try another approach. Further, it could be argued that my daughter, when she was coming home wearing her long face, was counting on the fact that I would respond to it in one of several familiar ways, and that she created a situation in which the probability of one of the responses which are favorable to her (for example my "attacking" question) would increase.

The point of this example is that every communication is based on the integration of all the relevant information about the recipient of that communication. The result of this integration is one or more hypotheses about the impact that communication will have on its recipient. Each of these hypotheses, in turn, would lead to one or more hypotheses about future behavior the recipient might choose to exhibit. In this way, soon after we have made the communication, we anticipate a number of possible alternative responses our partner may exhibit. It is important to notice that not all of the information which is needed to create these predictions exists in the immediate environment. For example, our partner's response may be based not only on our last comment, but rather on some combination of that and a previous comment. Information and knowledge about the recipient's personality based on previous learning is as well relevant data to be taken into account in the social-affective communication.

Remarkable simultaneous processing is required to adaptively communicate, requiring consideration of several hypotheses about the desired behavior that is expected or appropriate which is elicited by one's verbal behavior. Now we have the task of engaging our patient in a conversation so that he will be reinforced for the following behavioral dimensions. The first being, how many different hypotheses he has about the responses his communications may elicit and the second, to what extent his communication and hypotheses reflect the integration of the relevant information. This task in terms of the verbal content, should be similar to real situations in which the patient is having difficulty and is one in which requires therapeutic intervention. The purpose of this exercise is, however, to structure the dialogue in a manner which facilitates learning and understanding in patients with deficits in simultaneous information processing. Specifically, the exercise slows the verbal interaction such that all of the relevant information can be considered and requires the dialogue to be written so that all hypotheses can be overtly examined to determine which would be the most adaptive. Further, by writing the dialogue, deficits in memory do not impair the learning process.

For the purpose of this task, the patient and the therapist form a team which has to engage in meaningful conversation. After one of them has transmitted a communication, it is recorded by both in the protocol of the dialogue. Then the transmitter of the communication has to generate hypotheses about the different ways the recipient of the communication could respond. The hypotheses must be generated before the recipient responds. After all hypotheses have been generated, to which the recipient is not exposed, the recipient must respond. It is at this point that discussion can ensue as to the contextual appropriateness of the response can be discussed and evaluated. Further, a score can be given to the transmitter of the communication if the recipient's response correspondences to one of the hypothesized responses. An illustration of this technique concerning the conversation with my daughter would appear as follows:

Daughter's Protocol

| Dialogue | Hypotheses |
|---|---|
| Daughter - "I had a terrible day at school." | 1. Don't worry, You'll forget it tomorrow.<br>2. What happened?<br>3. Your room is in a mess, go clean it up and we'll talk later.<br>4. Would you like to talk about it over coffee?<br>5. Would you like to talk about it while I am having some food? |
| Father - "Would you like to talk about it?" | |
| Daughter - "Actually, it is not that important." | 1. Then why do you look so upset?<br>2. Okay |

Father's Protocol

| Dialogue | Hypotheses |
|---|---|
| Daughter - "I had a terrible day." | 1. No!<br>2. Would you really like me to? |
| Father - "Would you like to talk about it? | 3. I don't feel like talking about it now. |

This example illustrates a diversity of hypotheses, which are contextually appropriate given our relationship (father-daughter), and appropriate given the immediately proceeding communication. In other words, the hypothesized responses were based on past and present information and in context of our relationship. Generating hypothesized responses of this nature certainly requires simultaneous processing of information which is "external" (the communication) and "internal" (contextual information). Discussion which this technique generates is typically relevant for the social-affective difficulties each patient experiences and facilitates simultaneous information processing in these kinds of situations. Further, the quality of the hypotheses, in terms of their emotional structure, facilitate clinical intervention.

## The Mediating Technique

This exercise was designed for a group of four to six patients with two therapists. Each patient takes turns in attempting to mediate a social conflict situation played by two therapists. The mediator role was selected because it cannot be performed unless the mediator takes into account all relevant information on the total context of the situation. Another reason for choosing this particular task was to allow the patient to learn to improve the way he processes information regarding social behavior.

Learning to simultaneously attend to all aspects of a situational context involves several components and can be referred to as a contextual attitude. The contextual attitude involves:

1. Developing an objective attitude towards the information which is being processed: e.g., not imposing belief systems and habits on others. Differentiating between established facts and hypotheses.

2. Habitually generating hypotheses about information not known to him on the basis of information which is given, using any information as a springboard for getting more information, and forming a habit to engage in information-seeking behavior.

3. Developing a positive attitude towards feedback even when it disproves a hypothesis, benefiting from feedback so that either a specific hypothesis is followed further, or is rejected and replaced by another one, and assuming a positive attitude towards flexibility of thinking.

4. Forming a habit to reflect from time to time about one's own strategies, decisions and acts.

Further, learning theory and research suggests that the training should include the following features: (1) the solution is executed in small, well-defined steps, (2) Each step is immediately reinforced, (3) Erroneous information processing is clearly defined by the patient, is corrected, and the correction is positively reinforced, (4) Even though the task may be performed in a group, each individual proceeds according to his own pace and level, and (5) material around which problem situations are created is taken from patients' real life situations in order to facilitate generalization.

As stated earlier, the exercise is simultaneously performed by four to six patients with two therapists (T-1 and T-2). The therapists play the roles of two parties in a social conflict. Each patient's role is to mediate between the parties and to suggest a solution to the conflict to which they can both agree. The patient is given instructions as to the structured format through which the exercise is performed as well as a scenario outlining the nature of the conflict. An example of an appropriate scenario would be:

> You are one of John's best friends and you see John walking out of his fiancee, Sue's house on Friday night. He seems quite upset. You ask him what's wrong and he says that he has just had a fight with Sue. You want to help them resolve the conflict.

Further, the patient is presented with the following instructions:

1. You write your suggested communication (which is intended to either elicit relevant information or assist in the resolution of the conflict) on a yellow note pad. It is presented to either T-1 or T-2 for approval.

2a. If it is approved you are awarded 20 points. Then you copy your communication on a white pad (which is used for only approved communications) and present it to John or Sue (T-1 or T-2) in order to get their response.

2b. If your communication is not approved, you are fined 10 points and have to write on the yellow pad a statement beginning with the words "My mistake was that I...."

3. When you have correctly identified your mistake, you are awarded 15 points and you may then proceed to the next step which is a suggested communication to either John or Sue.

The background story of this problem situation, which is available to the therapists and which the patients have to uncover in order to be able to solve the problem, is as follows:

> John and Sue have plans to go out tomorrow afternoon (Saturday).

John, wanting to surprise Sue, has gotten two tickets to Annie, the very popular Broadway show. Sue, not knowing of John's plans, had made arrangements with their friends, Diane and Steve, to double date on Saturday. John and Sue have previously cancelled plans with Diane and Steve on several occasions because John doesn't particularly like them, although he can tolerate them. Sue is afraid of offending them if they cancel again. As she likes Diane very much, she does not want to risk endangering their relationship. John, on the other hand, has wanted to see this show for quite some time and the tickets were quite expensive. He doubts that he will be able to obtain such good seats for at least another six months. Sue feels that because it is possible to obtain tickets at any time, they should return these tickets, even if it means having worse seats in the future. John prefers to have good seats and does not want to return the tickets.

The Following is a Schematic Example of Part of a Written Dialogue Between One Patient and the Therapists:

| Patient (Yellow Pad) | Protocol (White Pad) | (Yellow Pad) T-1(John) | (Yellow Pad) T-2(Sue) |
|---|---|---|---|
| Hi, John, what did you fight with Sue about? | | /+20/COPY ON WHITE PAD | |
| | HI, JOHN, WHAT DID YOU FIGHT WITH SUE ABOUT? | | |
| | Sue does not want to go with me to a show. | | |
| John, you know how girls are. Don't get upset. | | /-10/IDENTIFY YOUR ERROR BY WRITING "MY ERROR IS THAT I..." ON YOUR YELLOW PAD | |
| My error is that I asked John not to get upset. | | TRY AGAIN | |
| I do not understand my error. | | T-1 EXPLAINS ORALLY | |

| Patient (Yellow Pad) | Protocol (White Pad) | (Yellow Pad) T-1(John) | (Yellow Pad) T-2(Sue) |
|---|---|---|---|
| My error is that I said to John that Sue is like other girls, but she is his fiancee. | | /+15/O.K. CONTINUE ON YELLOW PAD | |
| John, why doesn't Sue want to go with you to the show? | | /+20/COPY ON WHITE PAD | |
| | JOHN, WHY DOESN'T SUE WANT TO GO WITH YOU TO THE SHOW | | |
| | Sue wants to go to see her friend, Diane. | | |
| John, so go see Diane. | | /-10/IDENTIFY YOUR ERROR BY WRITING "MY ERROR IS THAT I...." ON YOUR YELLOW PAD | |
| My error is that I did not understand that they fight because John does not want to go to Diane. | | /+15/ O.K. CONTINUE ON YELLOW PAD | |
| John, why would Sue rather go to Diane's than to the show? | | /+20/COPY ON WHITE PAD | |
| | JOHN, WHY DOES SUE RATHER GO TO DIANE'S THAN TO THE SHOW? | | |
| | I was so upset with her that I did not ask her. Would you ask her? | | |
| Sue, I suggest you go to John and tell him that everything | | | /-10/IDENTIFY YOUR ERROR BY WRITING "MY |

| Yellow Pad | White Pad | T-1(John) | T-2(Sue) |
|---|---|---|---|
| is fine between you two and that you agree to go with him to see the show. | | | ERROR IS THAT I..." ON YOUR YELLOW PAD |
| My error is that I suggested to Sue to just give up her position. | | | /+15/O.K. CONTINUE ON YELLOW PAD |
| Sue, why don't you want to go with John to the show? | | | /+20/COPY ON WHITE PAD |
| | SUE, WHY DON'T YOU WANT TO GO WITH JOHN TO THE SHOW? | | |
| | I want to go but not on Saturday. | | |
| John, so go to Diane's with Sue. | | /-20/GRAVE ERROR! IDENTIFY BY WRITING "MY ERROR IS THAT I...." ON YOUR YELLOW PAD | |
| My error is that I always ask Sue and John to give up what they want. | | /+30/BEAUTIFUL! CONTINUE ON YELLOW PAD | |
| John, can you go with Sue another day? | | | |

ETC.

Following the previous individual mediation, the group of patients assumes the role of a mediator. Each member of the group suggests a communication which is evaluated in turn by the group and reinforced accordingly. The procedure is as follows.

1. Each member of the group will submit to the patient group one question or suggestion on the yellow pad.

2. The group will then decide as a whole whether each question

is acceptable. If the question is not acceptable to the group, the member who submitted it should identify the reason why, in writing, to the group's satisfaction.

3. An acceptable question is awarded 20 points, a rejected question is fined 10 points, and an acceptable identification of error is rewarded by 15 points.

4. After all the submitted questions are reviewed in this manner, the group will decide which of the accepted questions will be submitted to the therapists on the white pad for an answer.

5. After an answer has been received, proceed back to step one.

Having described the technique I would like to emphasize that even though the technique looks to be very complicated, most patients are able to learn what steps they are supposed to take at each time. The appearance of strict structure of the technique is very misleading. There is ample room for adjusting level of difficulty and content according to clinical considerations. Finally, we should mention the fact that the conflict in which the patient is mediating could be either one of a neutral quality, like the one used in the example, or one which is relevant to patients' emotional adjustment. An example of the latter kind is a story which we used which revolved around a war veteran who concealed from his future mother-in-law the fact that his leg has been amputated.

## SUMMARY

In summary, the contextual information processing principle can lend itself to the creation of many different training methods. It is our task, now, to collect quantifiable and objective data to test whether these techniques are not only theoretically interesting, but also helpful to train brain-damaged persons to readjust to real-life circumstances.

Interventive neuropsychology is a part of clinical neuropsychology, and indeed of clinical psychology. I do not think that we could deal successfully with theoretical justification of cognitive difficulties without dividing our attention, and that of our patients, in a functional and flexible way, between the various emotional ramifications associated with an impairment of cognition. The fact that the person we deal with has a limited capacity brain system puts him in very difficult situations; thus the brain damage may have secondary effects on that person's emotional processing. The possibility that a limited capacity brain system is less able to produce and express emotional experiences needs to be further investigated. There may be, in fact, a direct causal relationship between the cognitive consequences of brain damage and emotional deficiencies. It should be clear, therefore, that the treatment has to emphasize cognitive and emotional contents interchangeably, and in an integrative way.

## REFERENCES

1. Ben-Nachum, Z. Improving memory processes in brain-damaged people. Unpublished M.A. Thesis, Tel-Aviv University, Israel, 1978.

# THE RETRAINING OF FRONTAL LOBE DYSFUNCTION

James F. Craine, Ph.D.

Neuropsychology Service
Hawaii State Hospital
Kaneohe, Hawaii

The mystery and enigma of human frontal lobe cortical function has been a topic of fascination to a number of psychologists for many years. Unfortunately, information concerning function is usually best obtained as the result of a malfunction due to a known lesion. Goldstein (1944) reported a noticeable impairment of abstract attitude and that although these individuals appeared to have sufficient ability to handle routine work, they seemed to lack initiative, foresight, and the ability to handle new tasks. They were also frequently impaired in voluntary shifting of activity and choice, but because these are often rather subtle behaviors, he observed that these impairments would often be overlooked in everyday life. Similarly, A. R. Luria stated that the basic thought defect characteristic of patients with lesions of the frontal lobes does not consist of an absence of logical reasoning abilities, because they can reason from a logical basis and can find relationships and even solve problems in analogy (Luria, 1973). Instead, their defect appears when faced with the necessity of making a goal-directed choice from a number of equally probable alternatives.

Recognizing and then attempting specific remediation of frontal lobe dysfunction is of a relatively recent origin, and has proved to be a rather difficult and frustrating task. Endeavors in this direction quite frequently have had to be terminated with only a minimum of success. There is a general consensus that some restoration of function is possible in general (Hecaen & Albert, 1978) but there are severe limitations. Some very encouraging possibilities are indicated in cerebral blood flow studies (Lechner, Ott, Ladurner, 1979) in which mental activity composed of memorizing, reasoning, and abstract thinking, appears to result in increased cerebral blood flow, with special emphasis upon augmentation of flow in the prefrontal area. Of utmost significance and value in this work, however, are the specific suggestions and examples of methods for restoration of brain function following injury provided by A. R. Luria, with some special attention paid to remediation of defects of prefrontal lobe function (Luria, 1963). Additional suggestions and programs are provided in a later work (Luria, 1974) and we find these ideas also invaluable.

An imposing obstacle encountered in attempts at remediation is that frontal lesions appear to provide a bewildering multitude of behavioral and personality symptoms (Teuber, 1964). Fortunately, the state of the art of neuropsychological testing has evolved (Lezak, 1977) such that the nature of behavioral and cognitive impairment associated with cerebral dysfunction can informatively be described. Additional complications are noted, however, from recent studies with infrahuman subjects (Goldman, 1979) which document the extent to which subcortical and brain stem (thalamic and hypothalamic regions) lesions can have severe effects upon prefrontal lobe function due to extensive cortico-subcortical interconnections. Finally, we have to consider a number of additional variables such as type of lesion, extent of cortical area involved, and age of patient at onset of lesion.

Faced with this possible wide array of symptoms, many of them quite elusive, the question is raised as to how to proceed with a retraining program. From the beginning of our own retraining attempts with the brain damaged, we have recognized the problems inherent in attempting to work with frontal lobe patients (Gudeman, Golden, and Craine, 1978). We have frequently been rather reluctant to attempt to tangle with these problems because of the numerous difficulties involved. Despite our reluctance, however, we have managed to attempt to work with quite a few of these clients over the years, and by actual count I now note that of the 40 clients we have in training at the present time, nine are clearly labeled frontal lobe patients. We thus have been forced to find ways of dealing with these clients and are continually in the process of improving our methods. Fortunately, many of the techniques we use with our other clients who do not have involvement of frontal lobes appear to work equally well with our frontal lobe patients, except that we have to be aware of differences in emphasis.

## THE RETRAINING OF COGNITIVE DEFICITS ASSOCIATED WITH FRONTAL INJURY: A CASE EXAMPLE

In order to provide the flavor of a retraining program for frontal lobe patients, it should be helpful to provide an actual case example plus some anecdotal material. It is hoped that this method of presentation will illustrate the problems involved in dealing with these patients and at the same time indicate a number of possible solutions.

## The Individual Patient

This patient is called Mitchell and he was referred to us by his Vocational Rehabilitation Counselor. In keeping with the behavior frequently encountered in these patients, the counselor requested that we test Mitchell in our laboratory, because his behavior was "causing a great consternation to his care home operator, workshop supervisor, Handi-van driver, and myself, not to mention other workshop and agency staff personnel that come in contact with him." From the tone of this letter it was apparent that Mitchell was creating havoc wherever he went.

The injury incurred by Mitchell resulted from a fall from the 4th or 5th floor of a building, resulting in serious left frontal depression of the skull. The diagnostic impressions were as follows: (1) status left severe cranial bilateral injury with dementia, (2) mild left hemiparesis, (3) left frontal craniotomy defect, (4) blindness left eye; mild optic atrophy right eye. This injury had occurred nearly two years prior to our first contact with this patient.

This 27 year old male was found, on initial assessment to be excessively verbal, to have a tendency to express his excitement in a loud strange laugh associated with a clapping of his hands. His initial attitude toward testing was one of being non-committal as to whether he would condescend to cooperate or not. We found, however, that he was actually quite cooperative and seemed to need constant feedback as to his progress during testing. He responded well to praise and encouragement but also had a tendency to be quite impulsive whenever he ran into difficulty with the tasks. It was also noted that he was very distractible so that at times instructions had to be repeated and simplified in order for him to understand their meaning. Fortunately, his level of motivation was generally good, but at the times when he refused to cooperate, a method to secure cooperation was utilized to the effect that he was told he would receive a zero as his score unless he completed the task. This method was usually quite effective because it was very important for him to receive a good score. When told during testing that his loud laugh and hand-clap was quite inappropriate, he made a very conscious and obvious attempt to control it.

The neuropsychological testing revealed a level of mental ability that would be classed in the normal range, with indications of moderate brain dysfunction seen in both cerebral hemispheres but with focal difficulties in the left frontal area and the central portion of the right cerebral hemisphere. As would be expected, in view of the nature of the injury, it was noted that Mitchell had special difficulty with any complex reasoning or decision making task. He also had exceptional difficulty with a procedure which required him to repeatedly change his principal line of reasoning in order to solve the problem. Actually, any task that seemed to require intellectual flexibility was excessively difficult for him to handle. Our testing revealed that he did have the ability to learn a new task if properly motivated and that he was clearly not a fast learner, but instead seemed to proceed slowly and laboriously. In his favor, he showed evidence of being able to concentrate, to pay attention, and to discriminate auditory stimuli. He also had complete freedom from any sensory or perceptual disorder and appeared to understand things that were said to him without excessive difficulty.

In view of the results from the neuropsychological testing and from the report of his counselor, it was quite apparent that Mitchell was in need of therapeutic intervention. We offered to provide a training program for him in our laboratory providing he would be able to come in on a regular basis as an outpatient and work at the training program prescribed. We found him to be quite enthusiastic in regard to such a program and, in further discussion, found that he had a desire to be able to work in a photography studio. We thus elected to use as a long-range goal that Mitchell would be able to achieve employment in a photography studio as this choice seemed to be a reasonable possibility. This would mean some further education, but before he would be able to assimilate the necessary education, it would be necessary that we address ourselves to a number of shorter range goals in order to prepare him to cope with the additional education needed.

In view of the deficits noted during the testing, it was possible to select three areas that appeared to need special work in order to prepare Mitchell for achieving his long-range goal. These three areas involved visual memory, concept formation and ability to form abstractions, and intellectual flexibility. A number of specific exercises were formulated in order to achieve improvement in these areas, and the training was ready to commence.

## Problem-Solving

Our training program with Mitchell began approximately two years and three months after his injury. One of the first anomalies experienced was that as bright as he was verbally, it was incongruous to note the great difficulty he experienced when attempting to figure out where he should begin a solution for a given task. He seemed to have excessive difficulty organizing his method of approach. Whereas he could read easily and well on a word-for-word basis and could read a short paragraph and have no difficulty knowing what he had read, great difficulty became apparent when he attempted to answer questions asked about the short paragraph. In the beginning, he seemed to have no way of knowing how to begin to solve the problem presented.

For the purpose of training Mitchell in this particular area, we used the Thinklab, which is a reading and thinking kit frequently used for students from early adolescence to adult. The cognitive exercises in Thinklab require the reading and rereading of the short paragraph with the aim of finding the main idea, correlating facts given, and noting significant details, all on a graded basis from easy to difficult. Mitchell had no difficulty reading the short paragraphs aloud but when asked to answer the questions, he appeared to not understand what was being asked of him. In answer to the question, and as if this were the solution, he would simply read the whole paragraph aloud again. In attempting to get him to break it down into its elements so that he would be able to give answers, we tried to ask him to tell us for what the paragraph was asking. Again, his answer to this question would be to reread the entire paragraph aloud, word-for-word, verbatim, with no paraphrasing and no attempt to arrive at any other answer. At the completion, he would look at his trainer as if he were satisfied that he had given the answer. It was apparent that this was the only way he knew to give any of the information back that was contained in the short paragraph.

It was soon apparent that if any progress was to be made, something about this procedure had to be changed. It was thus necessary that we intervene in the task and make some alterations in order to induce learning. Assuming that he was being overwhelmed by the verbal aspects of this situation, we decided to help him by having him schematize and make some order out of the material. We asked him at this point to extract the information given in the paragraph by writing down the essential information. He had to be lead by the hand in this task by asking him first, for example, to tell how many people were involved in the problem. At this point he proceeded to count the names of the people and write down how many people were involved. Then he was asked to tell the names of these people. When he verbalized this, he was asked to write these down on his paper. In the process, it was demonstrated how to put the essence of the problem, piece by piece, on his paper schematically so that once he had this in front of him, he could look at it and study it. The expectation was that once he could observe this material in front of him schematically, he would then be able to solve the problem. This method of approach did prove to be effective because when he had all of the essential information gathered for him, he was finally able to make some order out of it.

After this procedure had been followed a number of times with a great deal of help from the trainer, it was apparent that Mitchell was seemingly incapable of breaking any of these problems down spontaneously in the manner we were requiring of him. The steps necessary in order to go through the sequence and order of putting them down on paper appeared to be something he could not comprehend without some additional help. The trainers continued to provide this help but it was apparent that he did not really know what he was doing, as he completed many of them purely by chance, consisting of the aimless manipulation of the matchsticks until the solution appeared. In other words, he did not plan his actions accordingly and arrive at the solution but instead worked in such a way that the solution arrived at him. At this point it was decided to repeat all of the matchstick problems and observe his reaction; so we began presenting these problems to him again from the beginning. He has a good memory and thus was able to recognize that these were problems he had previously completed, so he objected to having to do them again. We agreed with him that he was repeating the tasks; therefore, it should be quite easy for him, he was told, since he had solved each one of them before all he had to do was to repeat the same solution. It was immediately apparent to him, however, that he could not repeat them readily, as he had completed most of them previously purely by chance on a trial-and-error basis. Because he had not consciously derived a solution the first time, he was not able to remember how to proceed upon doing them again, and this was forcefully brought to his attention by his difficulty upon the repetition of the task. This method of repeating the task dramatically brought to Mitchell's attention that he was unable to follow the trail of his previous attempts because he had no trail to follow. He had not formulated a plan to follow and there were no labels upon his movements; so when he objected by saying that he had already done this, we could readily say, "Yes, you have, so do it again just like you did it before."

As it became very obvious to Mitchell that although he had solved the problems before, he did not have a solution to refer back to, it was possible to point out to him exactly where he went wrong. We were able to say to him, "Mitchell, you have to process and note exactly what you are doing in order to make sure you can solve the problem again. You cannot even take for granted that you are going to automatically remember the solution. You must tell yourself exactly how you are doing it, as you are doing it, so that you can solve the same problem again if it is presented." This made some sense to him; so in order to help him as he went through the solution, we required that he consciously use verbal cues in order to file the solutions away so that he would be able to retrieve them when needed. This also forced him to think rather consistently about the task and largely eliminated the trial-and-error behavior.

Because he had already been through the same puzzles previously, with constant urging to try other possible solutions, and because he already knew that solutions were possible, the task proceeded considerably faster the second time around. The difference, however, was that he recognized that he had to do some special work in order to store the solution so that he would be able to recall it if he were asked to do the same task again. The practice in putting verbal labels upon his moves and the emphasis upon planning before making the move, as well as labeling the moves, seemed to help him store these in his memory and thus made the task much more meaningful.

Verbal Fluency

As Mitchell was mastering the matchstick problems, this activity brought into focus another very definite problem which was observed to handicap him. When he was successful in his solution of a problem and we would ask him to tell us how he solved it, he would try to show us rather than tell us. We insisted that he tell us and at that point he would just say, "Like this, see, like this," and continue to demonstrate. As verbal as he was normally, he seemed totally incapable of verbally expressing the steps that were necessary to take in order to solve the problem. This demonstrated very clearly that he had excessive difficulty talking on demand and putting labels on each move he made. In order to help him with this problem, it was decided to initiate some activities involving verbal fluency.

The "Word Fluency" task is an exercise in which an individual is asked to give all the words aloud he can think of beginning with a given letter of the alphabet. We arbitrarily established the criteria for Mitchell that he would be required to say aloud thirty words in a two-minute period. It was thought that he would be able to produce 30 words in two minutes as he was typically exceedingly verbal. When he was required to produce words beginning with a specified letter of the alphabet, however, he experienced excessive difficulty. His typical response on the task was to proceed fairly rapidly for 20 or 30 seconds and then to remain blank for a rather long period of time. He would then resort to a randomness of response, repetition, or a production of nonsense words.

In terms of a strategy, Mitchell had a fairly good technique as he could select a category such as months of the year or states or countries and he could try to think of the words that began with the proper letter. In his eagerness to succeed, however, he had a tendency to confabulate. For example, when using the category "months of the year" and trying to produce words that began with the letter "f", he started out with February but could not locate any others. He then resorted to "Fune" and "Fuly" as if fulfilling the objective; then switching to countries he would produce the same mistakes such as starting out with France and moving to "Fain" (Spain) and "Fitaly." When utilizing states as a category, he produced Florida and then resorted to "Falifornia" and "Foregon." It was obvious that he understood what was expected of him and that he could monitor his output as he was aware of his confabulation.

One of the problems with Mitchell, in an activity of this type, was that he desperately needed to do well. The conclusion of his performing the Verbal Fluency task was always followed by his inquiry as to how he had performed. At that time he would be told, "Well, Mitchell, you only got 13 correct words." He would be amazed that his production was so low. Further, he was shown that his errors (repetitions and nonsense words) penalized him. It was apparent, however, that he had a high motivation to succeed, and that his memory was good such that he could remember words he had used in previous trials.

His main difficulty in the task, however, was that he could not seem to organize his activities properly. It was also recognized that the criterion of 30 words in two minutes was not an easy task to achieve but he continued to improve over time and eventually reached the point where he could consistently achieve 20 to 23 words before really getting stuck. At this point in the training, if for example he was on words beginning with the letter "m" and was stuck, he would break into the exercise and say, "I know some "T" words," and would want to change the letter of the alphabet. It was necessary to be very firm with him and stress that the goal was 30 words for each individual letter and that he was not to interrupt the task during the two-minute trial. It was also necessary to emphasize that he was not to waste any time or thought on anything other than the words on which he was working. Again, in view of the nature of the deficits, i.e., the frontal lobe dysfunction, it was important to restate the goal for him regularly in a very direct and explicit manner.

This strictness and continued redefinition and practice on the task began to yield progress. Once he was able to achieve 23 to 25 words in the two-minute period, it did not take him long before he was able to reach the criterion of 30 words. For an individual who spoke slowly, this high level would not be realistic; but for Mitchell it appeared to be a matter of thinking of the word, staying on track, and keeping his attention on the task.

An important step in the achievement of success for this particular activity was his discovery and utilization of better strategies to meet the criterion. We found it necessary to teach him the strategy of not letting himself get stuck in his solutions, but that if he were stuck, he should quickly move on and use other kinds of clues in his thinking. He finally became able to make use of a fairly large number of categories and some of them were quite extensive. He also began to make use of the alphabet in order to jog his memory for the desired words. Once he was able to voluntarily shift from one category to another when he became stuck at the task, he was finally able to complete this activity.

Intellectual Flexibility

The strategy that we were able to teach Mitchell of not letting himself get stuck but to move on to other categories was quite useful and he was aware of the improvements in his scores as he made use of this strategy. His problem with using this, however, impinged upon another area in which he had obvious difficulties. This is the area of flexibility or, more precisely, intellectual flexibility. Anyone who has a problem in this particular area would find it quite difficult to readily shift from one idea or thought or category to another. In order to help him with his obvious impairments with intellectual flexibility, we thus turned attention to another area of training.

This next problem, termed intellectual flexibility, is so typically encountered with frontal lobe dysfunction that it has been necessary to design a series of tasks or exercises to be used especially in this connection. We title these "Flexibility Exercises" and all of these have the advantage of being able to start at a very simple level and to progress in difficulty. Because Mitchell had problems in switching from one activity to another or from one frame of reference to another, it was immediately apparent that he was going to have an unusual amount of difficulty with our flexibility tasks. For example, the first activity we presented called, "Before and After," consists of a page of numbers in columns. The patient is first required to write the number that would occur before the number that is given on the page; e.g., if the number is eight, then he would write seven. He is then to continue down the page, in each case writing the number that comes before the given number until the trainer says, "Change." At that point he is required to circle the last number worked on and then proceed by writing the number that comes after the given number; e.g., six he would write seven. When the trainer again says, "Change" then he is again to circle the last number he worked on and begin writing the number that comes before the given number once again. As can be seen, this activity requires a patient to adjust to a pattern which differs from the preceding one and to repeatedly make these changes. This exercise also has the advantage that the trainer can require faster and faster changes as a patient becomes able to cope with this kind of activity.

The task of making the changes seemed to cause Mitchell to become extremely frustrated whereas he had no difficulty at all with the task as long as no changes were required. Because this 'changing' was such a problem, the first requirement was to have him do the entire page simply by writing all of the 'before' numbers and then have him do the same page writing all of the 'after' numbers, and keep track of how long it took him to perform this task. We then asked him to again do the task and imposed 15 second changes on the activity. His reaction to the change in direction every 15 seconds seemed to be that he started fast and then began slowing down so that the amount of work produced between changes became less and less. By this, we mean the total amount of numbers he could write down in the 15-second period became fewer and fewer. He appeared to have more trouble with each change and it was not long before he was making very little progress. He became progressively less efficient at the task, and in some instances it would take him so long to make the change that the time ran out before he could write down one number previous to making the next change.

After a considerable period of work with this particular task, however, he became more adept at making the changes and could cope with the task, so it was possible to reduce the period of change from 15 seconds down to ten seconds. This increased frequency of change adds more pressure to the individual performing, as he must become more efficient at making the switches if he is to continue to progress. When Mitchell progressed to the point where he could handle ten-second changes without undue difficulty, we shifted to another flexibility task called, "Add-and-Subtract." At this point we uncovered additional difficulties because the add-and-subtract activity involves increased verbal abilities and is definitely more complex than the before-and-after problems. He was able to add very well but had difficulty with subtraction, especially when he was required to 'carry' the number. This particular task requires two columns of numbers close together and a separate column for the addition and subtraction answers. Mitchell was first asked to perform addition operations on all of the numbers on the page and we kept track of how long it took him. Then he was asked to subtract each of the numbers on the page and we found that it required him considerably longer to do the subtraction. The length of time it took him to do the subtraction was used as the criteria for his completing the entire page with the addition of addition-subtraction changes.

As could be predicted, when the changes were imposed upon the activity (in terms of switching back and forth between addition and subtraction), Mitchell made many mistakes and the changes forced him to slow down considerably. After extensive work at this task, he was able to speed up in the activity but made many errors in the process. Scoring of the activity took into account not only time required to do the task, but also the number of errors, which were subtracted from the total number completed; thus the errors cut his score down considerably, even though he was finally able to speed up. At this point it was necessary to inform him that he was putting too much emphasis on speed in his work and thus was making an enormous number of errors. Too many mistakes were reducing his score whereas if he would work at a good speed, he had plenty of time to complete the task and meet criterion.

Before he was able to complete this task, it was necessary to convince Mitchell that he was able to work sufficiently fast to achieve criterion, but he would have to concentrate on not making mistakes. As in other areas, this convincing was not easy, but by continually calling attention to the scores wherein he was penalized for the errors, and by pointing out his ability to work rapidly and to make the changes satisfactorily, the idea finally got across to him that it was important for him to control his impulsive reaction and to think his way clearly through the task. Once he was able to thoroughly put the emphasis on accuracy, he was able to reach criteria quite quickly.

He progressed to another activity in the flexibility area as the "Odd-and-Even" activity was introduced. This exercise uses a sheet of paper with many numbers written in rows horizontally across the paper. The client has the task of starting at the top row and working across the page horizontally. He is told at the beginning of the task to cross out all of the even numbers and to continue until the trainer says, "Change." At that time he must circle the number he was working on and then proceed by crossing out the odd numbers until again the signal to change is given. In this way he continues to alternate between crossing out even numbers and odd numbers until the page is completed. This task seemed to bring in a totally different problem for Mitchell. Although he must have had the knowledge in the past, he did not seem to know what odd and even numbers were when we began to work with him on this task. The only way he knew whether or not a given number was odd or even was to divide the number by two and if there was no remainder, then it was even. If there were a remainder, he would call it odd. At this point, it was decided to let Mitchell divide the entire list of numbers on the page by two. In the process it was noted that although he had no trouble whatsoever handling the single digit numbers, he took a considerable time doing the double digit numbers. After he completed the task, we asked him what he noted about all these numbers; with some prompting, he was able to recognize that if the second number of double digit numbers is even, that would make the entire number even and he could thus treat it as if it were a single digit number.

The above-noted clarification seemed to be a great help to Mitchell in determining odd and even, but there was one other strange thing that happened in this process. If the number happened to be divisible by five, he would sometimes call it an even number even if it ended in five, which of course violated the rule when dividing by two. With a little more practice dividing these numbers by two, he was able to realize that the ability to divide it by five did not necessarily make it an even number. Considerable time had to be spent on this small item simply because if this were not clarified, Mitchell did not seem to be able to make any progress whatsoever with this portion of the task. It was necessary to be certain he had the right idea, because once he had an idea of the way to do something, he had great trouble changing.

While working with Mitchell on understanding whether double digit numbers were odd or even, work continued on the flexibility task by using single digit numbers only. In this case, the sheet of paper would have all single digit numbers on it; he was rather quick on this task. The problem that presented itself, however, was that he was too quick, as he would go across the two of numbers so fast that he would have to backtrack to make sure he had not skipped some along the way. He did this so regularly that it was apparent that when he reached the end of the line he recognized that he had gone too fast and must have skipped some of the numbers. Because his work was corrected in front of him and because he hated to see his mistakes counted, it was possible to use this as a motivator in helping him to place the emphasis upon slowing down and checking as he went along. It was emphasized to him that he was not to go back and check, as this was very wasteful of his time, but instead he should make a decision on every number one at a time, and check them as he went along. These instructions had to be repeated many, many times before we could get him to slow down and avoid having to repeat the task every time he finished a line.

Mitchell continued to argue vehemently on this particular matter of checking as he went along, as he said the method we were trying to suggest to him would make him go too slow. Because he continued to make an excessive number of errors using his own method, we asked him to try the suggestions and see if they would result in a better score. He stopped arguing long enough to try this particular strategy and although he was a little slower in completing the task, his total score turned out to be better because there were far fewer mistakes. It was also pointed out to him that as he made his decision faster, his overall time would improve. Once he absorbed this idea, he was able to work himself out of the single digit numbers and then into the double digit numbers.

By this time, the requirement of making the shifts from odd to even and back again all the way down the page did not seem to bother him as much as when he was originally presented the flexibility task. It was apparent that Mitchell was making some very good progress in this activity. We would judge that one of the keys to his progress in this flexibility activity was his use of verbalization to help him keep his focus. This verbalization was in the form of a self-instruction to the effect that when he originally brought this to bear on the add-and-subtract task, he would keep telling himself aloud, "Add, add, add." He performed the same kind of self-instruction for the odd and even so that whenever the change was introduced, he would repeat the new instruction and keep repeating it; if for example it were "even", he would say the same word over and over until it was time to make the next change, at which time he would repeat to himself "odd". It was thus found that this method of self-instruction proved to be a significant factor in his ability to master this particular kind of task.

It was rather surprising to note that Mitchell was able to invoke this kind of verbal aid to help him in this flexibility task.

It was 'surprising' because of the fact that verbal self-instruction is an activity that those with good or intact verbal ability might well use. But to find someone who was impaired in these abilities, and could still be able to benefit from this verbal self-instruction, was quite encouraging. Although he was weak in this area, he was able to use it quite well as long as he was able to do it for himself and make it very definite and specific so that he would not become confused while doing the task. Once he was sure of what was odd and what was even in terms of numbers, he was able to make the switch back and forth quite readily and this entire task proved no longer to be a problem for him. Once he was able to slow down and get the right answer for each problem by making sure that it was correct before proceeding to the next, he was able to work his way through the task and meet criterion.

## Impulsivity Problems

In order for Mitchell to reach criterion on the flexibility activities, it was apparent that he had to assume some definite control over his impulsivity. Whereas we had been able to help him indirectly with this problem, it was decided at this point to work directly on his impulsivity problems. In order to do this, an activity in which he must solve problems was introduced but it was structured in such a way that if he made a mistake in the solution, the entire problem would be called wrong, and correcting it would not help. This rule was invoked so as to force him to think ahead before he made any move. We wanted to force him to think before acting. The rule that he could not make a change and that any error would count against him, turned out to be a good motivator because he hated to have errors and very much wanted to be right all of the time.

An activity used for the retraining of Mitchell's impulsiveness is called "Attributes" and is useful for working on logical thinking, concentration, and planning. This is another activity that has the advantage of being able to be presented in a relatively simple form but can be made (progressively) more difficult until the task presented can be quite difficult to solve. The Attribute set consists of 32 blocks made up of four shapes (circle, square, triangle and diamond), of four colors (red, yellow, green and blue), and of two sizes (large and small). Eighteen-inch loops provide the arena for placing the blocks, and label cards are used in order to provide instructions as to what is to be put within the circle. This task can be quite easy if there is only one circle and, for example, one label card asking for square blocks or blue shapes, etc., but it can become more difficult if several label cards are used and/or if negative label cards are used (not blue, etc.). To add a substantial measure of difficulty to this task, however, it is possible to use two circles overlapping; then a decision must be made as to what is to be put in the parts of the circles that are shared in common. An because it was apparent that he was able to solve the problems once the steps were put down in front of him so that he could evaluate the facts for himself. After a while it was apparent, however, that he was not going to use this method spontaneously for himself, as he would continue to wait for the trainers to tell him what to put down on paper. The next step in the training was to refuse to give him the steps he needed and to make him work at extracting this material for himself. While Mitchell continued to work at the Think-lab exercises, slowly making progress, it was determined that this step in his training possibly could be more effective if at the same time we provided a non-verbal task in which he would be able to manipulate the parts individually and he could be observed in this manipulation. This brought us to the matchstick activity.

## More Problem-Solving

Most of us are familiar with the matchstick activity in the form of a puzzle in which a representation of a number of matchsticks in a precise geometrical configuration is presented. The requirement is then to form a different configuration with either the addition or subtraction of one or more matchsticks. As in keeping with our other activities, this task can begin at a very easy level and proceed in regular increments of difficulty to become a quite difficult activity. We want to see how long it will take for the patient to reach a predetermined criterion of success. It is recognized that this can be achieved simply by trial-and-error manipulation of the matchsticks or preferably, by an analysis of the problem, adequate planning, and a speedy and correct execution of the plan. The trainer can observe the various possible attempts at solutions being made and can evaluate the learning that is taking place in the process.

In his attempts to cope with this task, Mitchell would attempt one possible method for solution, and if it were correct, he was happy; if not successful, he would look at the trainer and say that he could not do it. At this point it was necessary to point out to him that all he did was to try one possible solution and because it didn't work, he was trying to tell us that it could not be done. Rather, we told him that it could be done and that we insisted that he try more than one possible solution. In this way it was redirected back to him such that he had to keep working at the task and find a solution. This particular kind of urging had to be repeated many, many times but was useful because it provided the idea to him that there are various possibilities that must be explored in order to arrive at a solution. This was the only hint that was given him, to the effect that there are other ways of doing the task, and we remained adamant that this was all the help that would be given him on this particular task.

Eventually Mitchell completed all of the matchstick problems increased level of difficulty again can be secured by using three circles overlapping. The use of negative cards also appears to substantially increase the level of difficulty.

A considerable amount of time daily was spent with Mitchell on the Attributes task as he was expected to do 15 different patterns per day. This requires a substantial amount of work and the activity was continued for a considerable period of time. He was fairly efficient in terms of solving the problems, as most of his mistakes were not in actual abstract reasoning but rather were mistakes as a result of not paying attention to what he was doing, in acting too fast, in mixing up the instructions, or in not properly understanding the instructions the first time they were given. The primary aim of this task, as stated before, was to help Mitchell control his impulsivity. The task was difficult enough that he had to carefully settle down and work at it. It also required that he keep his impulses under control for a fairly long duration of time.

It was clearly apparent that others had worked with Mitchell on his impulsivity because he was keenly aware of his tendencies. It would seem that the technique he used to combat his impulsivity was to try to establish a pattern of having everything being extremely well organized. It is probable that he was not like this before his accident. We would never see him other than very neatly dressed, with his hair combed just right, his lunch box with everything in a certain place and in perfect order. Everything in his daily life had to be organized and in its place and proper sequence. As would be expected, he brought his methods of organization to the "Attributes" task and it was apparent that when he could properly organize the task so he could approach it in a regular, orderly manner, he was better able to control his impulsivity. It was also very obvious that he felt much more comfortable in attacking any kind of a problem if he had it properly organized. His behavior tended to become quite random and out of control if he did not achieve proper organization. The excessively long time spent on the "Attributes" exercise served to help him learn further to keep his impulsivity under control. Because he used organization also in controlling the impulsivity on this task, the lengthy time spent on the exercises seemed to help him whenever it was necessary to teach him new techniques of organization.

## The Use and Misuse of Feedback

Interlocked with the excessively impulsive behavior was an inadequate and improper use of feedback. This is a problem that is so typically encountered in frontal lobe patients that it is almost always necessary to pay special attention to this deficit. These individuals can be bright enough and can obviously be receiving the information from their environment, but their behavior would appear to refute these facts and they appear to be quite variable in performance and at times appear incapable of learning. Close observation and work with these patients suggests that they often do not appropriately utilize information received.

It was quite apparent that Mitchell had difficulty benefitting from feedback. We observed numerous instances where he could obviously correctly perceive feedback information but was not making proper use of this information. Whereas he could solve problems quite adequately once he had all the essential portions of the problem, he did not seem to be able to query the information he received in order to extract what he needed. It was decided to use the Mastermind game as an activity for the purpose of helping develop the ability to process feedback information.

Because of the way it is constructed and played, the Mastermind game is ideal for excercising the use of feedback information. It also lends itself very well to patient progress monitoring. The game itself has a number of colored pegs and one person, in our case the trainer, arranges these pegs in a special sequence, which is the code, which is hidden from our patient. The patient then must attempt to arrange his pegs in the same color and same position as is contained in the hidden code. He regularly receives feedback information as to how accurate the colors and the positions of his pegs are in relation to the code he is attempting to solve. This game was completely new to Mitchell so he had to start from the beginning. Obviously, on his first row of pegs he has had no prior information so simply forms an initial hypothesis to be tested. He is then provided with the feedback information as to how accurate his pegs are in terms of color and position and he must sort out this information, discard the unneeded portion, and proceed ahead to make adjustments in his hypothesis. The game itself is very helpful in training an individual to use the feedback information and also to maintain a flexibility of thinking so that he can discard incorrect hypotheses and bring in new possibilities for testing. His method of solution has to be altered as the information he receives dictates a change.

As expected, Mitchell performed extremely poorly when we attempted to establish a baseline performance level on the Mastermind game. We were working with the simplest version of this game, using four colored pegs only, but because of his extreme difficulty with this task it was necessary to simplify it even further. We continued to use four pegs as the basic minimum but in order to make it easier, he was told the color of the pegs being used. This meant then that his task was simply to discover in which position these four colored pegs occurred. Even this extremely simplified version of the task was much too difficult at first. Despite the fact that after he laid down a row of pegs he would receive feedback information as to how many were in the correct position and could use this information in terms of previous rows laid down, he would sometimes tend to completely repeat one whole row in exactly the same color and order as in a previous row. He would not realize at the time that he was actually repeating something he had previously done and that such a mistake was unnecessary. This kind of behavior was repeated many times on this particular exercise. It had arbitrarily been decided that he should be able to complete this abbreviated task within four rows, so we adopted the policy of letting him attempt his solutions until he had completed the four rows before stepping in to begin to help him on the fifth and sixth rows. It was also decided that once he started to improve, it would no longer be necessary to provide extra assistance. The help we would attempt to give him from the fifth row on was in the form of pointing out to him the kinds of information that he was not utilizing in attempting to reach solution of the problem. Even with this kind of help, however, Mitchell frequently seemed to need several more rows of pegs before he was able to find the correct solution.

When a client fails to make proper use of feedback information, it is necessary to discover exactly why the difficulty is occurring. In this instance, while working the Mastermind problem, it was seen that Mitchell had two main areas of difficulty. The first was that he would repeat solutions simply because he was failing to recheck his previous work, therefore each new row he entered was like starting a game from the beginning. He was not using the information he had already gained in order to build a store of facts toward a solution and did not benefit from previous learning. The second problem involved his forgetting which hypothesis he was testing at the moment. This also could be disastrous as it did him no good whatsoever to come up with a good hypothesis and test it for solution then lose all of this work because he forgot the hypothesis. Once it was clearly established as to why the feedback was not being used, we were in a better position to help correct the deficit.

It was necessary to virtually take Mitchell by the hand and walk him through the various steps of forming a hypothesis and suggest the various kinds of logic that he could use. It was also necessary to go over and over with him the information contained in the feedback that he would receive. These had to be pointed out to him many, many times, with examples and demonstrations. Much of this work was done separately from the Mastermind game itself so that he could listen to the feedback and begin to understand what he was hearing. It was also necessary to insist that he verbalize aloud all of his ideas and his thoughts as he was going through this particular exercise. This enabled his trainer to follow his thinking and to denote when his problem-solving strategies became tangential. Verbalizing his strategies seemed to facilitate his cognitive organization and his approach to the task.

As he began to be able to formulate plans and to organize his thinking in order to solve these particular problems, he was able to learn how best to evaluate the kind of feedback he was receiving. He found he had to "zero in" on the specific question he was asking of the feedback information and to evaluate whether his hypotheses were right or wrong on this basis. In the early stages, even with suggestions and help, his solutions were very random with no logical trend, and it took him a great length of time in order to complete each problem. Because we greatly simplified the task, however, by asking only the position of the pegs and disregarding the color, the task was not nearly as complex as it could have been.

The second portion of his problem dealt with his forgetting of the hypothesis and thus not having an adequate plan of attack. Requiring Mitchell to verbalize his thinking aloud helped us to realize his problem in this area. In order to help him remember his hypotheses, we asked him to use a pencil and paper and write down his assumptions. To give additional help with the problem, we also explained to him the difference between an assumption and a given. By this, we explained that he could assume a certain idea was correct (an assumption) but when he received the feedback in relation to the moves he had made, he would then have received certain facts; if those supported his assumption, then it was no longer an assumption but was a given (a fact). Once he had established a peg as being in the correct position, a given, then he should make sure that that peg was kept in the same position on down the line as he proceeded with his solution. Again, it was necessary to have him verbalize aloud what an assumption was and what a given was for each of the positions of the pegs on the board.

As work proceeded on this exercise, Mitchell began to finally get the idea of what he was doing and was able to receive some enjoyment from the task. With the aids and the reminders, he began to remember his hypotheses, and also began to incorporate the information he was receiving from the feedback so as to test new hypotheses. He got to the point where there was no question that he was using the feedback information. As this occurred, he began to thoroughly enjoy the Mastermind game. We were then able to increase the complexity of the task, and as we did this, there was again observational evidence that he was making good use of the feedback information as he was able to generate various hypotheses, test them on the board, and either reject them if disproved, or accept them as a solution.

## DOES COGNITIVE TRAINING GENERALIZE?

The preceding description of cognitive training problems and solutions for a frontal lobe impaired patient touches on the major portion of the retraining program for this client. The narrative telescopes the many activities that took approximately a year into what appears to be a relatively short period of time. The actual amount of training time in our laboratory totaled 122 hours. There was no question that this patient improved considerably on the tasks which were presented to him and on which he worked so diligently. Our graphs of his daily scores attest to the progress he made over time. An important question remaining was whether he could generalize from the training experiences into other experiences of a similar nature but for which he was not specifically trained. Part of the answer was obtained when we retested Mitchell on the Halstead-Reitan Neuropsychological Battery and compared his scores on the Halstead Category Test. He had had excessive difficulty on this particular test on our initial examination, at which time he made 91 errors. On the retest, however, which was one year after his first taking the test, the 91 errors were reduced to 58. This is a noteworthy reduction in the number of errors and was achieved without any specific training on this particular task. Rather, these findings suggest that the cognitive skills learned through training generalized to another laboratory task. Some additional evidence was reported by the assessment technician, who noted that on the first administration, when he could not come up with a correct solution on this particular test, he did not seem able to generate a new or alternate hypothesis and would perseverate with wrong answers even though he was receiving information feedback that his responses were in error. On retest, however, this kind of behavior was not the case; instead, he was able to generate new hypotheses when the first or the second hypothesis he tried was proven to be incorrect. The available data was interpreted as suggestive of a least generalization of training from the training tasks themselves to performance on neuropsychological tests which proport to measure those cognitive functions in which training was oriented.

Mitchell is presently going to school to learn photography skills. At the present time he has enough knowledge to get a job in the field, but because he actually only knows how to develop film and doesn't know how to enlarge and print, he has decided to continue on in school and complete his instruction. We are confident that he will probably learn the necessary skills to obtain a job, but in the final analysis it will be his attitude and behavior, rather than skills, that determines his ability to get and keep a job. He recognizes now that he can handle ramdon, unplanned situations much better than he has been able to in the past. In recognition of his increased abilities, he has been given many more responsibilities at the boarding home where he is living, such as responsibility for many of the household chores and even responsibility for some of the other patients who are living at the boarding home. We have also been informed that his social worker plans to move him into an apartment of his own when he has a regular income from a job. He is looking forward to this step, does his own budgeting now and can think things through fairly well. It does worry him to contemplate being entirely on his own, however, but he has made excellent gains and feels he is capable of learning. He now recognizes the importance of planning and organizing his life.

## TYPICAL PROBLEMS AND SOLUTIONS ENCOUNTERED IN THE RETRAINING OF FRONTAL LOBE DYSFUNCTION

Whereas we have dealt at length with various problems and solutions in the retraining of one patient in the previous discussion, it has been our observation that most of our frontal lobe patients seemed to have many similar problems and need similar kinds of intervention. Before terminating the present discussion on this topic it should be useful to detail some of the most typical kinds of problems encountered with these patients, accompanied by some intervention strategies which have been found to be of value in dealing with these problems during the retraining program in our laboratory.

A list of the problems encountered with these clients could be very extensive if one wished to be highly specific. Eight problems characteristic of frontal lobe injury frequently appear and these are not listed in order of severity or importance in the training environment but merely as common problem areas that we have noted in our training laboratory.

(1) Lack of recognition of deficits: Frequently these patients have absolutely no awareness of the deficits which may be so apparent to others. Even when they do have an awareness of the deficits, however, they may know that something is wrong but in a rather vague way and have no idea of the precise difficulties they are encountering. In the training environment, we want to uncover the primary areas that are contributing to deficits because these are the areas we wish to train in order to help our patients cope with life situations. In this process we want to provide our patients with an awareness of these specific deficit areas by talking about them and by working on them, but at the same time we want to do this carefully. We don't want to overwhelm them with this recognition, but instead we can let their awareness grow while at the same time they are recognizing that they can make improvement in the same areas.

(2) Emotional problems: Lesions in frontal lobe areas most frequently will result in some definite personality and emotional changes. These changes may result in the patient becoming more emotional or, conversely, flatter in affect. In relation to this impairment, it is probable that more help needs to be given to the immediate family or important others in the patient's life. These patients can be extremely exasperating to those who are close to them and the patient often appears to have no awareness of the

effect of the behavior on others. These problems need to be discussed as a regular part of the training environment, but even more important, the family needs some help in understanding what has happened to their loved one who at times seems like a stranger in their midst. Psychological intervention for the family is often an important component of treatment.

(3) Impairment of ability to make proper use of feedback: This deficit would appear to be the single most commonly found problem occurring with our frontal lobe patients. Because they have great difficulty monitoring themselves adequately, we find we have to structure the tasks very specifically and monitor them very closely. It is necessary to train these patients intensively in how to make use of feedback. This needs to be done by discussion, by observation, by demonstration, and by intensive repetitive practice.

(4) Problems with planning and organizing: Impairments in these areas will almost always be seen but in varying degrees. Many exercises and much practice are needed in these particular areas, beginning at a level in which the individual is able to achieve success, and increasing in complexity so as to force learning to occur. It is helpful in this particular area to make use of overt verbal mediation for self-instruction. The advantage of verbal mediation is that it can be used by the individual when alone. Another advantage of verbal mediation and additional verbalization is that this allows more precise monitoring of our patients in our laboratory.

(5) Memory deficits, especially those involved in the organzing of memory functions: Because memory functions are susceptible to impairment by almost any type of brain lesion, it is not unexpected to find that a frontal lobe patient also has memory problems. Memory impairment associated with frontal lesions are frequently more subtle, however, than found with other kinds of lesions. This may be related to an inability to organize cognitive processes which entail the accessing of memory as most patients with known frontal lesions have relatively little difficulty with memory activities provided they are externally organized for them. They may have good recall in response to questions asked but cannot ask themselves the questions spontaneously. The retraining process must provide help in organization and these patients must also be taught to ask the questions of themselves that will result in production of the desired material from their memory banks.

(6) Impairments in intellectual flexibility: Because of deficits in this area, we will frequently see frontal lobe patients perseverating with poor responses. The problem is that they can work with one idea, but if this is not successful, they cannot seem to spontaneously generate new ideas or may have great difficulty in doing so. Training in this particular area can begin at an easy level and difficulty can be increased slowly so as to facilitate learning.

(7) A great variability in performance: Frequently, the frontal lobe patient is typically extremely variable in his performance. This may well be due to a combination of a number of the factors already mentioned. Recognizing that we have to deal with this variability, it is important to keep very strict controls on these clients in the retraining program. The trainer must be in charge at all times and set very definite limits. A well organized program will tend to restrict some of the variability in performance. Rewards for the good behavior or the good effort will also be helpful in restricting the variability. The entire training program should be designed to facilitate the patient's awareness of this variability as well as their control of overt and cognitive behavior.

(8) The problem of motivation: Whereas non-frontal lesion patients will usually have a keen awareness of their deficits and a desire to work hard to regain abilities, this is frequently not the case with lesions of the frontal regions. These individuals may have great difficulty properly assessing their condition, applying themselves conscientiously to a task, and modifying their behavior as necessary to achieve success in any given endeavor. If anything in their environment can be found to act as a motivator for them, this should be used in order to begin to achieve progress in training. Lacking good motivators, or perhaps in conjunction with weak motivators, it may be necessary to first supply an external control and direction to each step of an activity with this patient so as to ensure correct learning of response. Very gradually the external control of the behavior is supplanted by the patient's ability to assume an inner control. This process can be characterized as initially taking them by the hand and teaching them the "proper way to go" as a parent will do with a young child and gradually shaping a more sophisticated internal control of behavior.

## CONCLUSION

Our clinical experience and observation, along with some neuropsychological evidence, suggests that the behavioral and cognitive impairment associated with lesions of the frontal cortex are modifiable. The process of modifying these impairments is quite complex and often elusive and requires a sequential step by step approach beginning with minimally complex task requirements. There appear to be, however, some common cognitive characteristics of frontal cortex lesions which may suggest that some of the interventive strategies, such as those herein discussed, may be applicable to the treatment of frontal region patients in general. Throughout the training program it is necessary to keep very firm control of the situation and to monitor progress very closely. The training staff will also need special help with these patients as they will be encountering many problems and frustrations. More frequent case review is also necessary with these patients due to the complexity of the training needs. It is very gratifying, however, despite all of the difficulties, to note the progress that can be obtained on daily graphs over time, to observe the pleasure and pride these patients register as they achieve notable gains, and to recognize, finally that it is possible for these gains that are made in training to generalize to other situations and to all areas of these patients lives.

## REFERENCES

Goldman, P. S. Development and plasticity of frontal association cortex in the infrahuman primate. In C. L. Ludlow & M. E. Doran-Quine (Eds.), The neurological bases of language disorders in children: Methods and directions for research. NIH Publication No. 79-440, Aug. 1979.

Goldstein, K. The mental changes due to frontal lobe damage. Journal of Psychology, 1944, 17, 187-208.

Gudeman, H., Golden, C., & Craine, J. The role of neuropsychological evaluation in the rehabilitation of the brain-injured patient: A program in neurotraining. Manuscript Number 1693 Abstracted in the JSAS Catalog of Selected Documents in Psychology, 1978, 8 (2), 44.

Hecaen, H. & Albert, M. Human neuropsychology. New York: John Wiley & Sons, 1978.

Lechner, H., Ott, E., Ladurner, G. & Bertha, G. Static-dynamic aspects of cerebral blood flow in relation to brain function. In F. Hoffmeister & C. Muller (Eds.). Brain function in old age. Berlin: Springer-Verlag, 1979.

Lezak, M. D. Neuropsychological assessment. New York: Oxford University Press, 1976.

Luria, A. R. Restoration of function after brain injury. New York: The MacMillan Company, 1963.

Luria, A. R. The frontal lobes and the regulation of behavior. In K. Pribram & A. R. Luria (Eds.) Psychophysiology of the frontal lobes. New York and London: Academic Press, 1973.

Luria, A. R. The working brain. New York: Basic Books, 1974.

Teuber, H. L. The riddle of frontal lobe function in man. In J. M. Warren & K. Akert (Eds.). The frontal granular cortex and behavior. New York: McGraw-Hill, 1964.

# THE USE OF ELECTRONIC GAMES IN COGNITIVE REHABILITATION

William J. Lynch, Ph.D.

Director, Brain Injury Rehabilitation Unit
Veterans Administration Medical Center
Palo Alto, California

## BACKGROUND

In the early 1970's Atari, a once small electronics firm in Sunnyvale, California, developed and marketed the first commercially successful video game. Referred to as Pong, this video version of ping-pong paved the way for numerous other games which soon appeared in taverns, arcades, airport lobbies, and college dormitories throughout the country. Although Pong remains quite popular, there are now over 40 different Atari videogame programs varying from simple word games (Hangman) to complex games of strategy such as chess (Video Chess) or tic-tac-toe (3-D Tic-Tac-Toe). Each program contains variations both in number of players (1 to 4) and level of difficulty (slow or fast speed; larger or smaller light "paddle"). Some (Video Olympics) have as many as 50 variations from which to choose.

A recent issue of Mechanix Illustrated (Perry, 1980) was devoted to the topic of home computers and electronic games. It was revealed that, whereas in 1977 there were but six hand-held electronic games on the market, by 1980 the number had expanded to 420. The number of hand-held electronics games purchased in 1978 was over five million. By 1979 the number had nearly doubled to ten million; and by 1980, the total had increased to between 13 and 15 million. The amount of money spent for these games in 1980 was about 800 million dollars--and represented the largest total earned by any single toy type.

Although there have been occasional references to the use of video games in research, there have been no published reports of their use as rehabilitation techniques in a substantial series of patients. This chapter will discuss the use of video games in cognitive rehabilitation of patients with brain disorders. My intent is to familiarize the reader with what games are available and how they may be utilized in rehabilitation settings. My hope is that others will take an interest in gathering systematic data on a number of different patients so that more precise inferences about the efficacy of video games in cognitive rehabilitation may be possible.

## REASONS FOR POPULARITY OF VIDEO GAMES

There are at least five reasons for the rapid and widespread popularity of electronic games:

First, they are enjoyable to play for people of all age groups. Since they typically involve colorful and moving video displays, along with dramatic sound effects, they are attractive and reinforcing for the player. I have found that, with brain-injured patients, educational game programs presented on a TV screen are more readily accepted and attended to than standard classroom instruction. A final confirmation of this belief, however, must await controlled study.

A second reason is that electronic games are generally compact and portable. Since most games are constructed with microminiature silicon chips, there are a number of them which are pocket-sized and most are easily transportable. The player may be sitting at home, waiting for a train, or riding in a plane. Many games are available in standard, as well as portable, formats (such as Milton Bradley's Simon). Similarly, these games can be used and put away quickly with no troublesome disassembly or dismantling required. Thus, they may be picked up and used even if the player has but a few minutes of spare time.

A third reason is that of flexibility. Electronic games, especially home video games, have numerous variations and levels of difficulty. The player may compete against the computer or against another player. Most games have an element of apparent unpredictability about them, such that the player is rarely able to predict his or her opponent's (or the computer's) next moves. This inherent flexibility and variability prevents most home electronic videogames from being boring to the average player.

The fact that most electronic games are fairly inexpensive is a fourth reason for their popularity. As greater competition has brought down prices, the consumer can now choose among a number of systems that provide similar game formats. Currently, electronic sports games cost from \$20 to \$40, whereas certain challenging word or "thinking" games may cost between \$30 and \$70. As a general rule, the cost of an electronic game is a function of its complexity and the hardware required to play it. The more complex the game (such as Atari's Video Chess), the more built-in logic is required for the program. This built-in logic is termed "Read-only" memory or ROM, and thus is not modifyable by the user. The games which require a small computer and hand-held controllers are most costly than those which are wholly self-contained.

The final reason for the popularity of electronic games is the fact that many of them are educational and/or therapeutic. The games of Speak and Spell and Dataman by Texas Instruments for example, are designed for drills in the areas of spelling and mathematics, respectively. Milton Bradley's Simon, a very popular game commercially, is essentially a visual and auditory sequential memory task. Games requiring visual fixation and tracking (such as Atari's Breakout or Pong) are useful for eye-hand coordination.

In a sense, what electronic games have done is to make learning (and therefore rehabilitation) more enjoyable and challenging. Video games have made television viewing an active and interactive, rather than a totally passive and receptive, process.

## HOME VIDEO GAMES IN REHABILITATION SETTINGS

In this section, I would like to briefly describe the kinds of game programs which I have found useful in cognitive rehabilitation. While I will be discussing Atari videogames, the reader should be aware that other manufacturers--most notably Mattel, Inc.--have marketed similar devices of equal overall quality. A complete listing of Atari videogame programs can be obtained by contacting the manufacturer at:

Atari, Inc. Consumer Division
1195 Borregas Avenue
Sunnyvale, CA 94086

The present author has prepared a Guide for prospective users of Atari video games (lynch, 1981) which includes a listing of programs, their catalog numbers, controllers used, synopsis of the game, and suggestions as to the kinds of problems which could be treated with that game. Interested persons should write to the author at:

Brain Injury Rehabilitation Unit (205-B1-MP)
VA Medical Center - Menlo Park Division
3801 Miranda Avenue
Palo Alto, CA 94304

Atari's videocomputer programs may be divided for convenience of discussion into four broad types: (a) those which are verbal or mathematical games. (b) those which are memory games, (c) those which are spatial and perceptual-motor games, and (d) those which are table games.

## Verbal and Mathematic Games

Verbal skills are dealt with by a game called Hangman which requires the player to surmise a mystery word by guessing component letters. Each incorrect guess results in an additional portion of a hanging cartoon character being drawn in by the computer. This game is especially helpful for spelling and word finding problems.

Mathematics may be presented in a number of different forms. The Add Me game (part of Brain Games) requires rapid addition of four single digit numbers, whereas Fun with Numbers contains addition, subtraction, multiplication, and division problems which the player can initiate. Both simple single-digit numbers and complex two-digit numbers are included; and some problems involve carrying and remainders.

The Codebreaker game requires the player to guess a missing numeric code by trial and error. Finally, various card games such as Casino (includes poker and black jack) and Blackjack require the player to perform rapid calculations of both wagers and card values.

## Memory Games

The Brain Games program contains a number of useful memory tasks. Touch Me is quite similar to the Milton Bradley game of Simon. The player must recall sequences of highlighted rectangles (paired with tones) in a 3 x 2 or 3 x 3 matrix. With each new highlighted rectangle, the player must then recall all the previous ones in that series in order. Count Me is a visual version of the standard digit span task, and Picture Me is a visual memory task requiring the player to study and then reconstruct from memory a sequence of four geometric designs.

Concentration, a version of the old television game show, requires the player to recall the location of pairs or pictures revealed briefly--one at a time--on a matrix, and to then match them. The player who performs the most successful matches wins the game. This game is, obviously, a measure of "concentration" in general, but also of visual-spatial memory in particular.

## Spatial and Perceptual-Motor Skills Games

The various games included in the program Video Olympics require rapid eye-hand coordination, visual tracking, interception of a target. Breakout is based upon similar principles. However, the orientation of the moving dot of light is both vertical and horizontal, rather than simply horizontal.

There are numerous target games (such as Space Invaders, Air-Sea Battle, or Sky Diver) which involve coordination of visual input and motor output in order to guide the player toward a target or goal. Related to this category of games are those which emphasize strategy or searching, such as Adventure, Flag Capture, or Superman.

In many rehabilitation settings, the patient's suitability for driver's training needs to be determined before formal referral is made. As an adjunct to specific visual and motor skills testing, certain videogames may be helpful, either as a diagnostic aid or as a way of preparing the patient for actual driving training. The games of Night Driver, Indy-500 Street Racer, and Slot Racer may be useful in this regard.

Finally, the games which I would characterize as "sports games" (such as Basketball, Football, Golf, or Home Run) are helpful in retraining fine motor skills, reaction time, strategy, and judgment.

### Table Games

The so-called "table games" include Video Chess, 3-D Tic-Tac-Toe, Toe, Othello, and Backgammon. These programs require visual scanning, planning, and delay of responding. They involve a substantial spatial component, and, due to their complex rules, may be too difficult for most patients to learn initially. A new Atari Checkers program, which will be marketed soon, should prove simple enough for most patients to comprehend.

## RECORDING RESULTS OF VIDEO-GAME RETRAINING

It is essential that patient data be recorded so that progress can be documented. Although this may be accomplished in a number of ways, I have developed an all-purpose recording form which can be used with any of the Atari programs. A sample of a completed record form is shown in Figure 1.

The clinician first completes the top of the form by specifying the exact program name, game type, variation and level of difficulty. Although up to 10 trials or games may be recorded during each session, this may be varied according to need. The variable to be used as a criterion may be the total score for all trials, the mean score across all trials, the minimum or maximum score for each trial, or a certain number of consecutive trials of a certain value. Finally, following each block of five sessions, the therapist can decide to continue or discontinue the treatment, depending on the patient's progress toward the criterion.

Property of
VA Med. Ctr.
Palo Alto, CA

BRAIN INJURY REHABILITATION UNIT

RECORD FORM - VIDEO GAMES THERAPY

PROGRAM NAME: (Circle) Air-Sea Battle - Basic Math - Black Jack - Brain Games - (Breakout) - Code Breaker - Hangman - Hunt and Score - Indy-500 - Star Ship - Surround - Video Olympics

SPECIFIC GAME PLAYED: *Regular* (e.g., "Pong," "Touch me")

VARIATION: (if applicable) *two players* (e.g., 2 or 4 players with/without noise)

LEVEL OF DIFFICULTY: (Circle) A (B) Examiner: *Lynch*

GOAL/CRITERION FOR SUCCESS: *75 bricks, 3 trials* (be specific)

SCORE

| | TRIAL: | TRIAL: | TRIAL: | TRIAL: | TRIAL: |
|---|---|---|---|---|---|
| 1. | *30* | *39* | *65* | | |
| 2. | *26* | *42* | *73* | | |
| 3. | *19* | *53* | *75* | | |
| 4. | *39* | *60* | *69* | | |
| 5. | *41* | *61* | *78* | | |
| 6. | *40* | *69* | *70* | | |
| 7. | *35* | *50* | *79* | | |
| 8. | *39* | *63* | *85* | | |
| 9. | *46* | *68* | *89* | | |
| 10. | *52* | *70* | *-* | | |
| Total: | *367* | *575* | *683* | | |
| MEAN: | *36.7* | *57.5* | *75.8* | | |
| MIN/MAX: | *19 / 52* | *39 / 70* | *65 / 89* | / | / |
| DATE: | *2 /21/81* | *2/28/81* | *3/ 1/81* | / / | / / |

BASELINE

5-Trial Outcome: (Goal Met) - Goal Not Met
Plan: Continue - (Discontinue)

PATIENT: *8519*

Figure 1. Sample completed form for recording results of video game performance.

The raw data thus obtained is then transferred to a profile form. These are of two types: One (Figure 2.) is designed to record single session performance on a trial-by-trial basis; the other (Figure 3.) is designed to display performance across several sessions (up to five) on a day-to-day basis. Each form is designed so that the clinician can complete it according to his/her particular needs.

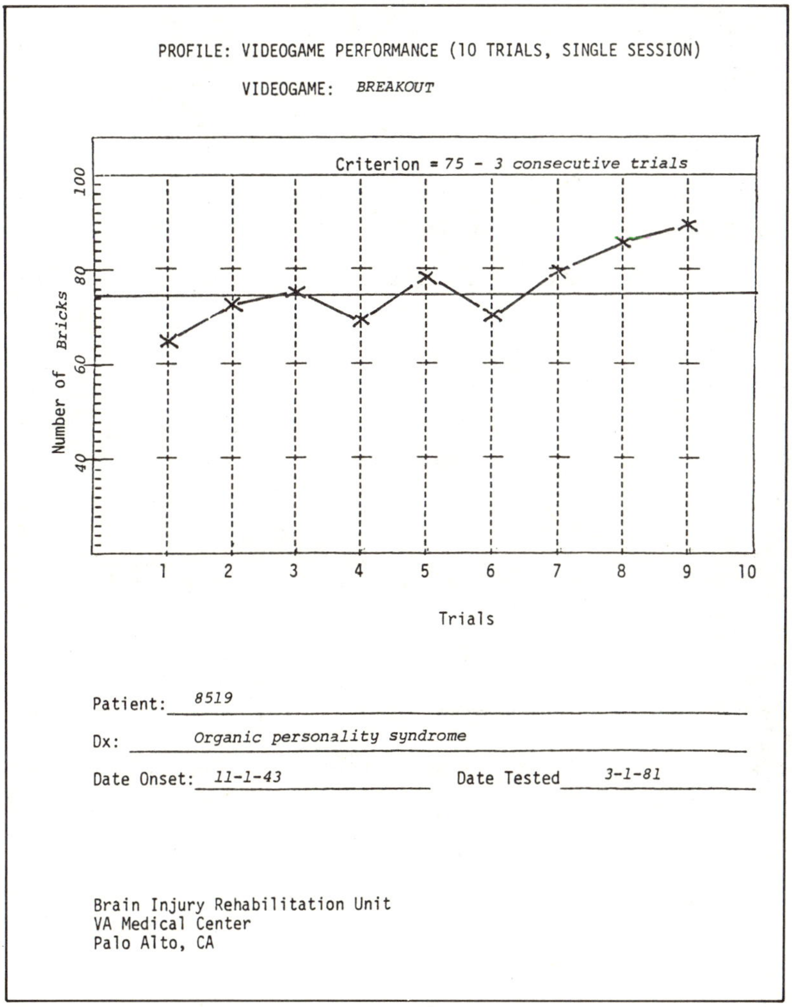


Figure 2. Sample profile for single session of video game training.

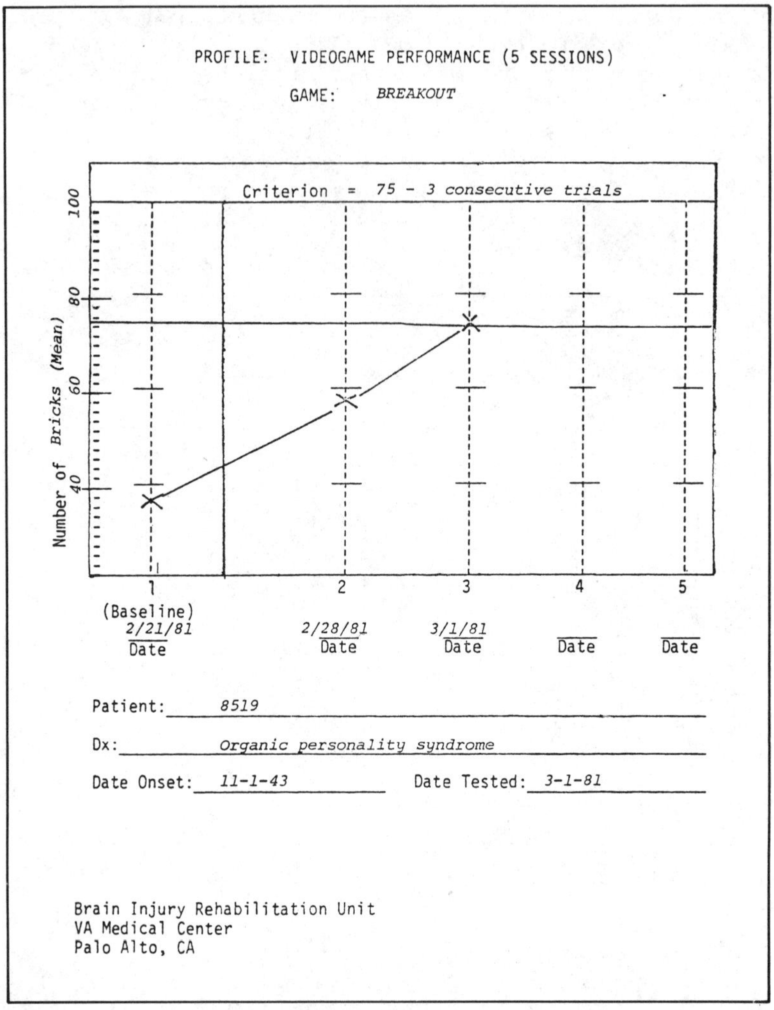


Figure 3. Sample profile for multiple sessions of video game training.

At the Brain Injury Rehabilitation Unit, the profiles are used for providing ongoing feedback to the patient and to provide both patient and staff member with a specific treatment objective for this form of cognitive rehabilitation. Copies of these forms will be provided on request to those wishing to use them.

## RESEARCH ON VIDEO GAMES

There is very little published research on the use of home video games as rehabilitation techniques. When I requested a computerized literature search in this area, I did not find a single relevant reference. I have recently learned from an official at Atari, Inc. that they have not gathered information on how persons perform, but only on how well they enjoy the games when they play them. Fortunately, I did happen upon one study which investigated the differential effects of complex visual and spatial performance upon brain electrical activity. This study (Rebert and Low, 1978) utilized bilateral EEGs recorded from central, temporal, and parietal scalp locations. The subjects--seven males and seven females--were recorded under six different conditions:

1. Resting - eyes closed
2. Resting - eyes opened
3. Listening to a verbal passage
4. Performing a visuospatial manipulation (counting piles of blocks)
5. Watching *Pong*
6. Playing *Pong*.

Each subject practiced *Pong* for eight trials on one day, and on the next day underwent for test trials. The authors found that females obtained a mean of 213 "hits" per trial, (i.e., interceptions of the light spot) whereas males attained a mean of 248. It should be noted, however, that these investigators required their subjects to play with both hands *simultaneously*, and that a "hit" was defined as either a deflection by a paddle or by the upper or lower margins of the video display area.

These authors expressed the view that proficiency at *Pong* requires that the player automatize his/her performance. To illustrate this, they noted that some subjects could attain 300 to 400 "hits" per game while engaging in simultaneous conversation. The results of the Rebert and Low study will be summarized briefly. Alpha power (a presumed index of "idling" or de-emphasis of a hemisphere during a task) was higher in the right cerebral hemisphere while the subjects listened to verbal material. Alpha power was higher in the left hemisphere during the imaginative block rotation task. When subjects either watched or played *Pong*, alpha power was supressed in the right hemisphere. Watching *Pong* was as effective as playing *Pong* with regard to parietal lobe alpha response; yet playing *Pong* enhanced the asymmetry of temporal and central alpha activity.

The right versus the left hemisphere contribution to the playing of *Pong* is not a simple one, however. It was observed, for instance, that subjects' performance first increased, then *decreased*, as alpha asymmetry became increasingly pronounced in favor of the right hemisphere. To further illustrate this complex alpha-task relationship, the authors state that the only difference noted between the "eyes open - resting" and "reading to subject" conditions was an increase in alpha in the right hemisphere during the latter. No change in left hemisphere alpha was observed during this transition.

Certainly, more studies of this and related types need to be conducted. Until such time as reliable data are available, the efficacy of video games in rehabilitation will, of necessity, remain in doubt. Care must be taken to use standard games in standard ways, and to gather date in an easily replicated manner. And finally, small sample studies--even single case studies--should be published, so that clinical literature in this field can begin to evolve.

## EXPANDING THE ROLE OF VIDEO GAMES IN REHABILITATION SETTINGS

I would expect video games to become a more integral part of many rehabilitation programs in the present decade. Some of the areas of increased utilization or application are summarized in the following overview.

### Diagnosis

Video games can be used to provide measures of alertness, attention, or concentration. Variables such as reaction time and resistance to action (inhibition of response) are likewise easily measureable with existing game programs. Sensory functions are measurable by video games as well. For example, visual detection, recognition, neglect, or field cuts can be quantified by existing or customized video game programs. In this same way, auditory neglect, discrimination, or recognition can be assessed.

Motor functions, such as speed, dexterity, or coordination are evaluated on a number of game programs. Finally, higher cognitive functions are currently measured by quite a few of the Atari game cartridges. Skills such as general knowledge, memory, judgment, mathematical reasoning, reading, vocabulary, and spatial relations are examples of these cognitive abilities.

### Treatment

In addition to being useful in diagnosis, video games can be used as methods for programmed retraining in each of the areas noted in the previous section. The videogame method has the advantage of being highly objective, both in the way in which stimuli are depicted and presented and in the way performances are evaluated or scored. Immediate and consistent feedback is an additional asset provided by the use of video games in treatment. Although personal contact is usually preferred, the fact that most video games can be played alone (or against the computer)--that is, without a therapist present--is another advantage. This would apply also to the assigning of certain video game training at home as an adjunct to in-clinic treatment.

Leisure Time and Recreation

It is likely that we will see an expansion of the use of video games as ways of relieving boredom while patients are awaiting appointments. Bedridden patients faced with the prospect of watching "soap operas" on their bedside television sets may be able to play video games, instead. Since the games are inherently interesing and challenging to most patients, patients can pass the time both enjoyably and therapeutically. The adaptation of video games to various kinds of physical handicaps is an area of concern for those who work with the brain-injured or spinal-cord-injured populations. Providing these populations with recreation can be a helpful contribution to their adjustment and recovery.

## THE FUTURE

It is inevitable that we will be seeing an increase in the variety and availability of home video games. Increasingly, the video "game" will be replaced by small computers with double or triple the built-in (ROM) memory capacity of existing units. Games will expand beyond simulations of traditional games (baseball, football, chess, etc.) to games which are designed especially for the computer. With the increase in availability of computer hardware and software (programs), the user will become more actively involved in customizing or designing his/her own programs to suit special needs.

More lifelike video displays are being developed in various centers. More dynamic, high resolution color images will become commonplace. There will be greater use of interactive programs which permit the player to respond to--and adjust--the game as he/she goes along. Computer graphics will continue to dazzle us with its precision and eerie, lifelike quality.

Perhaps the ultimate in video games will be reached when three-dimensional external images are perfected. There is talk of this being a possibility in the not-too-distant future for home televisions. Atari has already developed a series of game prototypes--to be marketed commercially in the fall of this year--which utilize holographic imagery for their video displays. To be sure, we have come quite a way from the humble beginnings of Pong.

## CONCLUSIONS

I hope that the foregoing discussion has brought home the point that the use of video games in rehabilitation is in its infancy. Research is sorely needed, and, of equal importance, an exchange of information about what is going on in the various centers using these games "informally" is essential. Even though the future seems clear, one should not neglect the realities of the present. Namely, the clinician would be well-advised to become involved in video games at whatever level he or she can afford in terms of departmental budgets and time commitments. Certainly, a $5,000 microprocessor with color videographics, high-speed printer and 48 K Random Access Memory (RAM) would be the preferred system for maximum efficiency and flexibility. Yet, a $20 hand-held Dataman might be equally as effective, given the fact that it is, in the end, not the hardware used by the clinician but the clinician using the hardware that ultimately determines the success or failure of cognitive rehabilitation.

## REFERENCES

Lynch, W.J. A guide to Atari videocomputer programs for rehabilitation settings (Revised Edition) (Unpublished document). Palo Alto, CA: Veterans Administration, 1981.

Perry, R. Mechanix Illustrated personal computers (No. 2). Mechanix Illustrated, 1980 (Oct.), 30-32.

Rebert, C., and Low, D. Differential hemispheric activation during complex visuomotor performance. Journal of Electroenchephalography and Clinical Neurophysiology, 1978, 44, 724-734.

## ADDITIONAL SUGGESTED READINGS

Furst, C.J. EEG alpha asymmetry and visuospatial performance. Nature 1976, 260, 254-255.

Galin, D. and Ornstein, R. Lateral specialization of cognitive mode: An EEG study. Psychophysiology, 1972, 9, 412-418.

Genkin, A. Asymmetry in phase duration of the encephalogram during intellectual activity. Electroencephalography and Clinical Neurophysiology, 1965, 18, 102-103.

McKee, G., Humphrey, B., and McAdam. Scaled lateralization of alpha activity during linguistic and musical tasks. Psychophysiology, 1973, 10, 441-443.

Rebert, C. Functional cerebral asymmetry and performance. I Reaction time to words and dot patterns as a function of EEG alpha asymmetry. Behavioral Neuropsychiatry, 1977, 8, 90-98.

Shepard, R., and Metzler, J. Mental rotation of three-dimensional objects. Science, 1971, 191, 701-703.

## CONCLUDING REMARKS

Lance E. Trexler, Ph.D.

Coordinator, Neuropsychology Service
Medical Psychology Department
Community Hospital of Indianapolis

The section on Interventive Strategies has provided a wealth of information on the treatment of neuropsychological deficits ranging from attentional disorders, syndromes of impairment associated with frontal lobe pathology and right hemisphere functions including neglect, visual organization and visual sequential analysis, to mention a few. The rehabilitation of these impairments has also been described from a variety of approaches, ranging from highly psychometric and reductionistic to relatively unstructured and dynamic. The methodology introduced by Lynch provides an innovative perspective on interventive strategies as well.

Assuming that the focus of cognitive rehabilitation is to facilitate learning, not only in the therapist's office but in the patient's natural environment, we need to delineate what the relevant parameters of learning are for a given patient with a given pattern of cognitive impairment. Further, these parameters need to be examined in context of their effect on various kinds of learning, whether it be perceptual, motor or language learning. As has been stated, it appears that the inherent goal of cognitive rehabilitation is to teach patients how to learn. Further, it may be one of our goals to teach the patient to recognize when he/she is and is not learning. However, in all of the foregoing chapters we hypothesize that presenting the patient with a structured stimulus of one type or another, depending upon the unique needs of the patient, will in one way or another facilitate learning. One potential problem with this basic assumption rests with reality that one's natural environment is not structured, organized or intrinsically cohesive. Rather, the perceiver organizes external stimuli, albeit in part as a function of the stimulus characteristics themselves, in a manner that brings about meaningfulness to that perceiver. Previous learning, the intent of the organism, and the status of ongoing cognitive processing all affect the way in which a given stimulus will be perceived, organized and made meaningful. Effecting these internal processes appear to be the goal of cognitive rehabilitation. As a consequence, perhaps we need to focus our efforts on assisting the patient decipher his/her intent with the situation at hand, organize the information available in a meaningful way, and deduce strategies which will operationalize that intent. Perhaps our thinking in rehabilitation is not dissimilar to that of early Greek neurologists who believed that the mind was like photographic paper which produces identical, internal copies of external stimuli. I am reminded of the faces of so many of our patients as they are wheeled from one therapy to another where we do all sorts of things to them, their look of initial quandary, eventual frustration in attempt to assimilate and make sense of all the incoming information, and finally passivity, as if to say "What are you going to do to me next?" I suspect, however, that we are not so passive in making sense of our environment or in successfully adapting to it. I am not sure that it is important what stimuli we provide to brain damaged patients as compared to the potential importance of what they do with that stimuli.

The information presented in this volume brings to bear much of the current state of the art effort in rehabilitation concerning cognition and abnormal cognition, as we know it. I believe that it is likely that we have come a full circle in asking ourselves how it is that we might rehabilitate the consequences of insult to the central nervous system, but perhaps with a deeper and richer perspective.

CONTRIBUTORS

Zila Ben-Nahum, M.A.
Unit of Neuropsychological Treatment and Rehabilitation
Givatayim, Israel

Yehuda Ben-Yishay, Ph.D.
Co-Director, Head Trauma Program
Institute of Rehabilitation Medicine
Associate Professor of Clinical Rehabilitation Medicine
New York University Medical Center
100 East 34th Street
New York, New York 10016

James F. Craine, Ph.D.
Head, Neuropsychology Service
Hawaii State Hospital
45-710 Keaahala Road
Kaneohe, Hawaii 96744

Leonard Diller, Ph.D.
Chief, Behavioral Sciences Department
Institute of Rehabilitation Medicine
Professor, Clinical Rehabilitation Medicine
New York University Medical Center
100 East 34th Street
New York, New York 10016

Yigal Gross, Ph.D.
Department of Psychology
Bar Ilan University
Ramat Gan, Israel
and
Unit for Neuropsychological Treatment and Rehabilitation
Givatayim, Israel

Chris Hagen, Ph.D.
Chairman, Speech-Language Pathology Department
Speech, Hearing and Neurosensory Center
8001 Frost Street
San Diego, California 92123

William J. Lynch, Ph.D.
Director, Brain Injury Rehabilitation Unit
Veterans Administration Medical Center
Palo Alto (Menlo Park Division)
3801 Miranda Avenue (MPD-205B1)
Palo Alto, California 94304

Diane L. Meeder, O.T.R.
Clinical Supervisor,
Occupational Therapy Neurology Services
Santa Clara Valley Medical Center
751 South Bascom Avenue
San Jose, California 95128

Gabriel Munk, M.A.
Rehabilitation Center
Shiba Hospital
Tel-Hashomer, Israel

Eugene B. Piasetsky, Ph.D.
Psychologist
Institute of Rehabilitation Medicine
New York University Medical Center
100 East 34th Street
New York, New York 10016

James D. Thomas, M.S.
Department of Psychology
Division of Clinical Neuropsychology
University of Houston
4800 Calhoun Street
Houston, Texas 77004

Lance E. Trexler, Ph.D.
Coordinator, Neuropsychology Service
Medical Psychology Department
Community Hospital of Indianapolis, Inc.
1500 North Ritter Avenue
Indianapolis, Indiana 46219

Joseph Weinberg, M.A.
Psychologist
Institute of Rehabilitation Medicine
New York University Medical Center
100 East 34th Street
New York, New York 10016

INDEX